Recent Advances in Family Medicine

Recent Advances in Family Medicine

Edited by Nora Ortega

AMERICAN
MEDICAL PUBLISHERS
www.americanmedicalpublishers.com

American Medical Publishers,
41 Flatbush Avenue,
1st Floor, New York,
NY 11217, USA

Visit us on the World Wide Web at:
www.americanmedicalpublishers.com

ISBN: 978-1-63927-453-6

Cataloging-in-Publication Data

Recent advances in family medicine / edited by Nora Ortega.
p. cm.
Includes bibliographical references and index.
ISBN 978-1-63927-453-6
1. Family medicine. 2. Medicine. 3. Physicians (General practice).
4. Clinical medicine. I. Ortega, Nora.

RC48 .F36 2021
610--dc23

Table of Contents

Preface

Every book is a source of knowledge and this one is no exception. The idea that led to the conceptualization of this book was the fact that the world is advancing rapidly; which makes it crucial to document the progress in every field. I am aware that a lot of data is already available, yet, there is a lot more to learn. Hence, I accepted the responsibility of editing this book and contributing my knowledge to the community.

The medical specialty that deals with the comprehensive health care for people of all ages is known as family medicine. It is a sub-field of primary care that is based on the knowledge of the patient's cultural and family background. Due to this, it emphasizes on preventing diseases and promoting health. It also focuses on providing continuous and comprehensive health care to individuals and families over all diseases, ages, genders and parts of the body. Various chronic, acute and preventive medical care services are provided under family medicine. It also includes routine check-ups, immunization, health-risk assessments, screening tests as well as personalized counseling to maintain a healthy lifestyle. This book provides comprehensive insights into the field of family medicine. It aims to equip students and experts with the advanced topics and upcoming concepts in this area. Coherent flow of topics, student-friendly language and extensive use of examples make this book an invaluable source of knowledge.

While editing this book, I had multiple visions for it. Then I finally narrowed down to make every chapter a sole standing text explaining a particular topic, so that they can be used independently. However, the umbrella subject sinews them into a common theme. This makes the book a unique platform of knowledge.

I would like to give the major credit of this book to the experts from every corner of the world, who took the time to share their expertise with us. Also, I owe the completion of this book to the never-ending support of my family, who supported me throughout the project.

Editor

1

Learning to use electronic health records: can we stay patient-centered? A pre-post intervention study with family medicine residents

Cédric Lanier[1,2*], Melissa Dominicé Dao[1], Patricia Hudelson[1], Bernard Cerutti[3] and Noëlle Junod Perron[1]

Abstract

Background: The Electronic Health Record (EHR) is now widely used in clinical encounters. Because its use can negatively impact the physician-patient relationship, several recommendations on the "patient-centered" use of the EHR have been published. However, the impact of training to improve EHR use during clinical encounters is not well known. The aim of this study was to assess the impact of training on residents' EHR-related communication skills and explore whether they varied according to the content of the consultation.

Methods: We conducted a pre-post intervention study at the Primary Care Division of the Geneva University Hospitals, Switzerland. Residents were invited to attend a 3-month training course that included 2 large group sessions and 2–4 individualized coaching sessions based on videotaped encounters. Outcomes were: 1) residents' perceptions regarding the use of EHR, measured through a self-administered questionnaire and 2) objective use of the EHR during the first 10 min of patient encounters. Changes in practice were measured pre and post intervention using the Roter interaction analysis system (RIAS) and EHR specific items.

Results: Seventeen out of 27 residents took part in the study. Participants used EHR in about 30% of consultations. After training, they were less likely to consider EHR to be a barrier to the physician-patient relationship, and felt more comfortable using the EHR. After training, participants increased the use of signposting when using the EHR (pre: 0.77, SD 1.69; post: 1.80, SD3.35; p 0.035) and decreased EHR use when psychosocial issues appeared (pre: 24.5% and post: 9.76%, $p < 0.001$).

Conclusions: This study suggests that training can improve residents' EHR-related communication skills, especially in situations where patients bring up sensitive psychosocial issues. Future research should focus on patients' perceptions of the relevance and usefulness of such skills.

Keywords: Electronic health record, Patient-Physician relation, Computer, Communication skills, Training

Background

The Electronic Health Record (EHR) is now widely used in clinical encounters and its use is promoted by national incentive programs [1–7]. The EHR improves the quality of biomedical data gathering and reduces the number of medical errors [8–13]. It also facilitates the sharing of medical information with the patient [14–16].

The literature shows that patients and physicians are mainly satisfied with the use of the EHR [13, 17–21]. However, some patients worry about the loss of confidentiality [18, 22] while some physicians express concerns about the negative impact of the EHR use on the physician-patient interaction [23–25].

Behavioral changes linked to the use of the EHR include the following: increased time spent with the EHR during the encounter, especially during the first minutes

* Correspondence: cedric.lanier@unige.ch
[1]Department of Community Medicine, Primary Care and Emergency Medicine, Geneva University Hospitals, rue Gabrielle Perret-Gentil, CH-1211 Geneva, Switzerland
[2]Primary care unit, University of Geneva, Centre Médical Universitaire de Genève, Geneva, Switzerland

of the encounter [26], increased moments of silence and a decrease in visual interaction between the physician and the patient [13, 27–31]. Such behaviours tend to distract physicians from picking up verbal or non verbal cues expressed by their patients [32]. Indeed, the time spent looking at the computer screen appears to be inversely correlated with physicians' interest for patient's psychosocial and emotional discourse [28–30].

Based on such observations, experts in medical communication issued several recommendations on the use of the EHR during the encounter in order to stay patient-centered (Table 1) [28, 33, 34]. Recommendations focus on physician's verbal and nonverbal communication skills especially during the first few minutes of the encounter. Indeed, physician-patient communication at the beginning of the encounter is particularly important as it sets the stage for a good relationship with the patient, and contributes to identifying the patient's emotional state and concerns, and to establishing a partnership with the patient [35, 36]; the way the EHR is used clearly affects the opening of the encounter [26]. Experts also highlight the importance of shifting away from the computer when patients express sensitive psychosocial issues [33, 34]. Other non communication elements also include physicians' typing and computer skills, spatial arrangement of the computer and screen, and personal style of EHR use [37–40].

Experts recommend integration of EHR skills in the undergraduate medical curriculum [41–44]. However, only a few studies have assessed the impact of training on the use of such recommendations and these report contrasting results. In a control-group study with first year medical students and standardized patients, Morrow and al. showed that a training course involving role-play increased the use of EHR-related communication skills such as introducing oneself before turning towards the computer, introducing the computer in the triadic relationship, alerting the patient verbally when the doctor turns his/her attention to the computer, and sharing visual information on the screen in the intervention group [45]. Reis et al. compared the impact of two different training formats (traditional lecture vs simulation-based) on resident-patient-EHR communication in a primary care training setting. Performances and attitudes improved in both groups. However, the simulation-based group evaluated the training experience more highly than did the traditional lecture group [46]. Han et al. reported a controlled pre-post intervention study in which medical students demonstrated more patient-centered skills than the control group after having attended an online self-study module on how to preserve the patient-centered relationship while using the EHR [47]. Silverman et al. showed that a specific course on ergonomic computer-use helped medical students to use the EHR in a more patient-centered way during clinical encounters with standardized patients [48].

Table 1 Recommendations on how to use the electronic health record (EHR). Adapted from [33, 34]

• To open the EHR before the patient enters the consultation room
•To set the agenda of the consultation before using the EHR/the keyboard
• To explore the patient's agenda
• To negotiate the agenda by taking into account the patient's agenda
• To allow the patient to have a visual access to the screen/EHR during the clinical encounter (when possible)
• To face the patient most of the time
• To signpost the use of EHR (to summarize what the patient said, to announce what is done with the EHR: documentation, EHR reading, etc....)
• To use verbal and non verbal attitudes to show the patient that the physician's attention is directed to the EHR or the patient (visual and/or verbal link)
• To involve the patient in reading the information or results displayed on the screen (to give information to help understanding)
• To stop using the EHR when patient expresses emotions or psychosocial issues (to stop typing, to look at the patient, listen, express verbal empathy)
• To use appropriate time sets to type (when the patient put on/off his cloths before or after the physical examination)

However, these interventional studies rarely involved real patients, assessed only short term effects (2–3 weeks) [27] and did not specifically study the impact of training on EHR use according to the content of the encounter.

The aim of our study was to assess the impact of training on EHR-related communication skills of residents with real patients during the first 10 min of the clinical encounter. We chose to focus on the first 10 min because we have observed that our residents tend to use the EHR mainly at the beginning of the encounter. In particular, we wanted to explore how EHR use changed when patients introduced psychosocial issues.

Method

Design, setting and participants

A pre-post study was conducted at the Primary Care Division of the Geneva University Hospitals, Switzerland between April and September 2013. The Primary Care Division provides approximately 13'000 medical consultations a year (a majority of follow-up consultations for chronically ill patients) to a diverse urban population, and is also a training center for 40 residents who spend 12 to 24 months training in primary care at the end of their general internal medicine residency training (after 2–4 years of hospital training) before moving to independent practice.

EHR implementation

In January 2012, a new electronic health record (EHR) was developed for primary care consultations, and all physicians in the division are now required to document patient encounters using this EHR. This new EHR is located within the hospital electronic health record, and reflects a problem-oriented medical structure [49]. Data can be entered in either free text fields or via pre-structured fields developed based on the French version of the International Classification of Primary Care (ICPC) [50].

Residents' and patients' perceptions regarding EHR use

In October 2012, as part of a needs assessment, a group discussion with 12 residents was conducted in order to explore their perceptions and difficulties regarding the use of the EHR during clinical encounters. They perceived several advantages such as rapid access to and visibility of the information documented in EHR for all health providers, facilitated billing and EHR-based drug prescription. They also reported several difficulties such as the need to master typing skills, the possible loss of confidentiality, and a negative impact on physician-patient communication which they described as altered and more distant, with a loss of visual contact. However, a small phone survey conducted by CL among a random sample of 20 patients who regularly attended the clinic for chronic conditions showed that they were not disturbed by the use of EHR (100% of the patients reported that their physician's use of EHR was beneficial and none was disturbed by such use).

Based on these results, we decided to develop and assess a training program on how to maintain patient-centered communication when using the EHR during clinical encounters. Residents from two clinics of the division, mainly new residents, were invited to take part in the study: the general primary care clinic ($n = 21$) and the primary care clinic for asylum seekers ($n = 6$).

Intervention

The 3-month training course included two large group sessions and 2–4 individual supervisions based on residents' own videotaped encounters (Fig. 1). During the first large group session which lasted 90 min, residents were asked to suggest and share strategies considered to be useful for overcoming the difficulties of EHR use during consultations. Based on this discussion and a review of the literature [33, 34], we elaborated nine recommendations for remaining patient-centered while using the EHR during the entire length of clinical encounters, which were subsequently provided to residents (Table 1).

During the next three months, pairs of residents had 2 to 4 1-h coaching sessions under the supervision of a clinical teacher in communication skills (CL, MDD or NJP). Residents were asked to videotape 1–2 new clinical encounters between the coaching sessions (those videos were not analysed for the study). At the beginning of the session, residents were first asked to reflect on their strengths and weaknesses on the basis of the nine recommendations developed during the large group session and provided during the coaching session; they then watched segments of videotaped clinical encounter (a segment chosen by participants or from the beginning, depending on their preferences) and analysed their EHR related behaviors together (the 2 residents and the teacher) ; individual difficulties were addressed through role-play followed by feedback. The focus depended on residents' needs but often included signposting when using the EHR (telling the patient what you are doing when you shift your attention to the computer) and stopping EHR use when patients expressed emotions or psychosocial issues. Objectives for improvement were identified and documented from one session to the next on a paper portfolio displaying the nine recommendations. The number of sessions varied according to the degree of improvement shown by participants but did not exceed 4.

During the second large group session which took place after three months, the residents involved in the training were asked to share their perceptions and experiences regarding the recommended strategies.

Data collection and outcome measures

Outcomes measures were

1) Residents' perceptions regarding the use of the EHR before and after the training intervention

Three weeks before and three weeks after the 3-month training period, participants were asked to fill in an 11-item, self-administered questionnaire (5-point Likert scales) about their perceptions regarding the use of the EHR during their clinical encounters (Table 3). This questionnaire was developed based on a review of the literature [23–25, 51–54].

2) Video-based analysis of the clinical encounters

Participants were also asked to videotape 3–4 of their own encounters during a half day three weeks before and three weeks after the training period. Eligible encounters were those conducted in French or English and without the presence of a third person (e.g. family member, interpreter). Before beginning the consultation, participants asked eligible patients to provide a written informed consent to being videotaped during the entire length of the consultation. The analysis was then performed only for the first ten minutes.

Content of the first 10 min of the clinical encounter before and after the training intervention

The content of the physician-patient verbal interaction was coded using the Roter interaction analysis system

Phase	Content	Timing
Needs assessment 2012	Group discussion with 12 residents about their perceptions regarding EHR implementation and use	
Pre-intervention phase April 2013	Measures - Self-administered questionnaire: Resident's perceptions on EHR use Objective analysis of the content of the medical encounters (RIAS coding) and the EHR use (4-5 videotaped medical encounters/per resident)	Month 0 (M0) to M1
Intervention phase	Training program : - 1. Small group training session (15/17 residents ; 90 min) : discussion and elaboration of nine recommendations for remaining patient-centered while using the EHR (personal experiences and review of literature) - 2-4 coaching sessions with a clinical teacher in communication skills (CL, MDD or NJP) (60 min) based on resident's own videotaped consultation recorded between the coaching sessions - Small group session (9/17 residents ; 90 min): sharing perceptions and experiences regarding application of the recommended strategies in real life	M2 to M5
Post-intervention phase September 2013	Measures - Self-administered questionnaire: Resident's perceptions on EHR use Objective analysis of the content of the medical encounters (RIAS coding) and the EHR use (4-5 videotaped medical encounters/per resident)	M5 to M6

Fig. 1 Overview of the intervention conducted and evaluation measures collected among residents

(RIAS), which is a well-known and validated tool used to capture patterns of verbal communication [55]. The physician and patient interaction was first coded using 7 content categories: 1) medical 2) therapeutic 3) lifestyle 4) psychosocial 5) positive talk 6) emotional talk 7) partnership. Other content codes, such as negative and social talk, were not used due to their minimal presence during clinical encounters. Within each content category and for each speaker, the type of utterance was also coded (closed or open-ended question, information-giving, counseling). Coding was performed by an experienced coder from a Canadian group who developed the French version of the RIAS, using MEDICODE software [56].

Objective use of the EHR during the first 10 min of the clinical encounter before and after the training intervention

The physicians' use of the EHR was coded using a scale we developed specifically for this study, based on initial observations and analysis of 15 videotaped encounters by the investigators, and a review of the literature [26, 28, 30, 40, 57, 58]. Coded behaviors included: use of signposting (telling the patient what you are doing when you shift your attention to the computer) when using the EHR and use of the keyboard and/or the screen with or without verbal or visual contact with the patient. Contact was coded as present when the physician displayed verbal, non verbal or visual contact with the patient at intervals of less than 5 s. Contact was coded as absent if the physician showed none of these behaviors during periods of 5 s or more (Table 2). This length of time was based on a study showing that pauses of at 5 s or more were more likely to break the conversation and to cause a change in the topic of the conversation [13, 59]. In order to evaluate whether EHR use varied according to the segment of the consultation (opening, history taking, physical examination, explanation/counseling, closing), a sub-sample of videotaped encounters (12 in the pre-intervention and 11 post-intervention) was coded during the entire length of the consultation.

The EHR coding, linked to both the RIAS utterances and to time (in seconds) was performed by DR on an excel file.

Table 2 Coding scheme for the electronic health (EHR) record communication

EHR use	Description
EHR signposting[a]	Signposting that he/she is starting to type or look at the screen
No EHR use	No use of keyboard or screen
EHR use with patient link	Verbal, non verbal (nodding) or visual link with the patient at least 1x during 5 s while • Typing on the keyboard • Looking at the screen • Typing on the keyboard and looking at the screen
EHR use without patient link	No verbal, non verbal or visual link with the patient during > 5 s while • Typing on the keyboard • Looking at the screen • Typing on the keyboard and looking at the screen

[a]Telling the patient what you are doing when you shift your attention to the computer

Patterns of EHR use

We coded patterns of EHR use as: "low" users (<30% of utterances/time linked to EHR use during the first ten minutes), "medium" users (30–40%) and "high" users (>40% of utterances/time linked to EHR use during the first ten minutes) on the basis of previous research [40].

Intra-rater reliability of RIAS coding, calculated on the basis of 18% videotaped encounters showed 95.5% of stability in utterance cutting and 80.5% of convergence in utterance coding and intraclass correlation coefficient was 0.97. The coder was regularly informed about the convergence rates. The categories for which the rate of disagreement was more than 20% were then discussed with another experienced coder in order to achieve agreement. Since all encounters were coded by the same rater, inter-rater agreement was not an issue in this study. However, a previous study has documented good inter-rater reliability of the RIAS [60].

Inter-rater reliability of EHR coding, calculated on the basis of 10% of the videotaped clinical encounters and performed by CL and NJP, was good (intraclass correlation coefficient = 0.91).

The study was approved by the Geneva University Hospital's research ethics committee.

Statistical Analysis

Descriptive statistics (frequency tables and relative percentages, means, standard deviations) were used to describe the residents' self-perceptions regarding the training course and its impact on their EHR use, content of physician-patient interaction and the use of EHR during videotaped encounters.

The residents' self-perceptions about the impact of the training were compared using paired t tests. The frequencies and relative frequencies of the use of EHR were compared using Chi-squared tests. All tests were performed with a significance level of 0.05. All analyses were run on R 2.15.3 (the R Foundation for Statistical Computing), and TIBCO Spotfire S + ® 8.1 for Windows (TIBCO Software Inc).

Results

Seventeen residents (63%) accepted to participate after having been contacted by email: 14 worked in the general primary care clinic and 3 in the primary care clinic for asylum seekers; 10 (59%) were female and mean age was 35 years old (SD 5.2). Five residents (29%) had obtained postgraduate certification in general internal medicine and fourteen (82%) had attended medical school in Switzerland. We did not record reasons for non-participation, but these included reluctance to be videotaped, lack of time/availability or interest.

Residents attended 2.8 (SD 0.57) individualized supervisions; fifteen residents (88%) took part in the first small group session and 9 (53%) in the second session. Reasons for non-attendance included being on vacation, on call or on sick leave.

1) Residents' perceptions regarding the use of the EHR

Residents generally felt the training helped improve their EHR-related skills and after the training course they were less likely to consider the EHR as a barrier to the physician-patient relationship (Table 3). However, they did not think the training had much impact on more general aspects of the patient-provider relationship (e.g. time dedicated to the patient, interest in their complaints, interruptions of patient talk...).

During the debriefing session, residents described what they learned about maintaining patient-centeredness when using the EHR, including: involving patients when using the EHR, indicating to the patient when using the EHR, documenting key words instead of writing sentences, maintaining contact with the patient during typing phases, and use strategic times to type.

2) Video-based analysis of the clinical encounters

One hundred fourty-two videotaped encounters were analysed (pre-intervention: $n = 73$ and post-intervention: $n = 69$).

Content of the first 10 min of the clinical encounter

The content of the first 10 min of the clinical encounter focused mainly on utterances in the following categories: medical (pre : 17% ; post : 18%), therapeutic (pre : 11% ; post : 13%), positive talk (pre : 22% ; post : 21%) or partnership (pre : 18% ; post : 20%). The lifestyle (pre: 3.5% ; post : 2.7%), psychosocial (pre : 6.6% ; post : 4.2%) and emotional talk (pre : 2.9% ; post : 2.8%) categories occurred less often during the first 10 min of the clinical encounter.

Table 3 Residents' self-perceptions about the impact of the training

Residents' self-perceptions	Number of residents $n = 17$		
(Likert 1 = completely disagree; −5 = completely agree)	Pre Mean (SD)	Post Mean (SD)	p
Training evaluation			
The training met my needs	-	4.11 (0.60)	
The training improved my communication skills related to the use of EHR	-	4.53 (0.52)	
The training improved my « general » communication skills	-	3.88 (0.78)	
I would recommend this training	-	4.43 (0.65)	
Self-perceptions on EHR use			
I feel comfortable using the EHR during the encounter	3.00 (1.23)	3.76 (1.20)	0.04
I have good typing skills	2.65 (1.12)	3.18 (0.88)	0.07
Using the EHR during the encounter increases the time dedicated to the patient	2.29 (1.26)	2.71 (1.16)	0.26
Using the EHR impacts negatively on the physician-patient relationship	3.65 (1.32)	3.41 (0.94)	0.51
Using the EHR decreases the visual link with the patient	4.00 (1.21)	3.81 (1.05)	0.57
Using the EHR is a barrier for the physician-patient relationship	3.53 (1.01)	3.00 (1.00)	0.03
I make the patient feel comfortable	4.18 (0.73)	4.41 (0.50)	0.22
I show interest for the patient's ideas	4.29 (0.77)	4.41 (0.51)	0.54
I pay attention to the patient	4.06 (0.75)	4.29 (0.69)	0.26
I let the patient talk without interruption	3.59 (0.94)	3.76 (0.97)	0.55

Objective use of the EHR during the first 10 min of the clinical encounter

In general, residents used the EHR about one-third of the utterances/time during the first ten minutes of the clinical encounter both intervention phases (pre: 27.9/26.2%; post: 30.4/28.2%), and used it more during medical and therapeutic talk and less for lifestyle or psychosocial matters (Table 4). EHR use with visual/verbal contact was 4 times more frequent than without visual/verbal contact.

After training, participants increased the use of signposting when using the EHR (Table 4). Although participants increased their use of the EHR after training (Table 4), it occurred only for medical or therapeutic talk (without verbal/visual contact) and positive talk (with verbal/visual contact). The use of the EHR significantly decreased during discussion of psychosocial issues (Table 4). Such changes were observed among different types of users of EHR (low: pre 57 utterances (10.6%) vs post 20 (4.6%) $p = 0.01$; medium: pre 27 (30.0%) vs post 12 (26.7%) $p = 0.01$; high: pre 162 (43.2%) vs post 24 (27.0%) $p = 0.01$).

Analysis of entire consultations confirmed that EHR was used more often during the opening and history taking phases (55 and 66% of the pre- and post-intervention phases) than during the explanation and counseling phases (40 and 32% of the pre- and post-intervention phases).

Patterns of EHR use

Five residents (29.4%) were high EHR users, 5 (29.4%) were medium users and 7 (41, 2%) were low users.

Discussion

Our study shows that before the training intervention, residents used the EHR about 30% of the time/utterances during the initial few minutes of the encounter and more often for medical than for psychosocial topics. They also used the EHR four times more often while maintaining visual/verbal contact.

Significant changes after the intervention included: more signposting of EHR use, increased link with patients while using EHR, more use of EHR related to medical and therapeutic topics and less use associated with psychosocial issues. Residents reported feeling more comfortable using EHR in the consultation, and perceived the EHR as less of a barrier to communication.

Our results confirm those previously published in adult primary care outpatient contexts. Two recent systematic reviews about the impact of the EHR use on the patient-doctor interaction report a mean use of EHR of 32% of the visit time with a range from 12 to 55% with experienced physicians using it less often [13, 27]. Most of the studies (76%) were conducted in adult primary care outpatient clinics but similar results were observed in specialities and in different clinical settings. Very few studies analysed the use of EHR among residents [13, 27]. One study which analysed screen gaze and use of typing among US residents showed increased EHR use (including both screen gaze and typing) among more experienced residents: 43 and 18% respectively among 3rd year residents vs 30 and 9% among 1st year residents. Screen gaze shared by both residents and patients was stable (10%) [61]. To our knowledge, no study analysed

Table 4 Use of Electronic Health Record (EHR) during the first ten minutes of consultation pre and post-training

Overall EHR use	All consultations ($n = 142$)		
	Pre ($n = 73$)	Post ($n = 69$)	
	Mean (SD)	Mean (SD)	p
EHR Signposting	0.77 (1.69)	1.80 (3.35)	0.04
	All utterances ($n = 29011$)		
	Pre ($n = 15181$) n (%)	Post ($n = 13830$) n (%)	p
EHR total use[a]	4237 (27.9)	4207 (30.4)	<0.01
• With link[a]	3215 (21.2)	3180 (23)	<0.01
• Without link[a]	800 (5.3)	726 (5.3)	0.96
Medical condition and therapeutic regimen[b]	1232 (28.5)	1322 (30.6)	0.04
Medical condition (without counseling)[b]	774 (29.8)	790 (31.8)	0.12
Therapeutic regimen (without counseling)[b]	458 (26.6)	532 (28.9)	0.14
Lifestyle and psychosocial[b]	307 (24.8)	114 (15.3)	<0.01
Lifestyle (without counseling)[b]	99 (25.5)	62 (24.8)	0.91
Psychosocial (without counseling)[b]	208(24.5)	52 (10.5)	<0.01
Positive talk[b]	821 (25.1)	871 (29.7)	<0.01
Emotional talk[b]	92 (21.2)	97 (25.5)	0.18
Partnership[b]	697 (25)	745 (27)	0.10

[a]% calculated with numbers of utterances while using EHR/all utterances
[b]% calculated with number of utterances per RIAS category while using EHR/number of utterances per RIAS category

EHR use with or without maintaining visual or verbal contact with the patient.

After training, our study participants felt more comfortable using the EHR and were less likely to feel that it interfered with the doctor-patient interaction. These findings are in line with studies conducted in encounters with standardized patients, and support the claim that specific training can improve EHR acceptance among medical students, residents and physicians [46, 48]. This is of importance since physicians are more reluctant than patients to use EHRs and are usually less satisfied than patients when using computers during clinical encounters [13, 27, 62]. The fact that increased EHR use among residents correlates with patient's dissatisfaction supports the need to train residents on the EHR use in a patient-centered way [61].

The training also impacted on residents' behaviour by increasing the use of signposting. Transition statements such as "signposting" are known to help the patient understand the structure and the meaning of the consultation, increase his/her participation and implication in the encounter and inform him/her when a new topic is introduced [35, 63, 64]. It is particularly important when using the EHR since the frequency of transitions statements is inversely correlated with the screen gaze [30]. Our results show that signposting, a strategy largely recommended by experts while using the EHR, can be taught effectively [13, 28, 33, 34].

We also found that the training course led to decreased use of the EHR when discussing psychosocial issues with patients, regardless of the resident's typing style (low, medium or high EHR users). This result is of interest since most experts recommend avoiding computer use when a psychosocial topic is addressed [33, 34].

Why residents increased their use of EHR during both medical and "positive talk" during the first ten minutes of the consultation post training remains unclear. Positive talk includes utterances such as laughter, agreement approvals and compliments and is considered to contribute to build the relationship [55, 65, 66]. Residents may still have difficulties postponing EHR use when biomedical issues are discussed. Residents may also use positive talk to enhance relationship-building while using the EHR. Further research should evaluate whether these changes also occur during the entire length of the encounter.

Limitations

Our study has several limitations. We were not able to conduct a controlled or randomized study given the small number of residents who accepted to take part into the study and the pre-post intervention design may threaten the validity of the results given a possible learning effect on use of EHR over time. However, since behavioral changes essentially focused on elements emphasized during training, such changes may be more related to the training than to natural progression over time. The timing and spatial disposition of the videotaping did not allow us to analyse the impact of training for two of the recommendations regarding EHR use: EHR opening was not systematically recorded and the screen position was not always entirely visible on all videotaped encounters. We also made no distinction between visual and verbal contact. Although previous studies have adopted different approaches [30, 67, 68], it is still unclear if verbal contact has the same "value" as visual contact during the physician-patient interaction. The importance of verbal and non verbal communication which has been emphasized by several authors should be further explored when related to EHR use [69, 70]. We did not assess patients' perceptions regarding the use of EHR, because prior studies have shown that patients were already very satisfied with their physician communication styles and that the introduction of EHRs did not change their satisfaction [17, 21, 62, 71]; given the results of our small phone survey on the use of EHR among chronically ill patients from our clinic, we did not expect to find any difference in patient's perceptions. We only analysed EHR use during the first ten minutes of the clinical encounter, and we may have missed important EHR related behaviors later in the consultations as well as changing patterns of EHR use. We based our study on the use of one type of EHR program and different EHR programs may yield different EHR behaviors. Finally, the fact that participants themselves asked their patients to participate and knew they were being videotaped may represent a limitation (through selection bias and Hawthorne effect).

Conclusion

Paying attention to both the patient and the computer is challenging and can modify the patient-physician relationship. Given the increasing use of EHRs in health care settings, physicians must find the best way to perform EHR-related tasks without negatively affecting the physician-patient relationship. This study suggests that training can improve residents' EHR-related communication skills, especially in situations where patients bring up sensitive psychosocial issues. EHR-related communication skills training should be integrated at all stages of medical training given the ongoing development of EHR in the health care system. More research is needed to further explore the EHR-related behaviours that patients expect or value from their doctor, in order to give more scientific evidence to expert recommendations on how and when to use the EHR. It would also be of interest to analyse which factors related to patients, physicians and computers influence the use of EHR during the clinical encounter.

Abbreviations

EHR: Electronic Health Record; ICPC: International Classification of Primary Care; RIAS: Roter interaction analysis system

Acknowledgments

The authors thank Denis Roberge from "Entre les lignes Inc." for the RIAS coding work.

Funding

The study was supported by a fund of the Faculty of Medicine of the Geneva University (Mimosa)

Authors' contributions

CL, MDD, PH, and NJP designed the study. BC, CL, NJP, carried out data analysis. CL and NJP wrote the first version of the article, which was then revised by all the authors. All the authors approved the definitive version of the article.

Competing interests

The authors declare that they have no competing interests.

Consent for publication

Not applicable.

Author details

[1]Department of Community Medicine, Primary Care and Emergency Medicine, Geneva University Hospitals, rue Gabrielle Perret-Gentil, CH-1211 Geneva, Switzerland. [2]Primary care unit, University of Geneva, Centre Médical Universitaire de Genève, Geneva, Switzerland. [3]Faculty of Medicine, University of Geneva, Geneva, Switzerland.

References

1. Als AB. The desk-top computer as a magic box: patterns of behaviour connected with the desk-top computer; GPs' and patients' perceptions. Fam Pract. 1997;14: 17–23.
2. Schoen C, Osborn R, Squires D, Doty M, Rasmussen P, Pierson R, Applebaum S. A survey of primary care doctors in ten countries shows progress in use of health information technology, less in other areas. Health Aff (Millwood). 2012;31:2805–16.
3. Xierali IM, Phillips Jr RL, Green LA, Bazemore AW, Puffer JC. Factors influencing family physician adoption of electronic health records (EHRs). J Am Board Fam Med. 2013;26:388–93.
4. Blumenthal D. Stimulating the Adoption of Health Information Technology. N Engl J Med. 2009;360:1477–9.
5. McConnell H. International efforts in implementing national health information infrastructure and electronic health records. World Hosp Health Serv. 2004;40: 33–7. 39–40, 50–52.
6. Lippert S, Kverneland A. The Danish National Health Informatics Strategy. Stud Health Technol Inform. 2003;95:845–50.
7. eHealth strategy for Switzerland. Federal Office of Public Health (FOPH). Available at https://www.bag.admin.ch/bag/fr/home/themen/strategien-politik/nationale-gesundheitsstrategien/strategie-ehealth-schweiz.html. Accessed 22 May 2017.
8. Hippisley-Cox J, Pringle M, Cater R, Wynn A, Hammersley V, Coupland C, Hapgood R, Horsfield P, Teasdale S, Johnson C. The electronic patient

record in primary care–regression or progression? A cross sectional study. Brit Med J. 2003;326:1439–43.
9. Kazmi Z. Effects of exam room EHR use on doctor-patient communication: a systematic literature review. Inform Prim Care. 2013;21:30–9.
10. Sullivan F, Mitchell E. Has general practitioner computing made a difference to patient care? A systematic review of published reports. Brit Med J. 1995; 311:848–52.
11. Burke HB, Sessums LL, Hoang A, Becher DA, Fontelo P, Liu F, Stephens M, Pangaro LN, O'Malley PG, Baxi NS, et al. Electronic health records improve clinical note quality. J Am Med Inform Assoc. 2015;22:199–205.
12. Chaudhry B, Wang J, Wu S, Maglione M, Mojica W, Roth E, Morton SC, Shekelle PG. Systematic review: impact of health information technology on quality, efficiency, and costs of medical care. Ann Intern Med. 2006;144:742–52.
13. Crampton NH, Reis S, Shachak A. Computers in the clinical encounter: a scoping review and thematic analysis. J Am Med Inform Assoc. 2016;23: 654–65.
14. Sullivan F, Wyatt JC. How computers can help to share understanding with patients. Brit Med J. 2005;331:892–4.
15. Hersh WR. Medical informatics: improving health care through information. J Am Med Assoc. 2002;288:1955–8.
16. Arar NH, Wen L, McGrath J, Steinbach R, Pugh JA. Communicating about medications during primary care outpatient visits: the role of electronic medical records. Inform Prim Care. 2005;13:13–22.
17. Chan W, McGlade K. Patients' attitudes to GPs' use of computers. Br J Gen Pract. 2003;53:490–1.
18. Garcia-Sanchez R. The patient's perspective of computerised records: a questionnaire survey in primary care. Inform Prim Care. 2008;16:93–9.
19. Garrison GM, Bernard ME, Rasmussen NH. 21st-century health care: the effect of computer use by physicians on patient satisfaction at a family medicine clinic. Fam Med. 2002;34:362–8.
20. Hsu J, Huang J, Fung V, Robertson N, Jimison H, Frankel R. Health information technology and physician-patient interactions: impact of computers on communication during outpatient primary care visits. J Am Med Inform Assoc. 2005;12:474–80.
21. Irani JS, Middleton JL, Marfatia R, Omana ET, D'Amico F. The use of electronic health records in the exam room and patient satisfaction: a systematic review. J Am Board Fam Med. 2009;22:553–62.
22. Ridsdale L, Hudd S. Computers in the consultation: the patient's view. Br J Gen Pract. 1994;44:367–9.
23. Doyle RJ, Wang N, Anthony D, Borkan J, Shield RR, Goldman RE. Computers in the examination room and the electronic health record: physicians' perceived impact on clinical encounters before and after full installation and implementation. Fam Pract. 2012;29:601–8.
24. Morton ME, Wiedenbeck S. EHR acceptance factors in ambulatory care: a survey of physician perceptions. Perspect Health Inf Manag. 2010;7:1c.
25. Shield RR, Goldman RE, Anthony DA, Wang N, Doyle RJ, Borkan J. Gradual electronic health record implementation: new insights on physician and patient adaptation. Ann Fam Med. 2010;8:316–26.
26. Pearce C, Trumble S, Arnold M, Dwan K, Phillips C. Computers in the new consultation: within the first minute. Fam Pract. 2008;25:202–8.
27. Alkureishi MA, Lee WW, Lyons M, Press VG, Imam S, Nkansah-Amankra A, Werner D, Arora VM. Impact of Electronic Medical Record Use on the Patient-Doctor Relationship and Communication: A Systematic Review. J Gen Intern Med. 2016;31:548–60.
28. Booth N, Robinson P, Kohannejad J. Identification of high-quality consultation practice in primary care: the effects of computer use on doctor-patient rapport. Inform Prim Care. 2004;12:75–83.
29. Greatbatch D, Heath C, Campion P, Luff P. How do desk-top computers affect the doctor-patient interaction? Fam Pract. 1995;12:32–6.
30. Margalit RS, Roter D, Dunevant MA, Larson S, Reis S. Electronic medical record use and physician-patient communication: an observational study of Israeli primary care encounters. Patient Educ Couns. 2006;61:134–41.
31. Warshawsky SS, Pliskin JS, Urkin J, Cohen N, Sharon A, Binztok M, Margolis CZ. Physician Use of a Computerized Medical Record System during the Patient Encounter - a Descriptive Study. Comput Methods Programs Biomed. 1994;43:269–73.
32. Sinsky CA, Beasley JW. Texting while doctoring: a patient safety hazard. Ann Intern Med. 2013;159:782–3.
33. Duke P, Frankel RM, Reis S. How to Integrate the Electronic Health Record and Patient-Centered Communication Into the Medical Visit: A Skills-Based Approach. Teach Learn Med. 2013;25:358–65.
34. Ventres W, Kooienga S, Marlin R. EHRs in the exam room: tips on patient-centered care. Fam Pract Manag. 2006;13:45–7.
35. Silverman J, Kurtz S, Draper J. Skills for Communicating With Patients. 3 Revisedth ed. Oxford: Radcliffe Publishing Ltd; 2013.
36. Stewart M, Brown JB, Donner A, McWhinney IR, Oates J, Weston WW, Jordan J. The impact of patient-centered care on outcomes. J Fam Pract. 2000;49:796–804.
37. Nemeth LS, Feifer C, Stuart GW, Ornstein SM. Implementing change in primary care practices using electronic medical records: a conceptual framework. Implement Sci. 2008;3:3.
38. Shachak A, Hadas-Dayagi M, Ziv A, Reis S. Primary care physicians' use of an electronic medical record system: a cognitive task analysis. J Gen Intern Med. 2009;24:341–8.
39. Ventres W, Kooienga S, Marlin R, Vuckovic N, Stewart V. Clinician style and examination room computers: a video ethnography. Fam Med. 2005;37:276–81.
40. Montague E, Asan O. Physician Interactions with Electronic Health Records in Primary Care. Health Syst (Basingstoke). 2012;1:96–103.
41. Triola MM, Friedman E, Cimino C, Geyer EM, Wiederhorn J, Mainiero C. Health information technology and the medical school curriculum. Am J Manag Care. 2010;16:54–6.
42. Lown BA, Rodriguez D. Commentary: Lost in translation? How electronic health records structure communication, relationships, and meaning. Acad Med. 2012;87:392–4.
43. Tierney MJ, Pageler NM, Kahana M, Pantaleoni JL, Longhurst CA. Medical education in the electronic medical record (EMR) era: benefits, challenges, and future directions. Acad Med. 2013;88:748–52.
44. Wald HS, George P, Reis SP, Taylor JS. Electronic health record training in undergraduate medical education: bridging theory to practice with curricula for empowering patient- and relationship-centered care in the computerized setting. Acad Med. 2014;89:380–6.
45. Morrow JB, Dobbie AE, Jenkins C, Long R, Mihalic A, Wagner J. First-year medical students can demonstrate EHR-specific communication skills: a control-group study. Fam Med. 2009;41:28–33.
46. Reis S, Sagi D, Eisenberg O, Kuchnir Y, Azuri J, Shalev V, Ziv A. The impact of residents' training in Electronic Medical Record (EMR) use on their competence: Report of a pragmatic trial. Patient Educ Couns. 2013;93:515–21.
47. Han H, Waters T, Lopp L. Preserving Patient Relationship-centered Care while Utilizing EHRs. MedEdPORTAL Publications. 2014;10:9729.
48. Silverman H, Ho Y-X, Kaib S, Ellis WD, Moffitt MP, Chen Q, Nian H, Gadd CS. A novel approach to supporting relationship-centered care through electronic health record ergonomic training in preclerkship medical education. Acad Med. 2014;89:1230–4.
49. Häyrinen K, Saranto K, Nykänen P. Definition, structure, content, use and impacts of electronic health records: a review of the research literature. Int J Med Inform. 2008;77:291–304.
50. WHO | International Classification of Primary Care, Second edition (ICPC-2). http://www.who.int/classifications/icd/adaptations/icpc2/en/. Accessed 26 May 2016
51. Rouf E, Whittle J, Lu N, Schwartz MD. Computers in the exam room: differences in physician-patient interaction may be due to physician experience. J Gen Intern Med. 2007;22:43–8.
52. Hackl WO, Hoerbst A, Ammenwerth E. "Why the hell do we need electronic health records?". EHR acceptance among physicians in private practice in Austria: a qualitative study. Methods Inf Med. 2011;50:53–61.
53. King J, Patel V, Jamoom EW, Furukawa MF. Clinical benefits of electronic health record use: national findings. Health Serv Res. 2014;49:392–404.
54. El-Kareh R, Gandhi TK, Poon EG, Newmark LP, Ungar J, Lipsitz S, Sequist TD. Trends in Primary Care Clinician Perceptions of a New Electronic Health Record. J Gen Intern Med. 2009;24:464–8.
55. Roter D, Larson S. The Roter interaction analysis system (RIAS): utility and flexibility for analysis of medical interactions. Patient Educ Couns. 2002;46:243–51.
56. Entre les lignes Inc. E, Montreal, Quebec, Canada H4A 3E8. www.ell-research.com. Accessed 22 May 2017.
57. Asan O, DS P, Montague E. More screen time, less face time - implications for EHR design. J Eval Clin Pract. 2014;20:896–901.
58. Ventres W, Kooienga S, Vuckovic N, Marlin R, Nygren P, Stewart V. Physicians, patients, and the electronic health record: an ethnographic analysis. Ann Fam Med. 2006;4:124–31.
59. Newman W, Button G, Cairns P. Pauses in doctor–patient conversation during computer use: The design significance of their durations and accompanying topic changes. Int J Hum Comput Stud. 2010;68:398–409.

60. Ong LM, Visser MR, Kruyver IP, Bensing JM, van den Brink-Muinen A, Stouthard JM, Lammes FB, de Haes JC. The Roter Interaction Analysis System (RIAS) in oncological consultations: psychometric properties. Psychooncology. 1998;7: 387–401.
61. Asan O, Kushner K, Montague E. Exploring Residents' Interactions With Electronic Health Records in Primary Care Encounters. Fam Med. 2015;47: 722–6.
62. Gadd CS, Penrod LE. Dichotomy between physicians' and patients' attitudes regarding EMR use during outpatient encounters. Proc AMIA Symp. 2000; 275–79. https://www.ncbi.nlm.nih.gov/pmc/articles/PMC2243374/.
63. Floyd M, Lang F, Beine KL, McCord E. Evaluating interviewing techniques for the sexual practices history. Use of video trigger tapes to assess patient comfort. Arch Fam Med. 1999;8:218–23.
64. Levinson W, Roter DL, Mullooly JP, Dull VT, Frankel RM. Physician-patient communication. The relationship with malpractice claims among primary care physicians and surgeons. JAMA. 1997;277:553–9.
65. Cole SA, Bird J. The Medical Interview: The Three Function Approach. 3rd ed. Philadelphia: Saunders; 2013.
66. Roter DL, Larson S. The Relationship Between Residents' and Attending Physicians' Communication During Primary Care Visits: An Illustrative Use of the Roter Interaction Analysis System. Health Commun. 2001;13:33–48.
67. Asan O, Young HN, Chewning B, Montague E. How physician electronic health record screen sharing affects patient and doctor non-verbal communication in primary care. Patient Educ Couns. 2015;98:310–6.
68. Farber NJ, Liu L, Chen Y, Calvitti A, Street RL, Zuest D, Bell K, Gabuzda M, Gray B, Ashfaq S, et al. EHR use and patient satisfaction: What we learned. J Fam Pract. 2015;64:687–96.
69. Zoppi K, Epstein RM. Is communication a skill? Communication behaviors and being in relation. Fam Med. 2002;34:319–24.
70. Ruusuvuori J. Looking means listening: coordinating displays of engagement in doctor-patient interaction. Soc Sci Med. 2001;52:1093–108.
71. Legler JD, Oates R. Patients' reactions to physician use of a computerized medical record system during clinical encounters. J Fam Pract. 1993;37:241–4.

2

Immigrant parents' experience with the Swedish child health care system

Elisabeth Mangrio* and Karin Persson

Abstract

Background: Immigration, particularly when it is involuntary, is known to be an emotional stressor, regardless of the reason behind it. It is always a challenge to be removed from the habitual and cultural action pattern of the person or family. This can make children more vulnerable, because they often arrive with an increased risk of poor physical health. Because of that, it is crucial that immigrant children have access to ongoing health care. The aim of this study is to shed light on the experience of non-European immigrants with Sweden's Child Health Care system.

Methods: Qualitative semi-structured interviews were conducted, with parents of children who were patients of one of the four child health care centres. The centres were in four areas in a town in southern Sweden in which there are substantial immigrant populations. The interviews were conducted, transcribed and then analyzed with content analysis.

Results: The results were divided into two main categories: The first is "the sense of being cared for in another way," which was divided into the following four subcategories: compare with the home country, getting a home visit, engagement and contentment and unfamiliarity with the language. The second main category. "The feeling of getting all the practical needs met through the child health care system" had the following four subcategories: The importance of advice and guidance, getting oral and written information, getting help when needed and getting support when needed.

Conclusions: The parents expressed contentment regarding the Swedish child health care and they were thankful for how it was organized, the engagement of the nurses, the information and advices given as well as for the opportunities of getting a home visit after birth. However, more research is needed in order to find out the extent to which the Swedish child health care system is culturally appropriate in the whole country.

Keywords: Migration, Qualitative research, Child health care, Support

Background

Immigration, particularly when it is involuntary, is known to be an emotional stressor [1]. Refugees have generally experienced high-stress conditions before the exodus, and the exodus itself may have been perilous. The arrival in the new country is usually followed by the asylum process, which is a time of uncertainty and possibly anxiety that can intensify any existing mental illness [1, 2]. Newly arrived families often settle in neighbourhoods with lower socioeconomic status; they often work in jobs with poor pay; and they may experience societal discrimination [1, 3, 4]. According to the qualitative study by Samarasinghe et al, the authors concluded that the stress parents experience during the residence-permission process is often transferred to their children and, as a result, the youngsters experience symptoms of stress [5].

Regardless of the reason behind the immigration, the absence of the person or family's cultural patterns—customs, values and attitudes toward males and females and the infirm and the healthy, ways to express feelings and solve problems—is a challenge. Learning a new culture and language patterns is gradual, and throughout process,

* Correspondence: elisabeth.mangrio@mah.se
Department of Care Science, Faculty Health and Society, Malmö University, Jan Waldenströms gata 25, 205 06 Malmö, Sweden

recent immigrants can experience significant stress, both physically and mentally [1, 6].

Immigrant children are not immune to the stress and, in fact, these circumstances can make children suffer from poor physical and mental health [6, 7]. According to studies by Hjern et al [8] and Schiariti [7], immigrant children need special attention since they have an increased likelihood of suffering from poor physical health. Special attention must be directed toward the lower breastfeeding rates among immigrant mothers, as well toward nutritional deficiencies among their children [8]. Earlier research has reported that migrant children face an increased risk of infections, behavioural problems, sleep problems and intentional and unintentional injuries. Immunisations are often delayed and hearing and vision and dental problems of many migrant children are neither assessed or treated [7]. It has been found that 40 to 50% of these youngsters suffer from psychiatric and psychosomatic disorders; this is mostly attributable to having been uprooted [8]. Therefore, it is crucial that these children receive social support because of the increased likelihood to suffer mental illness [8]. Providing appropriate services to migrant children will protect their physical health and their psychological and emotional well-being [7]. Since many immigrant children have been raised in societies where living conditions and child health care programmes differ considerably from those in Europe, these differences should be addressed in a structured way through the child health care program as soon as the children arrive in a new country [8].

A study that focused on primary health-care nurses' impressions of health among families who immigrated involuntarily revealed that nurses encountered family members suffering from depression and physical conditions such as eczema, gastritis and generalized body pain [9]. The nurses also noticed that the stress caused by the process of immigrating worsened the conditions of immigrants with chronic diseases such as diabetes and asthma. And as time passed, the women in particular were perceived to be feeling isolated and experiencing stress due to the unfamiliar demands and responsibilities. They suffered from tiredness, homesickness and resultant somatic symptoms [9].

Negative attitudes toward immigrants hindered the families from assimilating into society, and unemployment and inactivity intensified the situation and resulted in diminishing self-esteem [5]. Conflicts within immigrant families may occur because of the challenges parents face in adjusting to their roles in a new environment. A father who is unable to find employment may feel like a poor role model for the children, and this can lead to violent behaviour within the family. Language barriers often force children to act as translators for the parents and, this too, can make the parents feel inferior. It must be noted that a family's socio-economic background plays an important part in the family's ability to adapt to the new country; well-educated parents have been shown to adjust more easily than do parents with limited education [5].

In Sweden, 20% of all children have either one or two parents who were born abroad [10]. These children have an increased risk of ill health, usually in the form of poor dental health and greater likelihood of being injured at home or in the surrounding environment. Furthermore, the very act of uprooting children from their home countries can not only affect their health and well-being, but it can also negatively impact their family members [8].

Most of these families are in contact with Sweden's Child Health Care system [11]. Sweden has a tax-financed health system, and municipalities are responsible for providing general access to health care [12]. All children residing in Sweden legally are eligible, without charge, for CHC services and CHC is a well-established organisation with responsibility for reducing morbidity, mortality and disability in newborn and younger children. Through regular visits to the CHC, each child's weight and physical and developmental health are closely followed and vaccinations are given until the child is 5 years. Another purpose is to educate parents so that they can make the most of their child's developmental opportunities and that is done through parental groups offered during the child's first year. For all immigrants with low knowledge and fluency in Swedish, a translator is booked for the visits at CHC. Written information that is distributed at CHC is translated into the most common languages that are represented in Sweden [11].

Studies have shown health care professionals confront many challenges in working with immigrant families. In their work with immigrant children in the CHC, primary health nurses said they lack written guidance, emotional support and help with the workload. A majority of the nurses experienced difficulties in their interactions with children and parents of foreign origin, and a majority also said they lacked formal training in cultural competence [9].

Addressing children's health problems is mostly regarded as a difficult matter among nurses, especially if the nurse and parents do not share the same language and an interpreter is not available [9, 13]. According to Woodland et al [13], it is of great importance that the nurses at the CHC interact with immigrant families with cultural sensitivity and that they tailor the information provided to parents and children to facilitate comprehension. Therefore, there is a need to examine the child health-care-provision experience that immigrant parents encounter in Sweden from the CHC service. To the best of our knowledge, no previous studies have been conducted on this topic as it relates to services received by families from outside of Europe.

Methods

Design

A qualitative method was used, in which semi-structured interviews were conducted with parents of children attending any of the four participating CHC centres in a town in southern Sweden. The interviews were conducted, transcribed and then analysed with content analysis [14]. The first author (EM) has several years of working within a multicultural area within the field of child health care and have done previous research with populations of different nationalities.

Sampling frame

The sample consisted of 19 parents (14 females and five males) who, during the data-collection period, sought treatment for a child at any of the four participating CHC centre in southern Sweden. Families in which both parents immigrated from non-European countries and whose child was under the age of 5 years old met the sample criteria. Participating parents, who ranged in age from 21 years old to 45 years old were also required to either speak understandable Swedish or English to be included in the sample. The length of residency in Sweden for these families ranged from 2 years to 22 years.

Data collection

In the pre-data collection period, the chief administrators of 27 CHC centres were contacted by email to inform them of our study. Six showed an interest in taking part in the actual study. However, when registered nurses at these centres were asked about their willingness to act as gatekeepers, only one CHC was willing to participate. Therefore, the email canvassing process began anew in the same town, resulting in another three CHC centres becoming participating sites, because nurses from each were willing to participate as gatekeepers. Thereafter, continual contact was maintained with the gatekeepers, and they contacted the first author (EM) whenever eligible families were at the centres.

All interviews were conducted by the first author (EM) and the interviews were done either at a CHC facility or at the homes of participating families. An interview guide was used, see Additional file 1 and interviews were tape-recorded and transcribed directly after the interviews. After the pilot interview was completed, the second author (KP) read the interview and provided suggestions about ways to improve subsequent interviews. The interviews were conducted in Swedish ($n = 15$) and in English ($n = 2$). The interviews lasted between 5 and 15 min, with an average duration of 9,5 min per interview. Participating parents' countries of origin as well as the number of parents from each are shown in Table 1.

Table 1 Number of participants and country of origin

Countries of origin	Number of participants
Afghanistan	2
Chile	1
India	1
Iraq	4
Kurdistan	3
Kuwait	1
Lebanon	1
Pakistan	2
Palestine	1
Venezuela	1
Vietnam	2

Data analysis

Interviews were transcribed verbatim and checked against the original audio recording. The coding of the analysis was done by the first author, and the second author commented on the analysis. The interviews were analysed using content analysis with the purpose of identifying emerging themes and patterns, according to Burnard [14]. The analysis process was as follows:

1. Interviews were read and transcribed verbatim in either English or Swedish.
2. Open coding was performed, and used to create categories.
3. Matching subcategories were grouped into new categories.
4. The results were discussed by the authors, and adjustments were made continuously until all data were used.

When no data was suitable for more than one category, the process was considered complete. Then the titles of the categories and subcategories were evaluated to ensure that they provided a clear picture of the actual content. Table 2 provides excerpts (meaning units) from the interviews and the resultant, code, subcategory and category.

Results

After analysis, the results were divided into two categories: 1) The sense of being cared for in another way and 2) The feeling that all the practical needs were met through the child health care system.

The sense of being cared for in another way

This overarching category emerged from many of the parents who mentioned that when they compared Swedish

Table 2 Some extracts from the interviews, explaining the analysis through meaning unit-category

Meaning unit	Code	Category	Sub Category
We didn't know about the vaccination schedule, since it is different from India. The nurse helped us a lot, giving us information about all the different vaccinations that should be given to the kids, and she had a regular follow- up as well, so that was very good for us.	Didn't know about vaccinations and the nurse gave us information.	The feeling of getting all the practical needs met through the child health care system	The importance of advices and guidance
If I don't understand something, I tell the nurse and then she can explain for me, and explain if I misunderstood something. I am very content.	They explain for me when I don't understand.	The sense of being taken care of in another way	To not know the language

child health care provision with that of their countries of origin, they felt gratitude and thankfulness. They mentioned appreciation for the CHC system, the way the service was organized and how well children were cared for. Appreciation was also expressed for the interest that nurses showed for the children and that the nurses found ways to communicate with parents despite language differences and challenges. The following sub-categories emerged from this category: *comparison with the home country, having a home visit, engagement and contentment, unfamiliarity with the language.*

Comparison with the home country

Several interviewees expressed that the Swedish child health care system was good and that no similar health care could be found in their home countries. Some of them spoke about the lack of knowledge among women in their home countries regarding how to care for themselves and a newborn. They also mentioned equity in treatment compared with their home countries. They thought it was very good to have access to the Swedish CHC.

> *In Sweden, it is not like in our home country. It is not unpleasant and terrible like it is in my home country.* -Informant 5

Another interviewee expressed that hygiene, engagement and treatment from nurses in Sweden was better than that in the home county. A participant expressed the difference like this:

> *In my home country, the health care you get depends on money and which doctor you have and if you are poor you don't get the same treatment as the rest. It is better for my children to grow up here in Sweden.* -Informant 6

All parents interviewed had similar thoughts about the CHC; one parent expressed it like this:

> *There is a great difference here compared to my home country, and I am very content here. It wouldn't have been the same health care in my country.* -Informant 15

Having a home visit Getting a home visit from a nurse after delivery of a newborn was something that all interviewees expressed as quite different than their experiences in their home countries. Several expressed gratitude and appreciation for the home visits by the visiting nurse after their child's birth. They felt honoured and as though they were important persons when someone from the health care system took their time to visit in their home. Parents expressed that they appreciated the chance to sit down for a while and talk to the nurse during the visit. One of the interviewees expressed it this way:

> *It feels unbelievable! It is not like that in our home country and I felt so much of respect from the nurse when she came to our place. The nurses respect that a woman after birth feels tired and therefore they come to your place.* -Informant 9

Three participants expressed that they would have liked to have gotten a home visit, but it did not materialize. One woman mentioned that she had an appointment booked twice for a home visit, but it was cancelled each time, and she eventually needed to go to the CHC instead. Another mother said that she had not had any home visits for either of her two children and that she wished she would have gotten one. The third woman had enjoyed home visits when her first child was born, but the home visit for her second child was cancelled, and she felt disappointed.

Engagement and contentment

Almost every parent interviewed said that they were content with the level of involvement that the nurses exhibited when they visited a CHC centre. There was great appreciation for the nurses, who were described as nice, happy, and engaged with the families. The parents felt safe with the nurses and felt included while meeting with the nurses. Parents who brought their children to a CHC facility in a multicultural area characterized the entire staff as very nice. They attributed this ecumenical concern to the nurses' meeting people from many different cultures and that it created good encounters for them with the nurses. A mother spoke about their satisfying encounters with nurses like this:

> *You feel welcomed by the staff and we like especially the staff nurse in the waiting room and our own pediatric nurse. It is nice here and there is a warm atmosphere here.* - Informant 8

A few parents expressed that they were not as content as the interviewees above seemed to indicate. Some said that they would prefer to be reassigned to another nurse. In addition, another parent voiced contentment but mentioned that other parents not included in this study, were not as pleased. Some parents appreciated the doctors' visits that their children had, and they characterised the doctors as nice. Some parents believed that the nurses had genuine concern for their children and exhibited thoughtfulness about the children. And other parents mentioned that they believed that the CHC medical professionals respected their cultural background, and they had not experienced racism.

Unfamiliarity with the language

One mother mentioned her appreciation that the nurses explained and adjusted their language as soon as she told them that she didn't understand. However, she felt concern for the mothers with newborns if their Swedish-language proficiency was not as good as her own. Another mother explained that in the beginning, her Swedish was not good and, during that time, her interactions with nurses had not been as good as they were at the time of the interview. Other women did not get on well in the parental group meetings, and mothers had a difficult time understanding one other.

One father expressed the difficulties with language like this:

> *My wife gets a translator as soon as I am working, and through that way she gets a lot of information and understands.* -Informant 14

Other parents also got translation assistance and appreciated it. One father, whose experience of getting language help was satisfactory, expressed it like this:

> *Yes, my nurse came to our house and he is good and he talked in my language and first he called us and then we met at our house and he explained all the coming visits at CHC during the coming years.* -Informant 16

The feeling of getting all the practical needs met through the child health care system

This overarching category emerged from parents speaking about practical issues of child health care and that advice, guidance and information was provided to them when needed. The parents also expressed gratitude for practical help with referrals to other health care professionals as well as the support they got in their parenting roles, though some wished there had been more support and practical help available. From this, the following sub-categories emerged: *the importance of advice and guidance, getting oral and written information, getting help when needed, getting support when needed.*

The importance of advice and guidance

Several of the parents mentioned that they got advice about vaccinations, breastfeeding, growth, nutrition, child safety, as well as advice related to medical situations like as infections and diseases. One mother said the following:

> *She was having a bowel movement, and I didn't know that she would get that. It was happening every five minutes and we were wondering what it was and I went and asked my nurse and she gave me a prescription that could be got from the pharmacy. I didn't know where to go and whom to ask but she helped me.* Informant 1

One parent got advice at the parental group about nutrition and sleeping patterns:

> *They told us about nutrition at the parental group and that we could divide the portions six times a day and we have now tried that and the baby is sleeping much better after that.* -Informant 7

Several of the mothers and fathers thought that the nurses were good about giving proper advice and guidance, and when the nurses did not know what advice to give, they asked colleagues and came back to them with the information. Two parents mentioned disappointments due to having gotten wrong advice when seeking guidance on several topics.

Getting oral and written information

Several of the interviewed parents were content with the written and oral information given at the CHC facilities. Parents appreciated being told about information on the

Internet as well as handouts distributed at the centre. Other parents were content with materials mailed to them. One mother said this:

It has been very good, and we got letters home prior to every visit, and the nurse always gives oral information about the coming visit and what to expect, for example if there is going to be vaccinations given to the child -Informant 4

Another parent appreciated that they had communicated orally with centre personnel prior to vaccinations and, therefore, they knew what to expect and how it would be done. This type of information calmed them.

One mother who had recently arrived in Sweden mentioned that she would have liked more oral information about how the health care system works in Sweden and where to go if the child gets sick. She was also uncertain about the offerings of the various health care sectors in Sweden and did not know if other services were available for her and her child. Another parent would have liked more information about, for example, parental groups that could be joined, and one parent would have liked more oral information about food and proper nutrition:

The information about food and when to start giving different kind of food to the baby, that they could have explained a little bit more. They only gave a book and thought that I would read it. But I don't think all mothers read the book, so it would have been good with more oral information about nutrition. -Informant 10

Another parent who had just recently arrived in Sweden was very content with the information the nurse had told him and his wife. The nurse helped them understand about children's sleeping patterns and nutrition. They believed they needed the guidance, and they appreciated it.

Some of the parents in the sample mentioned that they appreciated help and guidance they received on a variety of childcare topics such as required vaccinations, check-ups and practical help with referring the child to other health services when needed. One parent expressed:

We have hearing deficit in the family and we were afraid that our child would have it as well and therefore we got help from the nurse to book an appointment for our child -Informant 11

Another mother expressed gratitude about the practical assistance provided her when the CHC referred her child for a developmental assessment, because the child was not doing well on age-appropriate cognitive testing at four-years-old. The referral revealed that the child was in need of extra support from the rehabilitation. The mother expressed gratitude that the nurse that was observant about the child's need for support and additional instruction or therapy. Another mother explained about the help that she got as a result of a social services referral:

They have a social worker here at the Family centre and I have got a lot of help from her. She helps me and explain for me how I should handle my child in the best and most proper way. -Informant 13

Another mother expressed feelings of thankfulness for the all help she gets:

Everyone here knows me well and they are fantastic people. I feel that I get all the help that I need and always gets it when I need and ask for it. -Informant 2

But a father expressed that, compared to 15 years before when he brought his now-older children to the centre, the CHC seems less helpful. The father said that he would have liked for young his children to be getting more check-ups and help than they are currently receiving. In a somewhat similar vein, one mother said that she would have liked a greater level of support with her second child, as she believed that she had received more with her first child.

However, this same mother was grateful for help she had gotten when the child had atopic eczema, and they needed to go to the emergency room. The nurse wrote a referral note which was accepted by the ER, and she was very thankful for that help.

Getting support when needed

Many of the study parents expressed gratitude for the nurses' support. One mother who had not been in Sweden very long said the support she got from her nurse was fantastic and that it was needed. Another woman explained that she didn't feel well after giving birth to her child, and she felt that the nurse was a great support. She continued by saying that she can visit or call the nurse whenever needed and that it is difficult to find such good support elsewhere. Another woman spoke of the support she is getting like this:

My nurse expressed that I could talk to her if needed, and since I got postnatal depression, I came to her and talked, and she said that it was normal to feel like that and that felt good to hear. -Informant 3

Other parents mentioned that the nurses were very supportive when they did not know what to do with their child. One parent expressed that when she became worried about a matter and told the nurse, the nurse listened with such interest that that she began to worry less.

Another mother expressed following support:

> *They always ask how I feel as a mother, and that feels good.* -Informant 12

Another mother felt good about getting support from the nurse through the Edinburgh Postnatal Depression Scale (EPDS) screening that took place at when her child was 2 months old. She stated that it felt pleasant as a mother to come for that meeting.

Discussion

The results showed that immigrant parents appreciated several components of the CHC's service. First, the parents were grateful for the Swedish health care system when comparing it to the health care that would have been given them in their home countries and, although some parents had had difficulties understanding Swedish in the beginning, they appreciated the availability of interpreters. Also appreciated was that nurses tried to speak with the parents in their native language whenever possible. They also mentioned appreciation of the practical help they got through advice and guidance, in both written and oral form, concerning different facets of child care and parenting. The parents also reported that they were satisfied with getting practical help when they needed it in general.

Parents who had home visits seemed to appreciate them as a first encounter, and the parents who did not have one were disappointed. Those who did have a home visit explained that it was nice to be able to sit down with the nurse, especially after giving birth and feeling tired. In addition, some were afraid of going out with the baby due to infection risks. When comparing Sweden's CHC to the health care their children would have received in their countries of origin, most agreed that they would not have gotten such visits there. A systematic review by Peacock et al [15] showed that home visits are important after birth from many standpoints: preventing illness, preventing a child's growth failure, providing parental support and preventing child abuse. Oddly, a few parents in the present study did not have any home visits, despite the directive that every CHC centre in Sweden must provide such visits [16]. This indicates that resources should perhaps be reallocated to ensure that all required home visits are carried out.

Many of the interviewed parents said that they were content and grateful for the encounters with the nurses and thought that they were engaged and showed respect for the families. They were also thankful for translators and, when comparing CHC services with the health care in their home countries, Sweden was well-rated. According to an Australian study, health care services that are sensitive to their clients' cultural and linguistic backgrounds are more likely to improve access and equity, health literacy and quality of care for immigrant children [13]. When health assessments are done with an appreciation for the client's culture, it can provide useful insights into cultural, dietary and health practices. This is also in line with findings of Shen et al. [17], who state that cultural competence is an essential component for providing relevant and culturally responsive health care to diverse populations. This type of cultural sensitivity can help reduce ethnic disparities in health care provision and potentially enhance the quality of care, patient satisfaction and health outcomes [17]. Health care professionals must take into account that refugees leave behind culture, language, environment, climate, family, friends, social system and norms of behaviour [18]. Another important part of this equation is availability of translators for newly arrived refugees, which is simply good practice in health care [13], and several of the parents interviewed noted its utility. The overarching theme "the sense of being taken care of in another way" was emerged from comments about the engagement of the nurses that was good rated according to the interviewees and was different from the one they remembered in the home country. It could probably be the cultural sensitivity that was evident for these families that Shen et al is mentioning [17], as well as the fact that the CHC offers good service when it comes to translation. This translation service is probably not so common in the home countries and was appreciated because of that. According to a systematic review by Berendes et al [19], the authors concluded that both private and public health care in low- and middle-income countries had poor quality in their provision, but the private had a better care when it comes to responsiveness, effort and being client oriented. An additional reason might be that Swedish child health care is free of charge [11]. Another reason that could have influenced the families' perceptions of the care given is that all children are offered the same national programme no matter where they come from [11]. Probably families comparing the Swedish child health care with that from the home countries could be related to these kind of aspects. All of this needs to be considered when working to improve the child health care system in Sweden.

Some of the parents in the sample expressed that they had gotten good support from the nurses regarding different matters, such as not feeling well after childbirth, especially after arriving in a new country and not knowing how to parent. As Samarasinghe et al mentioned, immigrant parents and their children experience stress in the new environment and, therefore, the support that the nurses provide can be essential to the families during this period in their lives [1, 5], especially because both parents and children may have experienced mental and physical challenges, and they typically need extra attention from health professionals [8].

The aim of the study was to cast light on the experience of non-European immigrant families with Sweden's the Child Health Care system. The participating CHC centres were in a multiethnic town in the southern Sweden and, although chief administrators of all 27 centres in this town were contacted by email, only four administrators responded. No explanations were given for the low response rate, but it is likely that it is due to a high workload. The four CHC centres were located in areas with substantial immigrant populations, so we had a good representation for the purposes of this study. However, a greater segment of the population could have been included if translators had been more available to us. Another limitation of this study is that the interviews were only conducted in Swedish or English and that could have affected the result of the present study. It could be assumed that newly arrived parents with greater health care need and greater need for support were excluded from the present study because of language barrier. If a translator was available, the result could therefore have been more nuance. However, there were a few parents with shorter stay in Sweden included in the present study.

The result that emerged in the present study was mainly positive comments about the CHC service and it must be considered that there is a possibility that the parents felt that is was difficult to share negative experiences during the interviews. Although the first author mentioned before every interview that all the information from the families should not be spread to the CHC service.

The interviews were conducted by the first author (EM), and after the pilot interview was completed, the second author (KP) read the interview and provided suggestions about ways to improve subsequent interviews. The coding of the analysis was done by the first author, and the second author commented on the analysis, thereby increasing the credibility of the results because the perceptions of both researchers were taken into consideration and were thoroughly processed [20].

The transferability of a qualitative study can be suggested, but in the end, this is something for individuals to decide for themselves [20]. Several findings in the data were recurring, which suggests that they may be transferred to comparable situations.

Conclusions

Non-European immigrant parents in Sweden expressed gratitude about receiving health care in a different way than they would have in their home countries. They were also grateful about the practical help they were afforded. Regarding childrearing, although the parents in this study seemed to get culturally sensitive and competent care, more research is needed in order to find out to what extent the Swedish child health care system is culturally appropriate to all peoples throughout the country.

Abbreviations

CHC: Child health care; EM: Elisabeth Mangrio; EPDS: Edinburgh Postpartum Depression Screening; KP: Karin Persson

Acknowledgements

Department of Care Science, Malmö University has supported the research.

Funding

No funding was needed for the study.

Authors' contributions

EM carried out the study design, the data collection and drafted the manuscript. KP provided critical methodological revision and supervision. Both authors read and approved the final manuscript.

Competing interest

The authors declare that they have no competing interests.

Consent for publication

Not applicable.

References

1. Samarasinghe K. En hälsosam anpassning: om ofrivilligt invandrade familjers hälsa under omställningen till Sverige och om hälsostödjande familjesamtal. 2010. Studentlitteratur. (In Swedish).
2. Fazel M, Stein A. The mental health of refugee children. Arch Dis Child. 2002;87(5):366–70.
3. Pitt RS, Sherman J, Macdonald ME. Low-income working immigrant families in Quebec: exploring their challenges to well-being. Can J Public Health. 2016;106(8):539–45.
4. Montgomery E, Foldspang A. Discrimination, mental problems and social adaptation in young refugees. Eur J Public Health. 2008;18(2):156–61.
5. Samarasinghe K, Fridlund B, Arvidsson B. Primary Health Care Nurses' conceptions of involuntarily migrated families' health. Int Nurs Rev. 2006;53(4):301–7.
6. Bhugra D. Migration and mental health. Acta Psychiatr Scand. 2004;109(4): 243–58.
7. Schiariti V. The moral needs of migrant children: a call for global action. Acta Paediatr. 2016;105(5):445–6.
8. Hjern A, Bouvier P. Migrant children–a challenge for European paediatricians. Acta Paediatr. 2004;93(11):1535–9.
9. Berlin A, Johansson SE, Tornkvist L. Working conditions and cultural competence when interacting with children and parents of foreign origin–Primary Child Health Nurses' opinions. Scand J Caring Sci. 2006;20(2):160–8.
10. Statistiska centralbyrån, Statistics Sweden. [http://www.scb.se/sv_/hitta-statistik/statistik-efter-amne/befolkning/befolkningens-sammansattning/befolkningsstatistik/] (In Swedish). Accessed 28 Jan 2017.
11. Magnusson M, Blennow M, Hagelin E, Sundelin C. Barnhälsovård-att främja barns hälsa. 2016. Liber (In Swedish).
12. Swedish Health Care [http://www.swedishhealthcare.com/about-sweden-and-swedish-healthcare/swedens-healthcare-system/]. Accessed 28 Jan 2017.
13. Woodland L, Burgner D, Paxton G, Zwi K. Health service delivery for newly arrived refugee children: a framework for good practice. J Paediatr Child Health. 2010;46(10):560–7.

14. Burnard P, Gill P, Stewart K, Treasure E, Chadwick B. Analysing and presenting qualitative data. Br Dent J. 2008;204(8):429–32.
15. Peacock S, Konrad S, Watson E, Nickel D, Muhajarine N. Effectiveness of home visiting programs on child outcomes: a systematic review. BMC Public Health. 2013;13:17–2458-13-17.
16. Ackreditering och avtal för barnavårdscentral i hälsoval Skåne: Region Skåne: [http://www.skane.se/Public/Protokoll/N%C3%A4rsjukv%C3%A5rdsberedningen/2014-12-03/Uppdaterade%20ackrediteringsvillkor%20f%C3%B6r%20barnav%C3%A5rdscentral%202015/BVC141201.pdf] (In Swedish). Accessed 28 Jan 2017.
17. Shen Z. Cultural competence models and cultural competence assessment instruments in nursing: a literature review. J Transcult Nurs. 2015;26(3):308–21.
18. Salaff JW, Greve A. Can Chinese women´social networks migrate? Women´s Studies International Forum. 2004;27:149–62.
19. Berendes S, Heywood P, Oliver S, Garner P. Quality of private and public ambulatory health care in low and middle income countries: systematic review of comparative studies. PLoS Med. 2011;8(4):e1000433.
20. Graneheim UH, Lundman B. Qualitative content analysis in nursing research: concepts, procedures and measures to achieve trustworthiness. Nurse Educ Today. 2004;24(2):105–12.

3

Primary palliative care team perspectives on coordinating and managing people with advanced cancer in the community

Julia Hackett[1*], Lucy Ziegler[2], Mary Godfrey[3], Robbie Foy[4] and Michael I. Bennett[2]

Abstract

Background: Primary health care teams are key to the delivery of care for patients with advanced cancer during the last year of life. The Gold Standards Framework is proposed as a mechanism for coordinating and guiding identification, assessment, and support. There are still considerable variations in practice despite its introduction. The aim of this qualitative study is to improve understanding of variations in practice through exploring the perspectives and experiences of members of primary health care teams involved in the care of patients with advanced cancer.

Methods: Qualitative, semi-structured interviews, focus groups, and non-participatory observations involving 67 members of primary health care teams providing palliative care. Data were analysed using a grounded theory approach.

Results: We identified distinct differences in the drivers and barriers of community advanced cancer care coordination, which relate to identification and management, and access to effective pain management, and go some way to understanding variations in practice. These include proactive identification processes, time and resource pressures, unclear roles and responsibilities, poor multidisciplinary working, and inflexible models for referral and prescribing. These provide valuable insight into how professionals work together and independently within an infrastructure that can both support and hinder the provision of effective community palliative care.

Conclusions: Whilst the GSF is a guide for good practice, alone it is not a mechanism for change. Rather it provides a framework for describing quality of practice that was already occurring. Consequently, there will continue to be variations in practice.

Keywords: Primary care, Palliative care, Gold standards framework, Qualitative research, Patient care

Background

Good provision of palliative care is a continuing clinical priority worldwide. People with advanced cancer are living longer and illness trajectories are changing [1, 2]. Prevalence of symptoms, such as complex pain, are likely to increase [3], requiring more input and support from a range of health professionals over longer periods of time. Receiving care at home is of great importance for most patients [4]. In the UK, primary health care teams (PHCTs) are multidisciplinary teams which are intended to provide the majority of palliative care to community based patients in the last year of life (see Table 1 for how the organisation of care across the PHCT is configured). High quality community-based palliative care requires good multidisciplinary teamwork [5–7] and close working relationships [8].

The Gold Standards Framework (GSF) describes and brings together a number of evidence-based principles of practice as a guide for the care of palliative patients and their families [9]. It was intended to help PHCTs

* Correspondence: julia.hackett@york.ac.uk
[1]Martin House Research Centre, Social Policy Research Unit, University of York, York YO10 5DD, UK

Table 1 The organisation of care across the PHCT

PHCT member	Role with patients with palliative care needs	Timing and type of involvement	How is involvement initiated	Method of involvement
GP	Provide general palliative care Assess patients' needs Prescribe and manage medications Identify patients approaching end-of-life Care planning and anticipatory prescribing Manage and coordinate end-of-life care	Prior to diagnosis Continuous however during period where patient is receiving treatment may be intermittent until later stages	Patient presents to GP Referral from oncology	Appointments in surgery Home visits Occasional phone calls to patient and family
District nurse	Provide general palliative care alongside GP, i.e.: management, coordination, and orchestration of services to enable good home care for dying patients Physical nursing needs, i.e.: wound management, continence care, catheter care, medication and syringe drivers	Last few weeks/days of life Often receive a referral soon after diagnosis of advanced cancer so will have initial meeting and then intermittent contact until later stages Continuous involvement in last few weeks/days of life	Referral from GP, oncologist, community matron, joint care manager, clinical nurse specialist	Always home visits Sometimes phone calls to patient and family
Clinical nurse specialist	Provide specialist psychological and physical symptom management that	Can be from diagnosis of advanced cancer Intermittent	Referral from GP, district nurse, oncologist Complex needs that cannot be managed by the GP and district nurse	Always home visits Often phone calls to patient and family
Community matron	Provide care and support to people with long-term chronic conditions to keep patients as healthy as possible and living independently Only involved if patient has a long-term chronic condition and cancer	From diagnosis of chronic condition Continuous	Referral from GP, district nurse, hospital team	Always home visits Sometimes phone calls to patient and family
Joint care manager	Provide a service to adults aged 65 years and over with complex health and social care needs and adults of all ages who have been identified as eligible for NHS Continuing Healthcare funding Assess health and social care needs; plan, coordinate, and review services required	Discharge from hospital At home but at risk of being admitted to hospital/care home when don't need to be In a Community Intermediate Care bed or at home with services to help you with personal care from Leeds Community Healthcare NHS Trust and need ongoing care Continuous	Referral from any health or social care professional	Home visits
Complex and palliative continuing care service	Provide bespoke packages of care to fast-track patients with highly complex continuing care needs	Last few days of life Continuous	Referral from district nurse	Home visits

identify, assess, and support patients with palliative care needs. It can be incorporated into general practice infrastructures at various levels (Table 2). Practices which achieve level 1, the maintenance of a register and regular palliative care meetings, are currently financially rewarded through the Quality and Outcomes Framework (QOF) [10]. Whilst the GSF is thought to have contributed to better-quality care, for example: in improving early identification of patients, there is still much room for improvement [11, 12].

Although the majority of practices in England have adopted the GSF in some form, to at least level 1, there are well-recognised variations in practice [6, 13] associated with shortcomings in the processes for coordinating, managing, and providing effective care [14, 15]. Whilst, there has been evaluation and measurement of the effects of using GSF at every stage, it is hard to describe exactly what the benefits have been for those who have used it and whether it has facilitated good multidisciplinary working. Previous research has shown that there is considerable variation between practices in the effectiveness of interprofessional communication [10]. Practices categorised as 'high performing practices' are reported to display a clear shared purpose among staff for palliative care, whereas those categorised as 'minimal performing practices' demonstrate little utilisation of basic processes recommended in the framework and deficiencies in interprofessional communication. Effective primary palliative care requires good team relationships and communication [6]. We therefore explored the

Table 2 The four levels of adoption of the GSF

Level 1	*Communication*	Compiling and maintaining a supportive care register to record, plan, and monitor patient care
	Coordination	Having a nominated coordinator to oversee implementation and maintenance of the framework
Level 2	*Control of symptoms*	Patients' symptoms, problems, concerns are assessed, recorded, discussed and acted upon to an agreed process. Advanced care planning tools are recommended
	Continuity	Systems to ensure continuity of care delivered by inter-professional teams and out-of-hours providers are used. Anticipatory care in place to reduce crises and inappropriate admissions
	Continued learning	Commitment to learning about end-of-life care and developing action plans to meet identified learning needs. Reflection on past events, what went well and why, and what did not go well and why
Level 3	*Carer support*	Work in partnership with carer and assess and support their needs for emotional, practical, and bereavement support
	Care of the dying	Appropriate care provided in the last days of life
Level 4	*Sustain, embed and extend improvements in end-of-life care*	Sustain and build on all developments as standard practice. Develop a practice protocol and extend to other settings, e.g.: care homes, non-cancer, ACP

perspectives and experiences of PHCT members who are involved in the multidisciplinary care of patients with cancer to see whether these can improve understanding of variations in practice.

Method

Design and participants

We conducted semi-structured interviews and focus groups with purposively selected PHCT members and non-participatory observations of multidisciplinary GSF meetings. We explored the perspectives and experiences of PHCT members who provide care to people with advanced cancer in the community to see whether these can improve understanding of variations in practice. For the purpose of this study, care provided in the community relates only to people with palliative care needs being cared for in the home. Advanced cancer is defined as active and non-curative. The research was conducted in Leeds, UK and was part of a research programme on the management of advanced cancer pain.

Data collection

First, L.Z. (an experienced psycho-oncology researcher) conducted five single-professional focus groups with key community professionals who covered the whole city: clinical nurse specialists (CNSs), community matrons, joint care managers, members of the complex and palliative continuing care service (CAPCCS), and GPs. These explored experiences of coordinating and managing people with advanced cancer in the community using a topic guide, which was based upon a review of the current literature at that time (Additional file 1). This provided a comprehensive picture of practice across the city and suggested that effective cancer pain management extended beyond individual professional practice, skills, or experience to broader barriers related to the organisations and systems within which professionals work.

Subsequently, as a sampling strategy, we asked practice managers and GP leads across all general practices in Leeds a series of questions based on the levels of the GSF to determine practice approaches to coordination and management. This allowed us to identify different models of advanced cancer care coordination. We purposively selected six of these practices, representing two different approaches to care, which we categorised as high and minimal performers according to their responses, and contacted them by letter/follow up telephone call. Three responded and gave written consent to allow non-participant observations of multidisciplinary GSF meetings (one at each practice). The aim of these observations was to build up a picture of how care of patients with advanced cancer is routinely organised, how decisions are made about assessment of pain, how this is communicated between professionals, how strategies for management are devised and which professionals are seen as key in delivering support and care. Notes on these aspects and non-verbal communication were taken by the observer (J.H., an experienced health sciences researcher) during these meetings and subsequently expanded. Interviews were conducted by J.H. with individuals identified during GSF meetings as being most involved in coordinating care. Interviews explored experiences of managing people with advanced cancer in the community using a topic guide, which was based upon a second review of the literature and findings from the initial focus groups (Additional file 2). Informed written consent was obtained from all individual participants included in the study. All focus groups and interviews took place in participants' place of work, during working hours, no one else was present. Participants were not known to the researchers prior to the study.

Data analysis

Interviews and focus groups were audio-recorded and transcribed verbatim. Data were collected over two periods, from June to August 2010 and April 2013 to

September 2014. Each participant was given a unique identifier to maintain confidentiality.

We adopted a grounded theory analytic approach [16, 17] as it provides an approach to construct theory driven understanding of health professionals behaviour and the factors that influence it. This combined concurrent data collection and analysis with modification to the topic guide to pursue emerging lines of enquiry. Debrief meetings for researchers took place after each interview providing space to reflect on the interview process and explore initial ideas. Further steps carried out by authors, separately and together, were familiarisation of the whole data set through multiple readings of transcripts, open and focused coding, memo writing and engagement with the literature, to facilitate the development of categories and concepts. Constant comparison and searching for negative cases were used throughout, whereby data segments and the developing codes and categories were compared both within cases to identify the sequencing of events, and how these were understood and acted upon, and between cases to examine variations between participants. Throughout data collection and analysis, data, codes and concepts were discussed within the research team (of varied disciplinary backgrounds: psychology, health sciences, sociology, and academic palliative care medicine) and with the wider steering group. The latter included patient representatives, clinicians and academics.

Results

In total, 67 health professionals took part. Five single professional focus groups comprised 27 health professionals: six GPs, eight CNSs, five joint care managers, four members of the Complex and palliative continuing care service, and four community matrons. Twenty-four general practice managers and/or GP leads responded to a series of questions about practice approaches to coordination and management of people with advanced cancer. Three practices were then selected (Tables 3 and 4) for non-participatory observation, involving a total of 32 health professionals. Eight interviews were then conducted with professionals: three GPs, three CNSs, and two district nurses. Mean focus group length was 31mins (range: 27 to 36mins) and mean interview length was 52mins (range: 27 to 64mins). Total observation time was 145 mins.

There were distinct differences in the drivers and barriers within the two models of community advanced cancer coordination. Each practice provided the system within which examples of multidisciplinary working, implementation of policy, and professional behaviours and attitudes could be mapped and subsequently compared. Drivers and barriers for these distinct models of operation include proactive identification processes, time and resource pressures, unclear roles and responsibilities, poor multidisciplinary working, and inflexible models for referral and prescribing. These are now presented within two key themes: identification and management, and access to effective pain management, with three subthemes: prescribing restrictions, home visits, and referrals.

Table 3 Practice characteristics for practices participating in observations and related health professional interviews

	Practice		
	A	B	C
List size range	5000–10,000	20,000–25,000	10,000–15,000
Deprivation decile	6	8	9
Full time GP partners	4	6	4
Part-time GP partners	1	4	4
Full time GP salaried	0	2	0
Part-time GP salaried	0	5	1
QOF achievement palliative care (%)	100	100	100
Number of staff at GSF meeting	10	13	9
Number of staff interviewed	3	2	3

Note: deprivation decile scores, 1 most deprived to 10 least deprived

Identification and management

A proactive approach, with early identification of and care planning for patients, was key to coordination and management. Proactivity demonstrated whether practices viewed people with advanced cancer as different, or not, from the general practice population and therefore requiring specific, flexible input. High performing practices, such as A and B, adopted formal proactive processes to ensure identification and monitoring of patients who were not previously known to GPs. They would initiate contact and, in doing so, commence assessment, monitoring and management of pain.

> If I receive a letter from the hospital that tells me somebody's got a new diagnosis, I make contact. Then the obvious triggers like multiple hospital admissions, we look at that, and because of the evidence you'll identify your 1% that way so if somebody's bouncing in and out of hospital... Over time we've found that the register's grown quite significantly, so we try to just discuss patients who are at the amber to red end of the traffic light system. (GP 8, Practice B)

These practices were engaged with and had ownership of the GSF, demonstrated through their management of the palliative care register and GSF meetings, and had clear roles and responsibilities within the primary palliative care

Table 4 Levels of GSF adoption for practices participating in observations and related health professional interviews

Key tasks	Practice A	Practice B	Practice C
Communication	Set up register Regular GSF meetings	Set up register Less regular GSF meetings	Set up register Regular GSF meetings
Co-ordination	Lead GP has special interest and is responsible for coordinating meeting and register DN input from DN team, no specific lead DN	Lead GP has special interest and is responsible for coordinating meeting and registerLead DN for practice	GP lead has no ownership, CNS is responsible for coordinating meeting and highlighting patients for register Lead DN for practice
Control of symptoms	Confident in symptom control and pool knowledge with other services Do not routinely use assessment tools	Lack of confidence in symptom control, but shared care with/supported by CNS and DN services Use assessment tools	Lack of confidence in symptom control and leave care to other services Lack of use of assessment tools
Continuity of care	Shared care with secondary care	Shared care with secondary care	Lack of continuity of care with secondary care, will not take responsibility of care or participate in shared care
Continued learning	Use of significant/after death analysis Identify and address knowledge gaps	Use of significant/after death analysis but infrequency of meetings impinges on this	Do not carry out continued learning unless instigated and led by CNS
Carer support	Carer support Extend care into bereavement phase	Carer support evident but infrequency of meetings impinges on this Extend care into bereavement phase	Carer and bereavement support left to CNS and not discussed within practice
Care in the dying phase	Involved in dying phase	Involved in dying phase	Reluctance to engage in dying phase

team. For example: in practices A and B, the palliative care lead GP, both of whom had a special interest in palliative care, was the nominated coordinator of the all work relating to the GSF, they led the meeting, and GPs generated and maintained the register personally, ensuring that all eligible patients were recorded. Patients mentioned at the meeting by the CNS or district nurse were already known to GPs and new referrals were noted down and recorded. Through this system they not only had ownership of the GSF, but achieved level 1. They also adopted flexible working practices, for example: a buddy system was used, whereby patients had a second named GP to account for periods of annual leave or part-time working. Meetings consisted of discussions on patients' status, managing needs, bereavement support, and significant event or after death review to re-appraise appropriateness of response. Therefore achieving levels 2 and 3 of the GSF.

Practice C did not differentiate between people with advanced cancer and other patients, did not regard them as requiring any special input, and therefore failed to adopt any flexible working practices. Observations highlighted a lack of ownership over the GSF and unclear roles and responsibilities within the primary palliative care team, for example: although they had a nominated coordinator to oversee all work relating to the GSF, this was the CNS, and not the palliative care lead GP, as a result the CNS led the meeting and identified patients for the register. Patients identified by the CNS and DN were not already known to the practice. There were no formal, proactive processes for identifying patients embedded as standard practice.

> I try and actively encourage them to look at the palliative care register in terms of getting additional people on. They really don't engage with that. I've asked several times "do you know if we've any other patients to discuss?" and they don't have a system. They do have a list, I'm just not sure how up to date that is and they've said they don't want a long list, there'd be loads of patients. And we're not really meant to lead the meeting, it should be the GP. I'm meant to be there as an additional person to contribute, and they just listen to me and chip in, it's meant to be the other way round. (CNS 9, Practice C)

Only patients already registered with the palliative care service were on their register. Although discussions about updates on patients' status and how to manage needs occurred, these were instigated by the CNS and district nurse, who felt these discussions were time limited and not seen as a priority. Consequently, although aspects of levels 2 and 3 of the GSF were covered, the impetus for them was led by specialist practitioners, demonstrating a lack of ownership from the practice.

Access to effective pain management

Patient access to effective cancer pain management was highly variable and influenced by professional priorities and complex practice level policies. The levels to which the GSF was adopted led to variations in effective pain management activities, in particular: prescribing restrictions, home visits, and referrals.

Prescribing restrictions

Many general practices operate a practice level policy whereby non-cancer patients are required to wait 48 h before prescriptions can be collected, however such policies may be flexible based on patient need. Practice C was relatively inflexible in its prescribing policy for people with advanced cancer. This limited the potential for a timely response to changing pain needs. The importance of this barrier is not only related to the need to offer fast, accessible services to cancer patients; but to the fact that some cancer patients only visit their practices to obtain repeat prescriptions and this represents their only encounter with primary care. This can influence their confidence in, and opinion of, their GP when care is transferred at a later stage of their illness.

> I had a very elderly lady on absolutely huge doses... but she still needed quite a lot of breakthrough analgesia, I went to see her and I rang the GP. "This is what I need, I need it today...", "Yes, it will be ready". When her husband went to pick it up, it wasn't ready and they said to him, "No, you will have to wait 'til Monday now". And then over that weekend they tried to struggle through with the OxyNorm and he had to get the emergency doctor out and his family had to drive round looking for a chemist that was open for these drugs. (CNS 8, focus group)

They also maintained a tight rein on prescribing budgets and minimised costs wherever possible. Medications prescribed on discharge from hospital were changed by GPs to explore whether a cheaper alternative might be effective. In an attempt to minimise potential wastage, patients were given limited supplies of anticipatory drugs. These universal cost saving prescribing practices were described in the context of patients with advanced cancer and demonstrated that despite such a diagnosis, the policy was not modified. Advanced cancer patients were treated in the same way as other patients in judgements made about prescribing.

> I reckon if someone isn't long for this world I would give them two vials of something to get them through the weekend and I'll see if they're still here on Monday. And then I'm more than happy to give them more. Otherwise I think there's too much wastage in the NHS. (GP 12, Practice C)

In contrast, others believed that there was no justification for trying to limit costs, particularly given the limited length of time the patient would require the drug and that the greatest costs to the NHS would be having to fast track a patient or an unplanned hospital admission. The ethos underpinning policy and practice here was that palliative care requires effective management of symptoms. In the multidisciplinary focus groups and interviews with CNSs, they agreed that patients with advanced cancer should be prioritised in terms of access to the most effective and tolerable pain control irrespective of cost. This suggests that minimising the cost of analgesia in advanced cancer patients is not a high priority for all and in this instance, the policy appeared to be generated and maintained at a practice level.

> I think cost does have a bearing, whereas I probably don't give a great deal of consideration to costing. I know that some GPs do, some of the drugs they're maybe not too keen to try and some will even suggest that they would prefer to go for something else as an alternative and they will mention costing. (CNS 7, focus group)

In instances where GPs were known to be difficult to work with, poor multidisciplinary working was evident as CNS's recounted times when they went around them instead of negotiating with them.

> There are always some GPs that you feel might be less amenable to prescribing for various reasons, if you felt that the GP wasn't willing to do what you thought was appropriate and couldn't give you a valid reason in your mind as to why, then in essence we would bypass the GP if we felt we couldn't negotiate with them. (CNS 8, focus group)

However, this then has repercussions for overall co-ordination and management, particularly monitoring of symptoms and care planning.

Home visits

Patient access to effective cancer pain management was highly variable and influenced by professional priorities and complex practice and service level policies and pressures. One such practice-level policy relates to GPs undertaking home visits, especially within the context of perceived increasing pressures and demands on time. Within practices A and B, GPs initiated and negotiated their involvement and viewed themselves as being involved in patient care from diagnosis to death.

> I think most people who are having palliative care at home will see their GP as the coordinator of that care. A GP is key to these patients, I do think we're very important. We ask them what they want, I don't force the issue, you know you can say to me if you want me to, "I would happily see you on a monthly basis" or whatever. In their last weeks to months of life when

> you have known them very well, I think you are a befriender as much as a clinician. (GP 8, Practice B)

In contrast, practice C were reactive in their approach to care, evidenced by their lack of initiating or actively maintaining involvement with patients. Home visits were only undertaken in exceptional circumstances and were identified as a nurse's responsibility rather than the GP's.

> We run more of a demand led system so it's up to the patient to ask, to make appointments, we don't have capacity really, if patients can come to the surgery we encourage it...Once they get more poorly, I think the district nurses and the Macmillan team take over more, we have more to do with people when they're able to come to see us. (GP 7, Practice C)

Others highlighted home visits as a high priority, with GPs and nurses proactively advocating for joint visits as a key component of effective pain assessment and management. Sometimes it was necessary to spend time with patients and their relatives, perhaps over consecutive days, to fully understand the nature of their symptoms. This also contributed to building a relationship, facilitating disclosure of the reality of patients' pain, and providing psychological support.

> I think personally it's nice to see them face to face. It's a lot nicer to see them in their own home, you probably feel like you've got more time, they're feeling more comfortable and a bit more secure to talk about things that they're not happy to talk about, it's more on their terms then. (GP 8, Practice B)

Referrals

GPs were highlighted by CNS's as the main referrer to their service. However, due to a lack of proactive identification processes, instances were recounted where patients had been missed and therefore not referred.

> Quite often they'll say on the letters 'may be worth involving palliative care' but it still relies on the GP seeing and deciding to do that. I'm thinking of that patient we saw at home, when you got the information from the oncologist the last two or three letters to the GP had suggested that there should be a referral to palliative care and the GP just hadn't done it. (CNS 4, focus group)

Poor multidisciplinary working was also evidenced by CNS's describing cases where patients were referred to their service without their GP knowing.

> By far the majority of the referrals come from GPs to the CNSs. There's occasional one that a consultant will refer direct to me from an outpatients and I will look at this and think why have you done that? (CNS 1, focus group)

This had consequences for patient access to other services, particularly district nursing, who are supposed to provide general palliative care alongside the GP. These services were then at a disadvantage as they have been brought in late to patient care.

> It just doesn't happen, we get the referral and then we then refer to the DNs. They're a really vital role of that consistent support monitoring and holistic care for them and we're coming in focussing on their specialist needs, not their general. If they don't have that district nurse, they often end up in crisis and then just come straight to us. Whereas, any district nurses then are deskilled in the palliative care. (CNS 9, Practice C)

Consequently, this lack of coordination and poor multidisciplinary working resulted in instances where there was no coherent pathway for patients to navigate through the services.

Discussion

We explored the perspectives and experiences of PCHT members who are involved in the multidisciplinary care of people with advanced cancer, to see whether these improved understanding of variations in practice. Within our research, Practices A and B were identified as high performing sites, whilst Practice C was identified as a minimal performer. Where this paper adds knowledge is that there were distinct differences in the drivers and barriers within these models of community advanced cancer coordination which help explain variations in practice. Practices A and B adopted formal proactive processes for identifying advanced cancer patients. They had clear roles and responsibilities with their primary palliative care teams which enabled good multidisciplinary working; and adopted flexible approaches to care, in particular evidenced by their attitudes to referrals, home visits, and prescribing. Within these practices, we identified that if professionals adopted a flexible approach to care then the scope to deliver effective individualised pain management was enhanced. Practice C however, were reactive in their approach to coordinating and managing care for these patients. There were no formal mechanisms in place for identifying patients; unclear roles and responsibilities within the team, which impacted upon multidisciplinary working; evidence of time and resource pressures at a practice level; and inflexible models for referrals and prescribing. This reactive, inflexible, and untimely approach to care meant that individualised care was difficult to achieve.

The extent to which a practice subscribes to a palliative care philosophy appeared to be fundamental to the provision of effective advanced cancer care coordination and management. We demonstrate how professionals within a multidisciplinary team work within an infrastructure that can both support and hinder the provision of effective community palliative care. Practice C operated within an ethos that did not differentiate the specific needs of people with advanced cancer and this inhibited a flexible approach to pain management. Adopting a universalist approach with people with advanced cancer had unintended consequences for coordination and management. The policies and procedures which they adhered to appeared to provide a structured mechanism for decision making in relation to pain management and diverted practice away from the subjective and interactive processes related to pain management evident in Practices A and B. However, when such a policy is formalised within a practice setting, the scope for individual professional perspectives and subsequent variation in practice becomes limited, even when the professional was not part of the devising body. In addition, the operation of inflexible prescribing restrictions, is a policy that could result in unintended consequences that are potentially more costly to the NHS, such as unplanned hospital admissions. Practice C illustrates how a not uncommon set of external and internal constraints [18] can have unintended consequences for pain management. Any strategy to support practices in improving pain management must be informed by an understanding of such constraints.

Challenges to effective multidisciplinary team working are evidenced by nurses' accounts of the difficulties in working with GPs, reporting power relationships, and implicit and explicit rules governing the process of inter-professional work [6, 18]. These dynamics sit at the core of providing effective primary palliative care. Professional identities and organisational structures affect coordination and management because these are key aspects of effective teamwork. The GSF may have been intended to provide a framework to guide care and provide a toolkit for the coordination and management of advanced cancer care, however our data illustrates that, despite the financial incentives associated with it, it is inadequate in recognising the complexity of practice and implementation of change. Instead of providing a mechanism for change, we suggest that it provides a framework for describing quality of practice that was already occurring. It is a guide for good practice, but fails to describe an implementation approach, therefore cannot itself change practice.

In high performing practices, GPs were proactive in identifying and coordinating care in order to aim for continuity with patients [19, 20]. They were engaged with and took ownership of the GSF and had clear roles and responsibilities. Although engagement and continuity are key, the workload of primary care is growing [20, 21], with more GPs are working part-time, and out-of-hours care more frequently occurring with health professionals who are unfamiliar with the patient [22]. Our findings show how these developments can be overcome by providing proactive care and putting flexible systems in place to take account of these changes, for example: having a second named GP to cover periods of annual leave or part-time working. Future developments must recognise the changing landscape of primary care to enable adaptation.

Timely referrals were highlighted as enabling professionals to develop relationships with patients and their families earlier, enhancing the ability to deliver effective individualised patient care and enabling continuity [6]. The current focus of the GSF in the last year of life doesn't take account of the shifting trajectory of advanced cancer, including the increasing need for input and support over longer periods of time [1]. We question how care should be initiated and coordinated when different members of the PHCT enter and exit patient care at different points, therefore have different levels of engagement, and view the meaning of palliative care from the perspective of their input. Standardised definitions of roles and responsibilities are needed [20, 23].

The way professionals, policies, and services within the UK primary care system interact is dynamic and complex, with many aspects of exactly how this occurs remaining unclear. This lack of clarity is likely to be due to the considerable variability in how the three components of the system interact, specifically the variability in the level of engagement between: generalists and specialists; professionals and patients; and professionals, policies, and service level initiatives. This means that although we are beginning to understand the component parts of this system, we do not fully understand the whole. For example, one of our study practices clearly recognised or perceived strong pressures to control costs and demand, and is unlikely to be atypical in doing so. This has implications for developing and targeting interventions. The recognition that advanced cancer coordination and management cancer-pain management in primary care occurs within a multidisciplinary team suggests that an intervention to improve this that was embedded at a professional or service level alone will struggle to be effective. Further measures to improve continuity and coordination need to be developed through close working with a range of practices, with varying abilities to respond to clinical policy frameworks.

Strengths and limitations

Exploring the involvement of all members of the PHCT, allowed us to gather a wide range of views and subsequently focus on those most involved in care. A limitation is it took place in one UK city and we were unable to recruit more practices to take part in the observations and associated interviews, particularly from more deprived areas. Future research could explore these drivers and barriers within a larger number of practices, representing a wider range of deprivation. Whilst this could be a potential limitation of the analysis, the themes that emerged concerning the organisation of care resonate with those reported more widely [24, 25]. We identified two key contrasting approaches, although these may not be the only models of advanced cancer coordination and management, and illustrate and highlight drivers and barriers that can shape variation in practice. Secondly, our study spanned a change in the structure of primary care, when clinical commissioning groups replaced primary care trusts. Local priorities may have changed, however this was not evident within our findings. The significance of our study is that it provides insight into specific practice cultural and organisational factors that shape interpretation of policies and subsequent practice.

Conclusion

We identified distinct differences in the drivers and barriers within these models of community advanced cancer care coordination. These provide valuable insight into how professionals work together and independently within an infrastructure that can both support and hinder the provision of effective community palliative care. Whilst the GSF is a guide for good practice, it fails to describe an implementation approach, therefore is not a mechanism for change. Consequently, there will continue to be variations in practice. If general practices remain purely reactive in their approach to care, then this will have unintended consequences for coordination and management. Overcoming these issues is key to ensuring the provision of effective community palliative care.

Abbreviations

CAPCCS: Complex and palliative continuing care service; CNS: Clinical nurse specialist; GP: General practitioner; GSF: Gold Standards Framework; PHCT: Primary health care teams; QOF: Quality and Outcomes Framework

Acknowledgements

We would like to thank all those who participated in the research and are grateful to the general practice managers who helped coordinate recruitment.

Funding

This work was supported by the National Institute for Health Research under its Programme Development Grants scheme and its Programme Grants for Applied Research programme ("Improving the Management of Pain from Advanced Cancer in the Community" (IMPACCT): [RP-DG-1108-10010] and [RP-PG-0610-10114]). The views expressed in this report are those of the authors and not necessarily those of the NHS, the National Institute for Health Research or the Department of Health. The funder was not involved in the design, collection, analysis, and interpretation of the data; nor in writing the manuscript.

Authors' contributions

MB and MG proposed the idea for the study. MB, MG, and RF contributed to the design of the study. JH and LZ carried out the data collection. JH coded and analysed the data. JH wrote the first draft of the manuscript and all authors contributed to the writing of the final version.

Competing interests

The authors declare that they have no competing interests.

Author details

[1]Martin House Research Centre, Social Policy Research Unit, University of York, York YO10 5DD, UK. [2]Academic Unit of Palliative Care, Leeds Institute of Health Sciences, University of Leeds, Level 10 Worsley Building, Clarendon Way, Leeds LS2 9NL, UK. [3]Academic Unit of Elderly Care and Rehabilitation, Bradford Institute for Health Research, Temple Bank House, Bradford Royal Infirmary, Duckworth Lane, Bradford BD9 6RJ, UK. [4]Academic Unit of Primary Care, Leeds Institute of Health Sciences, University of Leeds, Level 10 Worsley Building, Clarendon Way, Leeds LS2 9NL, UK.

References

1. Hackett J, Godfrey M, Bennett MI. The process of managing advanced cancer pain toward the end of life: the patient and carer perspective. Palliat Med. 2016;30:711–9.
2. Murray S, Kendall M, Boyd K, Sheikh A. Illness trajectories and palliative care. BMJ. 2005;330:1007–11.
3. Portenoy RK. Treatment of cancer pain. Lancet. 2011;377:2236–47.
4. Higginson I, Sen-Gupta G. Place of care in advanced cancer. J Palliat Med. 2004;3:287–300.
5. Forrest S, Barclay S. Palliative care: a task for everyone. Br J Gen Pract. 2007; 48:1297–8.
6. Mahmood-Yousuf K, Munday D, King N, Dale J. Interprofessional relationships and communication in primary palliative care: impact of the gold standards framework. Br J Gen Pract. 2008;58:256–63.
7. Goldschmidt D, Groenvold M, Johnsen A, et al. Cooperating with a palliative home-care team: expectations and evaluations of GPs and district nurses. Palliat Med. 2005;19:241–50.
8. Momen N, Hadfield P, Harrison K, Barclay S. Managing pain in advanced cancer: a survey of United Kingdom general practitioners and community nurses. J Pain Symptom Manag. 2013;46:345–54.
9. The Gold Standards Framework. A programme for community palliative care. [http://www.goldstandardsframework.org.uk/].
10. Munday D, Mahmood K, Dale J, King N. Facilitating good process in primary palliative care: does the gold standards framework enable quality performance? Fam Pract. 2007;24:486–94.
11. Shaw K, Clifford C, Thomas K, Meehan H. Improving end-of-life care: a critical review of the gold standards framework in primary care. Palliat Med. 2010;24:317–29.
12. Thomas K, Clifford C, Armstrong Willson J. Summary evaluation of effectiveness for gold standards framework Primary Care; 2016.
13. More care, less pathway: a review of the Liverpool Care Pathway. Independent review of the Liverpool Care Pathway [https://gov.uk/government/uploads/system/uploads/attachment_data/file/212450/Liverpool_Care_Pathway.pdf].
14. Kendall M, Boyd K, Campbell C, Cormie P, Fife S, Thomas K, Weller D, Murray S. How do people with cancer wish to be cared for in primary care? Serial discussion groups of patients and carers. Fam Pract. 2006;23:644–50.

15. Dale J, Petrova M, Munday D, Koistinen-Harris J, Lall R, Thomas K. A national facilitation project to improve primary palliative care: impact of the gold standards framework on process and self-ratings of quality. Qual Saf Health Care. 2009;18:174–80.
16. Charmaz K. Constructing grounded theory. 2nd ed. London: SAGE pUblications Ltd; 2014.
17. Corbin J, Strauss A. Basics of qualitative research: techniques and procedures for developing grounded theory. 3rd ed. London: SAGE; 2008.
18. Jacobsen R, Moldrup C, Christrup C, Sjogren P. Patient-related barriers to cancer pain management: a systematic exploratory review. Scand J Caring Sci. 2009;23:190–208.
19. Beernaert K, Deliens L, De Vleminck A, Devroey D, Pardon K, Van den Block L, Cohen J. Early identitification of palliative care needs by family physicians: a qualitative study of barriers and facilitators from the perspective of family physicians, community nurses, and patients. Palliat Med. 2014;28:480–90.
20. Mitchell S, Loew J, Millington-Sanders C, Dale J. Providing end-of-life care in general practice: findings on a national GP questionnaire survey. Br J Gen Pract. 2016;66:647–53.
21. Roland M, Everington S. Tackling the crisis in general practice: if general oractice fails, the whole NHS fails. BMJ. 2016;352:i942.
22. Borgsteede S, Deliens L, Francke A, van Eijk JTM, Willems D. Good end-of-life care according to patients and their GPs. Br J Gen Pract. 2006;56:20–6.
23. Gardiner C, Gott M, Ingleton C. Factors supporting good partnership working between generalist and specialist palliative care services: a systematic review. Br J Gen Pract. 2012;62:353–62.
24. Linklater G, Leng M, Tiernan E, Lee M, Chambers W. Pain management services in palliative care: a national survey. Palliat Med. 2002;16:435–9.
25. Aranda S, Yates P, Edwards H, Nash R, Skerman H, McCarthy A. Barriers to effective cancer pain management: a survey of Australian family caregivers. Eur J Cancer Care (Engl). 2004;13:336–43.

4

Evaluation of an educational intervention to increase HIV-testing in high HIV prevalence general practices

Charlotte F. Davies[1], Joanna M. Kesten[2,3,4], Mark Gompels[5], Jeremy Horwood[3], Megan Crofts[6*], Annette Billing[7*], Charlotte Chick[1] and Margaret T. May[1,4]

Abstract

Background: HIV-infected patients often present to primary care several times with HIV-indicator conditions before diagnosis but the opportunity to test by healthcare professionals (HCPs) is frequently missed. Current HIV testing rates in primary care are low and educational interventions to facilitate HCPs to increase testing and awareness of HIV are needed.

Method: We implemented a pilot feasibility stepped-wedged randomised controlled trial of an educational intervention in high HIV prevalence practices in Bristol. The training delivered to HCPs including General Practitioners (GP) aimed to increase HIV testing and included why, who, and how to test. The intervention was adapted from the Medical Foundation for HIV and Sexual Health HIV Testing in Practice (MEDFASH) educational tool. Questionnaires assessed HCP feedback and perceived impacts of the intervention. HIV testing rates were compared between control and intervention practices using 12 monthly laboratory totals.

Results: 169 HCPs (from 19 practices) received the educational intervention. 127 (75%) questionnaires were completed. Delivery of the intervention was received positively and was perceived as valuable for increasing awareness, confidence and consideration of testing, with HCPs gaining more awareness of HIV testing guidelines. The main pre-training HIV testing barrier reported by GPs was the patient not considering themselves at risk, whilst for nurses it was a concern about embarrassing or offending the patient. Most HCPs reported the intervention addressed these barriers. The HIV testing rate increased more in the control than in the intervention practices: mean difference 2.6 (95% CI 0.5,4.7) compared with 1.9 (− 0.5,4.3) per 1000 patients, respectively. The number of HIV tests across all practices increased from 1154 in the first 6 months to 1299 in the second 6 months, an annual increase in testing rate of 2.0 (0.7,3.4) from 16.3 to 18.3 per 1000 patients.

(Continued on next page)

* Correspondence: Megan.Crofts@UHBristol.nhs.uk; Annette.Billing@nhs.net
[6]Genitourinary medicine, Unity Sexual Health, Bristol Sexual Health Services, Tower Hill, Bristol BS2 0JD, UK
[7]NHS Bristol, North Somerset and South Gloucestershire CCG, South Plaza, Marlborough Street, Bristol BS1 3NX, UK
Full list of author information is available at the end of the article

(Continued from previous page)

Conclusion: There was a small increase in HIV testing rates over the study period, but this could not be attributed to the educational intervention. More effective and sustainable programmes tailored to each practice context are needed to change testing culture and HCP behaviour. Repeated training, supported by additional measures, such as testing prompts, may be needed to influence primary care HIV testing.

Keywords: General practice, HIV testing, Primary care, Step-wedged RCT, Education intervention, Feasibility study, Implementation study

Background

Approximately 101,200 people in the United Kingdom (UK) are living with human immunodeficiency virus (HIV), of these 13% are undiagnosed and unaware of their infection [1]. The majority of HIV transmissions are from untreated (often undiagnosed) individuals. Patients are unlikely to transmit HIV to sexual partners if they are diagnosed and treated with effective anti-retroviral therapy (ART) [2]. In 2015, 39% of newly diagnosed adults were diagnosed late in England [3, 4]. Late diagnosis of HIV is associated with increased hospitalisation, decreased life expectancy [5–7] and higher treatment and care costs [8].

Recent audits and reviews show a clear need to increase and improve HIV testing in the UK particularly within primary care [9, 10]. Routine testing in general practice in the UK is recommended in areas with > 2 per 1000 population diagnosed prevalence [11] based on cost-effectiveness studies of HIV testing in the USA and France [12–14]. Healthcare professionals (HCPs) in primary care have opportunities to initiate HIV testing in at risk individuals and thereby reduce the proportion of undiagnosed infection in the UK [15, 16]. Patients with HIV often see their General Practitioner (GP) with an HIV indicator condition (IC) (a sign, symptom or diagnosis that is more commonly found in those with HIV) several times before their HIV is detected [15–22]. Due to the stigma surrounding HIV there are often barriers to testing experienced by both the HCP and the patients. Literature reviews reveal that the barriers HCPs experience barriers to HIV testing including lack of confidence or anxiety around offering a test, concern about offending or upsetting patients [23], privacy and confidentiality issues [23] and insufficient knowledge or training [24, 25]. There are also structural and organizational barriers such as lack of time during consultations and limited resources allocated to HIV testing [26]. A more proactive offer of a test by the HCP could increase HIV testing rates [25] and thereby reduce undiagnosed infection and late diagnosis in the UK, as recommended by national HIV testing guidelines [18, 27]. Routine testing of HIV could also help reduce the stigma attached to HIV [28].

Interventions to address these issues in primary care include expanding HIV testing by screening all newly registered patients [29–31]. Opt-out testing in 8 pilot studies (including 2 within primary care) were shown to be feasible, acceptable and cost-effective [32]. A recent cluster randomised controlled trial (RCT) in Hackney (London UK) offered opt-out rapid point of care testing (POCT) alongside education sessions to newly registered adults in comparison to usual care, resulting in increased rates of HIV diagnosis [31]. The study was shown to be cost-effective in the medium term in settings with extremely high HIV incidence, defined as > 5 /1000 population [33]. Educational interventions for GPs and nurses within primary care aimed at increasing HIV testing rates have also shown encouraging results [34–36]. However, most of these studies have taken place in extremely high HIV prevalence cities in the UK such as London and Brighton. Therefore, it is not known whether similar results will be obtained in high diagnosed prevalence practices (defined as > 2 per 1000) in a city with estimated HIV prevalence similar to the national average for England, currently 2.3/1000 population aged 15–59 years [37].

This implementation study aimed to investigate the feasibility of a stepped-wedge RCT to evaluate an educational intervention's appropriateness, usefulness and effectiveness on increasing HCPs HIV testing rates in high HIV diagnosed prevalence practices in Bristol, a city with an overall estimated HIV prevalence of 2.5/1000 population aged 15–59 years [37]. Qualitative interviews with HCPs were also undertaken at least 3 months post-intervention to explore how the training was experienced by HCPs and to understand the perceived impacts of the intervention on HIV testing and explore the barriers to testing in more detail. These results are reported elsewhere [38].

Methods

Design of pilot feasibility stepped-wedged RCT

This was a pilot feasibility stepped-wedge RCT which invited 26 GP practices in Bristol, South Gloucestershire and North Somerset with high practice population HIV diagnosed prevalence (> 2 per 1000) to take part. Practices that agreed to take part were randomised to either the intervention arm (first to receive training) or to the control arm (second group to receive training) using a Stata random allocation program (Fig. 1). Training sessions were delivered between October 2015 and March 2016 in

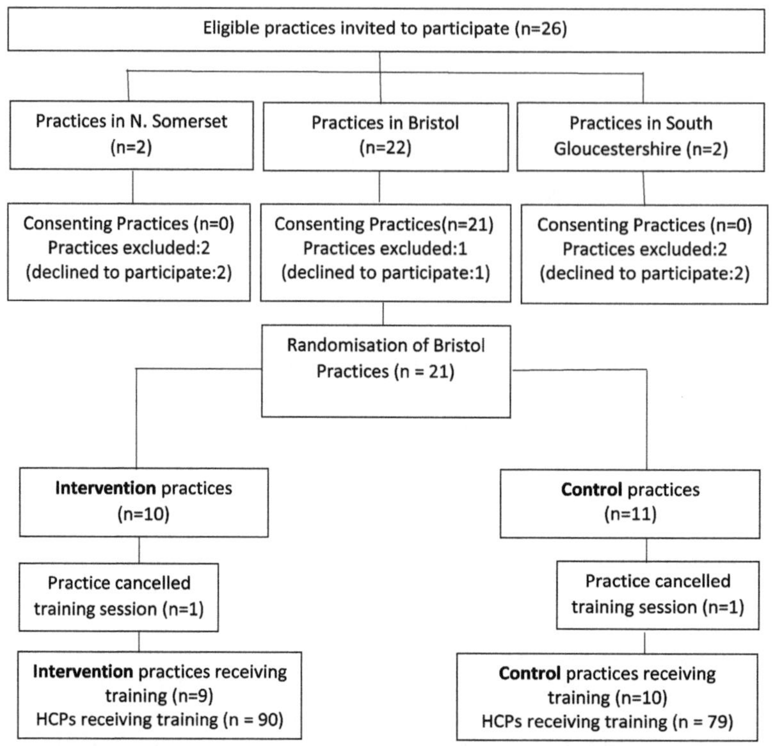

Fig. 1 Practice recruitment into the stepped wedged RCT of the HIV testing education intervention

the intervention arm and from April to July 2016 in the control arm. The intervention was delivered at a rate of approximately two practices per month over roughly 10 months. The first two practices acted as pilots which informed tailoring of the training before further roll out.

Details of intervention

We chose the format of the intervention, a one-hour interactive workshop delivered within general practices by a genito-urinary medicine (GUM) specialist registrar, in consultation with GPs who indicated that due to workload pressures they would only be able to commit to attend to a single short session. All staff at the practice were invited to attend, not just clinical staff with a particular interest in sexual health. The content of the training was designed to increase testing and was based on the Medical Foundation for HIV and Sexual Health (MEDFASH) HIV Testing in Practice (TIPs) educational tool (http://www.medfash.org.uk/welcome-to-hiv-tips) which was adapted for local use, for example, by using locally relevant statistics and signposting to local services. TIPS was already a nationally-approved training programme and therefore we thought that, if successful, it could be easily rolled out in other areas. The training provided a short knowledge assessment quiz, an update on current BHIVA and NICE HIV testing recommendations and HIV associated clinical ICs and covered barriers to HIV testing that the practice team had or may have encountered and explored ways to overcome these. The presentation included a summary of all the ICs, but highlighted those that occur more commonly in primary care, such as seroconversion illness, rash, oral and gut conditions, dermatology, respiratory and other "non-specific" weight loss/sweats/abnormal blood count presentations. Conditions were grouped "syndromically" to reduce confusion and increase memorability. The training also included the following topics: why test and the importance of testing, who to test, how to do a test including the discussion with the patient, how to handle both negative and positive results and linkage to care. The training concluded with a discussion about how the practice could increase testing, which included case study examples. After the training, each practice received a summary sheet on the information covered which included references to useful resources (including the MEDFASH TIPs website link).

Analysis

Quantitative evaluation of HIV testing

Numbers of HIV tests at the practice level and their results were obtained from the Public Health England (PHE) South West laboratory at Southmead Hospital. These were aggregated monthly by practice. Routine tests done by midwives for antenatal screening were excluded. Data on practice population size were obtained from the primary care commissioners and used to convert frequencies to annualised rates per 1000 patients. The month of the intervention was coded as zero, with number of months pre-intervention and post-intervention labelled negative and positive, respectively (Fig. 2).

We calculated the difference in HIV testing rates by practice and overall in 6-month blocks. For the randomised comparison we compared the differences in pre- and post-intervention rates in the intervention practices with the differences in rates in the matched time periods in control practices (all prior to intervention) and tested for a difference in differences between the arms to account for variation between practices. We estimated the positivity rate for the HIV tests in the intervention and control practices combined.

Questionnaire evaluation of education intervention

A questionnaire evaluation was also undertaken immediately after the training by participants to obtain feedback on the appropriateness and usefulness of the intervention. The questionnaire format involved scoring statements and providing open text responses. An example questionnaire is shown in the Additional file 1. Mean scores for seven statements were calculated using a 4-point Likert scale (1 = strongly disagree, 2 = disagree, 3 = agree, 4 = strongly agree).

Results

Of the 26 General Practices invited to participate, 21 agreed to take part and were randomized (10 to intervention and 11 to control arms). Of note, none of the four practices outside Bristol agreed to participate. One practice in each arm did not receive training because of logistical issues (no convenient time available) and therefore training sessions were delivered to 9 practices in the intervention arm and later to 10 practices in the control arm (Fig. 1).

Quantitative evaluation of HIV testing

Practice HIV testing rates were compared pre-and post-intervention and between control and intervention practices using a randomised comparison. Figure 2 shows the timeline for the randomised comparison. In the intervention practices, the number of HIV tests in the 6 months pre-intervention was 574 which increased to 631 in the 6 months post intervention, corresponding to an increase in annual HIV testing rate from 17.4 to 19.1 per 1000 patients (Table 1). The number of HIV tests in the control arm also increased from 580 to 668 in the same time period, corresponding to an increase in annual HIV testing rate from 15.3 to 17.6 per 1000 patients. Over all the practices the increase in annual HIV testing rate per 1000 patients was 2.0 [95% Confidence Interval (CI) 0.7, 3.4] and was similar in the intervention [1.7 (− 0.3, 3.8)] and the control [2.3 (0.5, 4.1)] practices. The mean difference in testing rates was 1.9 (− 0.5, 4.3) and 2.6 (0.5, 4.7) across the intervention and control practices, respectively, a difference of differences of − 0.7 ($p = 0.68$) in favour of the control arm which could have been due to chance. Any increase in testing was likely due to secular trend rather than to the education intervention. In the intervention arm, there were 6 positive tests, 3 pre- and 3 post-intervention. In the control arm there were 9 positive tests, 7 in the first and 2 in the second period. During the 12 months of the study there were a total of 2453 HIV tests recorded of which 15 were positive, a positivity rate of 6.1 per 1000 tests which exceeds the 2 per 1000 threshold for prevalence of undiagnosed HIV considered to be cost effective in primary care HIV screening [39].

Questionnaire evaluation of education intervention: HCPs feedback on training

In total, 169 HCPs (93 GPs, 53 nurses and 23 `others') received the training. The 'other' group consisted of healthcare assistants (HCA), practice managers, assistant practice managers and medical students. On average 9.3 HCPs per practice received the training (range 4 to 17). Feedback was available from 127 evaluation questionnaires out of a possible 169 (75% response rate) which participants completed immediately after the training.

The month in which the intervention took place is labelled 0. The randomised comparison used data from 6 months pre-intervention (-6 to -1) to 6 months post-intervention (1 to 6) in the intervention practices, and from 12 months pre-intervention for the control practices (in two blocks -12 to -7 and -6 to -1).

Months in the study																		
1	2	3	4	5	6	7	8	9	10	11	12	13	14	15	16	17	18	19
Randomised comparison																		
Intervention practices																		
pre-intervention						Int.	post-intervention											
-6	-5	-4	-3	-2	-1	0	1	2	3	4	5	6						
Control practices																		
pre-intervention (pre 1)						pre-intervention (pre 2)						Int.						
-12	-11	-10	-9	-8	-7	-6	-5	-4	-3	-2	-1	0						

Fig. 2 Timeline

Table 1 Randomised comparison between intervention and control practices. Number of HIV tests, annual rate of HIV testing per 1000 patients, and difference in rate by practice and randomisation arm and overall, and number of positive tests. Data for 6 months pre and post intervention for intervention practices, and for corresponding time periods (both pre-intervention) for the control practices

		Randomised comparison				
	Total population	No. of HIV tests		Annual rate of HIV tests per 1000 patients		
		Pre	Post	Pre	Post	Difference
Intervention practices		−6,-1	1,6	−6,-1	1,6	post-pre
1	5547	99	90	35.7	32.4	−3.2 (−13.0, 6.5)
2	6295	112	122	35.6	38.8	3.2 (−6.3, 12.7)
3	12,794	103	105	16.1	16.4	0.3 (−4.1, 4.7)
4	8506	52	44	12.2	10.3	−1.9 (−6.4, 2.6)
5	7206	40	47	11.1	13.0	1.9 (−3.1, 7.0)
6	7203	48	57	13.3	15.8	2.5 (−3.1, 8.1)
7	6304	60	67	19.0	21.3	2.2 (−4.8, 9.2)
8	5496	15	21	5.5	7.6	2.2 (−2.1, 6.5)
9	6710	45	78	13.4	23.2	9.8 (3.4, 16.3)
Mean difference $n = 9$						1.9 (−0.5, 4.3)
TOTAL intervention	66,061	574	631	17.4	19.1	1.7 (− 0.3, 3.8)
Positive tests		3	3			
		Pre 1	Pre 2	Pre 1	Pre 2	Difference
Control practices		−12,-7	−6, −1	−12,-7	−6, −1	Pre2-Pre1
10	9081	36	36	7.9	7.9	0.0 (−3.7, 3.7)
11	4133	16	22	7.7	10.6	2.9 (−2.9, 8.8)
12	10,833	63	76	11.6	14.0	2.4 (−1.9, 6.7)
13	14,547	149	159	20.5	21.9	1.4 (−3.4, 6.1)
14	2878	38	41	26.4	28.5	2.1 (−10.0, 14.2)
15	4711	18	27	7.6	11.5	3.8 (−1.8, 9.4)
16	12,456	108	115	17.3	18.5	1.1 (−3.6, 5.8)
17	6945	92	132	26.5	38.0	11.5 (3.1, 20.0)
18	3334	16	18	9.6	10.8	1.2 (−5.7, 8.1)
19	6960	44	42	12.6	12.1	−0.6 (−5.8, 4.6)
Mean difference $n = 10$						2.6 (0.5, 4.7)
TOTAL control	75,878	580	668	15.3	17.6	2.3 (0.5, 4.1)
Positive tests		7	2			
All practices						
Mean difference $n = 19$						2.3(0.7, 3.8)
TOTAL all (pooled)	141,939	1154	1299	16.3	18.3	2.0 (0.7, 3.4)
TOTAL positive tests		10	5			

Some HCPs left the session early and were too busy to complete the questionnaire. Questionnaire participant characteristics are shown in Table 2.

All mean scores were above 3 ('agree') for the statements shown in Fig. 3. The following statements '*I can apply the information gained from the training in my practice setting*' and '*The trainer actively involved me in the learning process*' scored the highest mean level of agreement (both statements scoring 3.7). The following statements '*The training met my professional educational needs*' and '*As a result of the training I feel more confident in my ability to discuss HIV testing with a patient*' and '*more confident in my ability to conduct HIV testing*' had a mean score of 3.6. Statements that attendees were '*more aware of the BHIVA and NICE guidelines on HIV testing*' scored the lowest mean level of agreement (both scored 3.4).

Table 2 Evaluation Questionnaire and interview participant characteristics

General Practice Number	Evaluation Method	GP (*n*)	Nurses & Other[a](*n*)	Gender of HCP interviewed Male/Female	Questionnaires Total (*n*)
1	Interview	1	1	1/1	10
	Questionnaire	4	6		
2	Interview	0	1	0/1	12
	Questionnaire	8	4		
3	Interview	0	1	0/1	4
	Questionnaire	2	2		
4	Interview	2	2	0/4	6
	Questionnaire	4	2		
5	Interview	0	2	1/1	9
	Questionnaire	3	6		
6	Interview	2	0	1/1	5
	Questionnaire	4	1[b]		
7	Interview	1	0	0/1	6
	Questionnaire	4	2		
8	Interview	0	1	0/1	9
	Questionnaire	3	6		
9	Interview	6	1	2/5	10
	Questionnaire	7	3		
10	Interview	0	1	0/1	6
	Questionnaire	4	2		
11	Interview	1	0	0/1	6
	Questionnaire	4	2		
12	Interview	2	0	0/2	7
	Questionnaire	6	1		
13	Interview	1	0	0/1	7
	Questionnaire	3	4		
14	Interview	0	0	0/0	5
	Questionnaire	3	2		
15	Interview	0	0	0/0	8
	Questionnaire	7	1		
16	Interview	0	0	0/0	3
	Questionnaire	2	1		
17	Interview	0	0	0/0	4
	Questionnaire	2	2		
18	Interview	0	0	0/0	6
	Questionnaire	4	2		
19	Interview	0	0	0/0	4
	Questionnaire	3	1		
		Overall totals			127

([a]Advanced Nurse Practitioner and Healthcare Assistants, [b]Questionnaire completed by a Clinical Pharmacist, HCP: Healthcare Professional. Practices 14 to 19: no interviews took place at these practices, only evaluation questionnaires were completed)

The four most frequently cited barriers to HIV testing reported in the questionnaire by GPs prior to training were: 1) *"The patient doesn't consider themselves at risk"* 2) *"Concern about embarrassing or offending the patient"* 3) *"I don't want to scare my patient when their symptoms probably aren't HIV related"* and 4) *"There isn't time to discuss HIV"*.

The four most frequently cited barriers reported by nurses were 1) *"Concern about embarrassing or offending the patient"* 2) *"The patient doesn't consider themselves at risk"* 3) *"I don't know how to manage HIV"* and 4) *"What would I do if I found an HIV positive"* and *"I don't want to scare my patient when their symptoms probably aren't HIV related"*.

When GPs and nurses were asked *"Did the training session adequately address the barriers that apply to you and/or your practice and how to overcome these?"* the majority of GPs (94%) and practice nurses (78%) replied that the intervention had adequately covered the barriers as well as ways/techniques to overcome them.

Questionnaire data showed that delivery of the HIV training was received positively by the majority of HCPs,

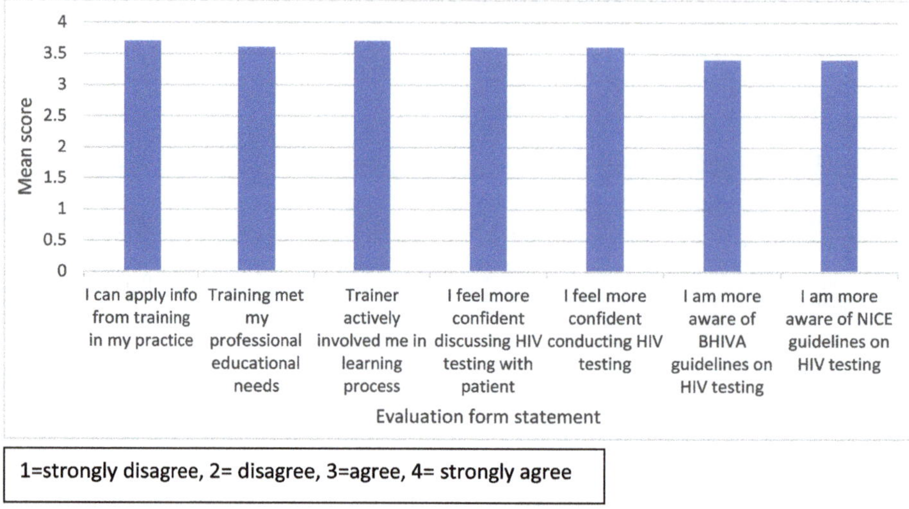

Fig. 3 Results of evaluation questionnaire completed by healthcare professionals attending the intervention

it was perceived as valuable for increasing awareness of HIV ICs, confidence and consideration of testing and HCPs gained more awareness of BHIVA and NICE HIV testing guidelines. HCPs scored highly for feeling more confident around discussing and conducting an HIV test immediately post training.

Discussion

This study has shown that although an HIV testing educational intervention was received very positively by HCPs this did not result in increased HIV tests. We showed that HIV testing rates did increase over the study period, but this was a secular trend rather than due to the intervention and occurred in both control and intervention arms of the trial. Possible explanations for the lack of effect of the education intervention on testing rates include weak design features such as one-off training compared to more sustainable programmes with regular reinforcement training and performance feedback, the focus on information rather than skills-based training which may have failed to overcome communication barriers experienced by HCPs in offering HIV tests, and that chosen practices may have already reached saturation point for HIV testing because they were those with the highest diagnosed prevalence of HIV in Bristol. Organisational and structural barriers included severely limited resources available for delivering this intervention due to local authority budget restrictions. Furthermore, GP practices were very limited in their available time to dedicate to further training even if it had been affordable. There is increasing pressure on GPs to undertake more health surveillance with less resource which has probably contributed to GPs prioritising other areas above testing for HIV [26]. Inadequate consideration of the local context may have thwarted implementation of the desired behaviour change needed to increase HIV testing in general practice, even when evidence of the benefit of increased testing in reducing late diagnosis was clearly presented [40].

Strengths and limitations

A stepped-wedged RCT is a novel way to evaluate the effects of an educational intervention. It incorporates a fair process of determining the order of intervention rollout where there are logistical constraints, as it cannot be delivered to all practices simultaneously. The RCT approach also has advantages over audit as it minimises selection bias as to which practices received the intervention and which were controls. We compared testing rates in a randomised comparison that accounted for trends in testing over time. As this was a pilot feasibility study, the number of general practices was small, and the data collection time period was relatively short. In particular, there were too few positive tests recorded to inform whether the education intervention improved targeting or appropriateness of testing. Furthermore, tests were anonymised therefore we could not determine for those who tested positive whether they had a prior HIV diagnosis or whether they linked to care.

We targeted delivery of the training to practices with a high diagnosed HIV prevalence (2–5 per 1000 population) in the practice population which may mean that these findings are not generalisable to practices with different diagnosed HIV prevalence rates [41]. The practices in our study had very high testing rates before the intervention (16.3 per 1000 population), which were much higher than the national average for general practice (10.1 per 100 and 4.4 per 1000 population in very high and high prevalence areas, respectively). Therefore, the capacity to increase testing rates in participating practices may have been smaller than in practices not in the study that test less. In East London where there have been interventions to increase HIV testing [39], there were pre-existing local sexual health enhanced services, but this was not the case in Bristol. However, the practices with higher diagnosed prevalence in Bristol would have had an increased awareness of testing due to having registered HIV positive patients which may explain their already high testing rates.

The testing data is at the practice level and therefore it was not possible to examine variation in testing at the HCP level. The effects of the intervention may have been diluted if only a small proportion of HCPs in the practice attended the training. A one-off session may have limited attendance rates compared to training sessions given frequently, which would have allowed more HCPs the opportunity to attend. However, a one-off session reduces the burden on HCPs which may have encouraged more to attend.

In the UK, the population of pregnant women is very low risk for HIV, with testing rates around 96%. Therefore, this population is different from those who are offered an HIV test during usual primary care consultations. We excluded HIV tests that were known to be carried out by midwives, but some tests that were carried out as part of ante-natal screening may have inadvertently been included. This would tend to raise testing rates, but result in fewer positive tests, but this should not have been differential between the arms of the trial. We considered positive HIV tests to be newly diagnosed patients, but it is possible that the result could have been from a repeat test after a positive test during ante-natal screening, or a patient with diagnosed HIV that was transferring from another practice or had not declared their HIV status to the GP.

Our study in context

Other sexual health testing educational interventions have been undertaken in the UK [35, 42]. HIV testing rates increased in general practices receiving a multifaceted educational intervention (Sexual Health in Practice -SHIP) in an extremely high diagnosed HIV prevalence area in London [35] and that these were sustained over 8 years [43]. This study used five rounds of training over a 24-month period which differs to the one-off training used in the current study, potentially illustrating the benefits of repeated training sessions over time. Other differences included a broader focus on sexual health, separate peer led training for GPs and practice nurses, and a focus on practicing skills, particularly rapid sexual risk assessment and verbal strategies to overcome barriers to testing.

A national pilot of an educational intervention known as 3Cs and HIV study was undertaken by PHE to improve general practice staff skills and confidence to increase chlamydia testing rates, provide condoms with contraceptive information and carry out HIV testing according to national guidelines [42]. Similarly, to our study, results of this pilot showed that the short educational sessions had no impact on chlamydia testing and that there remained barriers preventing testing intentions being translated into measurable changes in test numbers [42]. There were also many barriers to testing reported by GPs and nurses in our study which need to be actively addressed to reduce undiagnosed infection. Similar barriers were reported from qualitative interviews which took place after the HIV testing workshops in the 3Cs and HIV study which revealed that staff still lacked confidence and experience of offering HIV tests in routine consultations [44].

As part of our study a qualitative researcher carried out interviews with HCPs who attended the training approximately 3-months post-training. The HIV training was experienced positively and improved perceived awareness, confidence, and consideration of HIV testing whilst perceptions of testing rates were mixed. Continued barriers to testing included perceived lack of opportunity to consider HIV during consultations. The study, which is reported more fully elsewhere [38], concluded that repetition may be needed to sustain the impact of the education intervention.

Implications for research and/or practice

Increasing the uptake of HIV testing across healthcare settings [3] and reducing the stigma surrounding HIV testing is still a major priority in the UK because of late HIV diagnosis with advanced disease [15, 45, 46]. However, we cannot tell from our data whether the rate of HIV testing in our study practices was sufficiently high already to meet the requirements of guideline testing. For the level of HIV testing to reach saturation in areas of high diagnosed HIV prevalence, all new patients registering with a GP, those having a blood test who have not tested for HIV in the previous 12 months, those from high risk groups, those who have travelled to endemic regions, and those with HIV indicator conditions should be offered an HIV test in accordance with BHIVA and NICE recommendations [3]. Opt-out testing can facilitate increased testing as has been evident with the successful national policy recommendation introduced in 1999 that all pregnant women should have an HIV test alongside other antenatal screening tests (via an opt-out approach). The policy has a 96% acceptance rate in antenatal settings and has had a dramatic effect on reducing the number of women with undiagnosed HIV post-delivery and mother-to-child transmission [32]. Studies promoting IC-based testing [43] have shown a relatively low increase in testing compared to HIV screening studies such as the RHIVA trial of rapid HIV testing [31], although positivity rates tend to be higher in targeted interventions [10].

The findings from this study have implications for policy-makers. Training on its own is not an effective behaviour change technique and future interventions to increase HIV testing should consider using behaviour change theory to develop a complex intervention. This might be based on the behaviour change wheel known as the "COM-B" system which considers capability (psychological and physical), opportunity (physical and social), and motivation (reflective and automatic) to change behaviour [47]. Single training sessions on HIV testing, although perceived positively by HCPs, are likely to require repetition and support from additional interventions or strategies to help encourage increased HIV testing rates. Computer prompts based on risk algorithms are one strategy to support HIV testing. Prompts would notify the HCP when patients show HIV ICs or behavioral risk factors (e.g. drug use, unprotected sex). Studies using clinical reminders or computer prompts based on HIV risk factors have shown the benefits of this type of intervention, impacting significantly on HIV testing rates [48–53]. A recent initiative in the UK assessed the feasibility of an electronic clinical decision support system, prompting HIV testing based on doctors and nurses selecting certain other tests (e.g. hepatitis serology). The system was found to be useable and acceptable by hospital doctors, GPs and nurses and there was a 6% increase in testing rates over the 3-month study period [54]. A recent literature review has provided evidence that HIV ICs have the potential to be used more effectively as triggers for earlier HIV testing [55].

Conclusions

Interventions to improve general practice HIV testing rates remain a priority. A single educational training session did not increase HIV testing rates in 19 practices in Bristol with high diagnosed HIV prevalence, despite HCPs reporting that the training was useful and that they felt more confident to offer testing. Commissioners and Public Health Officials need to understand the pitfalls and risks of a one-off training intervention in general practice and consider implementation of more effective and sustainable programmes. Better designed complex interventions tailored to the context of each practice are required to change HIV testing culture and HCP behaviour. Further educational sessions would need to be supported by different strategies to help reinforce and facilitate any long-term impact on HIV testing rates.

Abbreviations

ART: Anti-retroviral therapy; BHIVA: British HIV Association; GP: General Practitioner; GUM: Genito-Urinary Medicine; HCAs: Health Care Assistants; HCP: Healthcare professional; HIV ICs: HIV Indicator conditions; HIV: Human immunodeficiency virus; MEDFASH: Medical Foundation for HIV and Sexual Health; MSM: Men who have sex with men; NHS: National Health Service; PHE: Public Health England; POCT: Point of care testing; RCT: Randomised controlled trial

Acknowledgements

We would like to thank all the HCPs from the participating practices that attended the one-hour interactive workshop over the course of the 18 months of the study and who also completed the study evaluation questionnaires. PHE for the provision of the testing data. We would also like to thank Dr Sarah Jahfar (GP) for her help during the study set up and design stage of the intervention.

Funding

This research was partly funded by the NIHR Health Protection Research Unit in Evaluation of Interventions at University of Bristol. MM is supported by the NIHR Biomedical Research Centre at University Hospitals Bristol NHS Foundation Trust and the University of Bristol. JH's time is supported by the National Institute for Health Research (NIHR) Collaboration for Leadership in Applied Health Research and Care West (CLAHRC West) at University Hospitals Bristol NHS Foundation Trust. JK is partly funded by NIHR CLAHRC West at University Hospitals Bristol NHS Foundation Trust and NIHR Health Protection Research Unit in Evaluation of Interventions.
The views expressed are those of the author(s) and not necessarily those of NHS England, NHS Improvement, the NIHR or the Department of Health and Social Care.
Payment to HCPs for participation in qualitative interviews were funded by Bristol City Council. Transcriptions costs for HCPs interviews were funded by North Bristol NHS Trust HIV Research Fund.

Authors' contributions

MM, MG, AB, and CD, and conceived the study. CD, CC and MM performed statistical analyses. CD, JK, MM and MG drafted the manuscript which was critically revised for important intellectual content by all authors. All authors have read and approved the final version of the manuscript.

Consent for publication

Not applicable.

Competing interests

The authors declare that they have no competing interests.

Author details

[1]Bristol Medical School, University of Bristol, Canynge Hall, 39 Whatley Road, Bristol BS8 2PS, UK. [2]Bristol Medical School, University of Bristol, Oakfield House, Oakfield Grove, Bristol BS8 2BN, UK. [3]National Institute for Health Research Collaborations for Leadership in Applied Health Research and Care West (NIHR CLAHRC West), University Hospitals Bristol, NHS Foundation Trust, 9th Floor, Whitefriars, Lewins Mead, Bristol BS1 2NT, England. [4]National Institute of Health Research (NIHR) Health Protection Research Unit (HPRU) in Evaluation of Interventions, Bristol Medical School, University of Bristol, Oakfield House, Oakfield Grove, Bristol BS8 2BN, UK. [5]Department of Immunology, Southmead Hospital, North Bristol NHS Trust, Westbury-on-Trym, Bristol BS10 5NB, UK. [6]Genitourinary medicine, Unity Sexual Health, Bristol Sexual Health Services, Tower Hill, Bristol BS2 0JD, UK. [7]NHS Bristol, North Somerset and South Gloucestershire CCG, South Plaza, Marlborough Street, Bristol BS1 3NX, UK.

References

1. Public Health England. HIV in the UK 2016 Report .https://www.gov.uk/government/uploads/system/uploads/attachment_data/file/602942/HIV_in_the_UK_report.pdf. Accessed 14 Feb 2017. 2016.
2. Rogers A, Bruun T, Cambiano V, Vernazza P, Estrada V, Van Lunzen J, et al. HIV Transmission Risk Through Condomless Sex If HIV+ Partner On Suppressive ART: PARTNER study (CROI abstract 153LB). Abstracts from the 2014 Conference on Retroviruses and Opportunistic Infections. Top Antivir Med. 2014;22(e-1):34.
3. National Institute for Health and Care Excellence (NICE). HIV testing: encouraging uptake. Quality standard [QS157] 2017.
4. Antinori A, Coenen T, Costagiola D, Dedes N, Ellefson M, Gatell J, et al. Late presentation of HIV infection: a consensus definition. HIV Med. 2011;12(1):61–4.

5. Girardi E, Sabin CA, AdA M. Late diagnosis of HIV infection: Epidemiological features, consequences and strategies to encourage earlier testing. J Acquir Immune Defic Syndr. 2007;46:S3–8.
6. Chadborn TR, Delpech VC, Sabin CA, Sinka K, Evans BG. The late diagnosis and consequent short-term mortality of HIV-infected heterosexuals (England and Wales, 2000-2004). AIDS. 2006;20(18):2371–9.
7. May M, Gompels M, Delpech V, Porter K, Post F, Johnson M, et al. Impact of late diagnosis and treatment on life expectancy in people with HIV-1: UK Collaborative HIV Cohort (UK CHIC) Study. BMJ. 2011;343(d6016):1–11.
8. Beck EJ, Mandalia S, Sangha R, Sharott P, Youle M, et al. The Cost-Effectiveness of Early Access to HIV Services and Starting cART in the UK 1996–2008. PLoS ONE. 2011;6(12):e27830. https://doi.org/10.1371/journal.pone.0027830
9. Hartney T, Kennedy I, Crook P, Nardone A. Expanded HIV testing in high-prevalence areas in England: results of a 2012 audit of sexual health commissioners. HIV Med. 2014;15(4):251–4.
10. Elmahdi R, Gerver SM, Guillen GG, Fidler S, Cooke G, Ward H. Low levels of HIV test coverage in clinical settings in the UK: a systematic review of adherence to 2008 guidelines. Sex Transm Infect. 2014;90(2):119–24.
11. National Institute for Health and Care Excellence (NICE). Guidance 60. 2016. Available: https://www.nice.org.uk/guidance/ng60/chapter/recommendations#offering-and-recommending-hiv-testing-in-different-settings.
12. Walensky RP, Weinstein MC, Kimmel AD, Seage GR 3rd, Losina E, Sax PE, et al. Routine human immunodeficiency virus testing: an economic evaluation of current guidelines. Am J Med. 2005;118(3):292–300.
13. Paltiel AD, Weinstein MC, Kimmel AD, Seage GR 3rd, Losina E, Zhang H, et al. Expanded screening for HIV in the United States--an analysis of cost-effectiveness. N Engl J Med. 2005;352(6):586–95.
14. Yazdanpanah Y, Sloan CE, Charlois-Ou C, Le Vu S, Semaille C, Costagliola D, et al. Routine HIV screening in France: clinical impact and cost-effectiveness. PLoS One. 2010;5(10):e13132.
15. Burns FM, Johnson AM, Nazroo J, Ainsworth J, Anderson J, Fakoya A, et al. Missed opportunities for earlier HIV diagnosis within primary and secondary healthcare settings in the UK. AIDS. 2008;22(1):115–22.
16. Read P, Armstrong-James D, Tong CYW, Fox J. Missed opportunities for HIV testing-a costly oversight. QJM. 2011;104(5):421–4.
17. Goodall L, Leen C. Late diagnosis of HIV: could this be avoided? Scott Med J. 2011;56(2):84–6.
18. British HIV Association. UK National Guidelines for HIV testing; 2008. https://www.bhiva.org/HIV-testing-guidelines. Accessed 04/2016.
19. Scognamiglio P, Chiaradia G, De Carli G, Giuliani M, Mastroianni CM, Barbacci SA, et al. The potential impact of routine testing of individuals with HIV indicator diseases in order to prevent late HIV diagnosis. BMC Infect Dis. 2013;13:473:1–10.
20. Wellesley R, Whittle A, Figueroa J, Anderson J, Castles R, Boomla K, et al. Does general practice deliver safe primary care to people living with HIV? A case-notes review. Br J Gen Pract. 2015;65(639):e655–61.
21. Joore IK, Arts DL, Kruijer MJ. Moll van Charante EP, Geerlings SE, Prins JM, et al. HIV indicator condition-guided testing to reduce the number of undiagnosed patients and prevent late presentation in a high-prevalence area: a case-control study in primary care. Sex Transm Infect. 2015;91(7):467–72.
22. Damery S, Nichols L, Holder R, Ryan R, Wilson S, Warmington S, et al. Assessing the predictive value of HIV indicator conditions in general practice: a case-control study using the THIN database. Br J Gen Pract. 2013; 63(611):e370–7.
23. Bradshaw P. Four ethical issues to consider before offering HIV tests to your patients. Pulse. 2016. http://www.pulsetoday.co.uk/your-practice/four-ethical-issues-to-consider-before-offering-hiv-tests-to-your-patients/20033417.article. Accessed 12/2016.
24. Deblonde J, De Koker P, Hamers FF, Fontaine J, Luchters S, Temmerman M. Barriers to HIV testing in Europe: a systematic review. Eur J Pub Health. 2010;20(4):422–32.
25. Davies C, Gompels M, May M. Public and Healthcare Practitioner attitudes towards HIV testing: Review of the evidence in the UK. Int STD Res Rev. 2015;3(3):991–1022.
26. McMullen H, Griffiths C, Leber W, Greenhalgh T. Explaining high and low performers in complex intervention trials: a new model based on diffusion of innovations theory. Trials. 2015;16:242.
27. Public Health England. Addressing late HIV diagnosis through screening and testing: An evidence summary; 2014. https://webarchive.nationalarchives.gov.uk/20140722054022/, http://www.hpa.org.uk/webc/HPAwebFile/HPAweb_C/1317141126407. Accessed 04/2016.
28. Orkin C. BHIVA response to Pulse article (12 Dec 2016) 'Four ethical issues to consider before offering HIV tests to your patients': British HIV Association BHIVA; 2016 [Available from: http://www.bhiva.org/BHIVA-response-to-Pulse-article-12-Dec-2016.aspx.
29. Prost A, Griffiths CJ, Anderson J, Wight D, Hart GJ. Feasibility and acceptability of offering rapid HIV tests to patients registering with primary care in London (UK): a pilot study. Sex Transm Infect. 2009; 85(5):326–9.
30. Bryce G, Wilkinson P, Nicholson S, Jeffery A, Hankins M, Jackson D. A study to assess the acceptability, feasibility and cost-effectiveness of universal HIV testing with newly registering patients (aged 16-59) in primary care. HIV Med. 2011;12:3–4.
31. Leber W, McMullen H, Anderson J, Marlin N, Santos AC, Bremner S, et al. Promotion of rapid testing for HIV in primary care (RHIVA2): a cluster-randomised controlled trial. Lancet HIV. 2015;2(6):e229–35.
32. Health Protection Agency. Time to test for HIV: expanded healthcare and community HIV testing in England; 2011. https://www.bhiva.org/file/gMSwfxmXnFQeb/Time_to_test_final_report__Sept_2011.pdf. Accessed 04/2016.
33. Baggaley RF, Irvine MA, Leber W, Cambiano V, Figueroa J, McMullen H, et al. Cost-effectiveness of screening for HIV in primary care: a health economics modelling analysis. Lancet HIV. 2017.
34. Dhairyawan R, Hutchinson J, Deayton J, Estcourt C. Educating East London primary care providers to improve rates of HIV testing and HIV recognition in an area of high HIV prevalence and late presentation. HIV Med. 2010; 11(Suppl. 1):114–5.
35. Pillay TD, Mullineux J, Smith CJ, Matthews P. Unlocking the potential: longitudinal audit finds multifaceted education for general practice increases HIV testing and diagnosis. Sex Transm Infect. 2013;89(3):191–U25.
36. Majewska W, Pakianathan M, Bassant L, Howland C, Forsyth R, Marett B. Increasing HIV testing in non-GUM settings - a new training resource. HIV Med. 2012;13:62–3.
37. Brown A, Kirwan P, Chau C, Khawam J, Gill O, Delpech V. Towards elimination of HIV transmission, AIDS and HIV-related deaths in the UK – 2017 report. November 2017, Public Health England, London; 2017. https://assets.publishing.service.gov.uk/government/uploads/system/uploads/attachment_data/file/675809/Towards_elimination_of_HIV_transmission_AIDS_and_HIV_related_deaths_in_the_UK.pdf.
38. Kesten JD, Davies C, Horwood, J, May, M, Gompels, M, Billing A, Coleman B, Crofts M. Qualitative evaluation of an education intervention for healthcare professionals on appropriate HIV testing in higher prevalence general practices in a city in the southwest of England. 23rd Annual Conference British HIV Association; 2017 5/4/2017; Liverpool, UK: HIV Medicine.
39. Leber W, Beresford L, Nightingale C, Barbosa EC, Morris S, El-Shogri F, et al. Effectiveness and cost-effectiveness of implementing HIV testing in primary care in East London: protocol for an interrupted time series analysis. BMJ Open. 2017;7(12):e018163.
40. Bokhour BG, Saifu H, Goetz MB, Fix GM, Burgess J, Fletcher MD, et al. The role of evidence and context for implementing a multimodal intervention to increase HIV testing. Implement Sci. 2015;10:22.
41. Nash S, Furegato M, Gill O, Connor N. Public Health England (PHE), London. HIV testing in England: November 2017 report; 2017. Available: https://assets.publishing.service.gov.uk/government/uploads/system/uploads/attachment_data/file/759270/HIV_testing_in_England_2017_report.pdf.
42. Town K, McNulty CA, Ricketts EJ, Hartney T, Nardone A, Folkard KA, et al. Service evaluation of an educational intervention to improve sexual health services in primary care implemented using a step-wedge design: analysis of chlamydia testing and diagnosis rate changes. BMC Public Health. 2016;16:686.

43. Pillay K, Gardner M, Gould A, Otiti S, Mullineux J, Barnighausen T, et al. Long term effect of primary health care training on HIV testing: A quasi-experimental evaluation of the Sexual Health in Practice (SHIP) intervention. PLoS One. 2018;13(8):e0199891.
44. Allison R, Ricketts EJ, Hartney T, Nardone A, Town K, Rugman C, et al. Qualitative impact assessment of an educational workshop on primary care practitioner attitudes to NICE HIV testing guidelines. BJGP Open. 2018. https://doi.org/10.3399/bjgpopen18X101433.
45. Kober C, Dowson L, Maher T, Perry N, Fisher M, Richardson D. A qualitative study to explore why individuals who are late presenters with HIV infection do not test sooner. HIV Med. 2010;11(Suppl.1):1–119.
46. Lowbury R. A roadmap for eliminating late diagnosis of HIV in England. Halve It position paper [Internet]. 2018 1/11/2018:[1–75 pp.]. Available from: http://halveit.org.uk/wp-content/uploads/2018/10/halve_it_position_paper_FINAL.pdf.
47. Michie S, van Stralen MM, West R. The behaviour change wheel: A new method for characterising and designing behaviour change interventions. Implement Sci. 2011;6.
48. Goetz M, Hoang T, Bowman C, Knapp H, Rossman B, Smith RD. A system-wide intervention to improve HIV testing in the Veterans Health Administration. J Gen Intern Med. 2008;23(8):1200–7.
49. Schrantz S, Babcock C, Theodosis C, Brown S, Mercer S, Pillow M. A targeted, conventional assay, emergency department HIV testing program integrated with existing clinical procedures. Ann Emerg Med. 2011;58(1 Suppl 1):S85–8.e1.
50. Federman D, Kravetz J, Vasquez L, Campbell S. Improving human immunodeficiency virus testing rates with an electronic clinical reminder. Am J Med. 2012;125(3):240–2.
51. Dosekun O, Perera S, Sanghera T, Hayes M, Bexley A, Goubet S, et al. HIV testing in clinical indicator diseases in outpatient settings: offer and uptake rates and impact of educational and active interventions. HIV Med. 2013;14:45.
52. Avery AK, Del Toro M, Caron A. Increases in HIV screening in primary care clinics through an electronic reminder: an interrupted time series. BMJ Qual Saf. 2014;23(3):250–6.
53. Marcelin JR, Tan EM, Marcelin A, Scheitel M, Ramu P, Hankey R, et al. Assessment and improvement of HIV screening rates in a Midwest primary care practice using an electronic clinical decision support system: a quality improvement study. BMC Med Inform Decis Mak. 2016;16:76.
54. Chadwick DR, Hall C, Rae C, Rayment M, Branch M, Littlewood J, et al. A feasibility study for a clinical decision support system prompting HIV testing. HIV Med. 2017;18(6):435–9.
55. Davies C, Gompels M, May M. Use and effectiveness of HIV indicator conditions in guiding HIV testing: A review of the evidence. Int STD Res Rev. 2017;6(2):1–27.

5

Potential for substitution of mental health care towards family practices

Tessa Magnée[1*], Derek P. de Beurs[1], Richard Boxem[2], Dinny H. de Bakker[1,3] and Peter F. Verhaak[1,4]

Abstract

Background: Substitution is the shift of care from specialized health care to less expensive and more accessible primary health care. It seems promising for restraining rising mental health care costs. The goal of this study was to investigate a potential for substitution of patients with psychological or social problems, but without severe psychiatric disorders, from Dutch specialized mental health care to primary care, especially family practices.

Methods: We extracted anonymized data from two national databases representing primary and specialized care in 2012. We calculated the number of patients with and without psychiatric disorder per 1,000 citizens in three major settings: family practices, primary care psychologists, and specialized care. Family physicians recorded psychopathology using the International Classification of Primary Care, while psychologists and specialists used the Diagnostic and Statistical Manual of Mental Disorders, 4th Edition.

Results: Considerable numbers of patients without a diagnosed DSM-IV psychiatric disorder were treated by primary care psychologists (32.8%) or in specialized care (20.8%). Over half of the patients referred by family physicians to mental health care did not have a psychiatric disorder.

Conclusion: A recent reform of Dutch mental health care, including new referral criteria, will likely increase the number of patients with psychological or social problems that family physicians have to treat or support. Enabling and improving diagnostic assessment and treatment in family practices seems essential for substitution of mental health care.

Keywords: Family practice, Mental health, Psychiatric disorders, Primary care, Health services

Background

Substitution is the shift of care from specialized health care to less expensive and more accessible (primary) health care. This method seems promising for restraining rising health care costs [1]. The urgency for substitution in Dutch mental health care is high, as costs have increased significantly in the last years in the Netherlands [2]. Presumably, some patients treated in specialized mental health care do not have a severe psychiatric disorder, do not genuinely need treatment from specialists, and could be treated in a primary care setting instead. Previous studies suggest that up to one third or even one half of the patients who receive treatment in mental health care do not meet the formal criteria for a psychiatric disorder [3–5], although they may have other need indicators which justify treatment.

The WHO underlines the importance of integrating mental health care into general health care settings [6]. However, the consequences of enhanced primary mental health care for health care utilization and costs remain unclear. Previous reviews on consultation of mental health professionals by primary care professionals suggest that it is as effective as care as usual in improving clinical outcomes [7], but that it may also reduce utilization of health care services [8]. A Cochrane review on counselling provided in primary care in the UK [9] concluded that patients were satisfied, and that counselling was associated with enhanced clinical effectiveness

* Correspondence: t.magnee@nivel.nl
[1]Netherlands Institute of Health Services Research (NIVEL), PO Box 15683500 BN Utrecht, The Netherlands

compared to care as usual (but only in short-term). However, counselling in primary care did not seem to reduce overall healthcare costs. A Cochrane review on mental health workers integrated in primary care concluded that their presence might decrease consultation rates of other primary care professionals, prescriptions of psychotropic drugs, and referrals to specialists [10]. However, effects were modest and results were not consistent amongst all included studies. Moreover, economic significance of the results remained unclear. Some studies in the UK and the US suggest that enhanced primary mental health care is cost-effective [11, 12], but also that it requires (extra) direct financial investments over the short-term [13].

In 2014, the Dutch government introduced a reform of mental health care to promote the substitution of mental health care towards general health care settings, especially towards family practices. According to new referral criteria (Fig. 1), all patients with only mild psychological symptoms or social problems should be treated within family practices. Family physicians (FPs) are no longer allowed to refer patients without an actual psychiatric disorder to mental health care, consisting of primary care psychologists (PCPs) and specialized mental health care. Patients with a psychiatric disorder and non-complex problems (no comorbidity with for example a personality disorder or complicating psychosocial problems) should be referred to primary care psychologists (since the reform labeled as 'basic mental health care') for short-term care, while patients with complex problems should be referred to specialized mental health care for (longer term) treatment by a multidisciplinary team.

To prepare FPs for the treatment of more patients with mental health problems, the function of the mental health nurse (MHN) was introduced. Increasing numbers of Dutch FPs collaborate with an MHN: a nurse with mental health expertise, or a psychologist. MHNs can perform diagnostic research and provide short-term care [14], but they may also indirectly improve FPs' knowledge and skills in the field of mental health. Short-term psychological interventions provided in the primary care setting are accessible, seem effective, and lead to high patient satisfaction [9, 15–19]. Examples of such interventions are self-help programs, counseling, problem solving therapy, and brief cognitive behavior therapy.

Although many previous studies have evaluated the integration of mental health care into primary care, it is not clear what effects a national reform aimed at a shift of patients from specialized care towards primary care might have. The aim of this study was to investigate the potential for substitution of Dutch mental health care in the context of the new referral rules for FPs. Our central

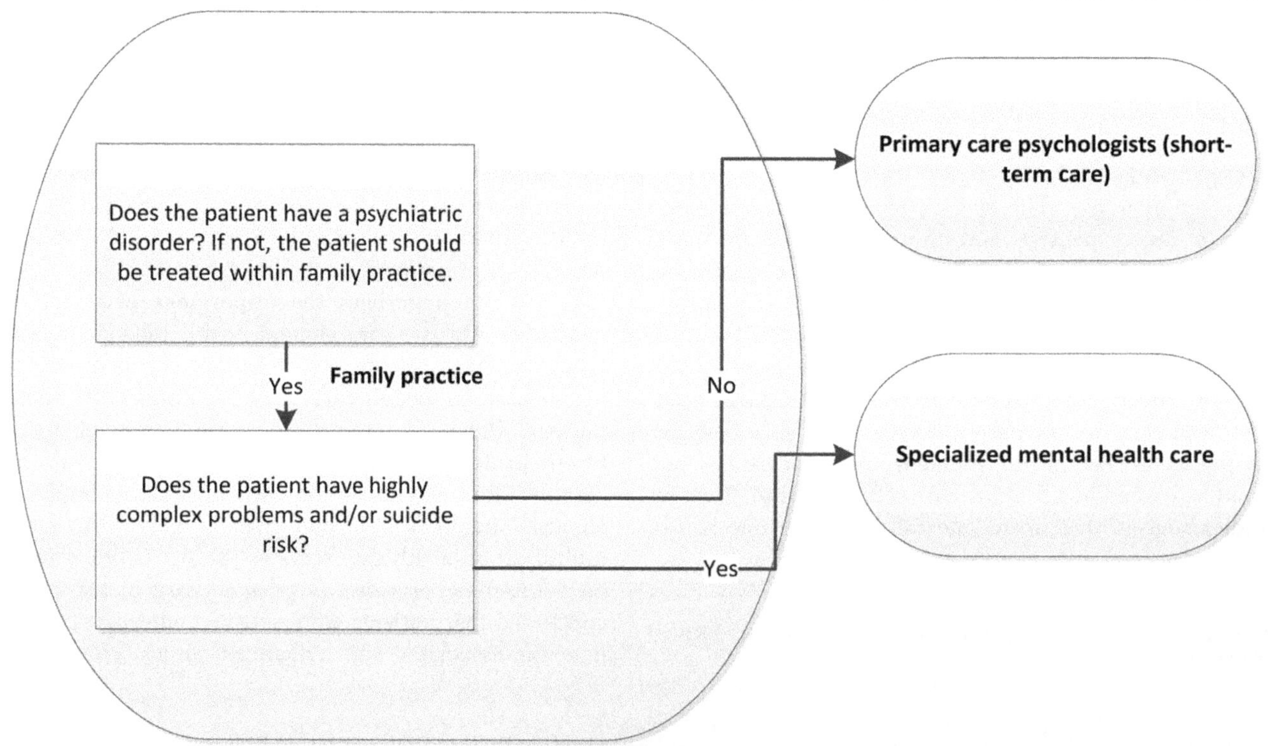

Fig. 1 Mental health care in the Netherlands: referral rules. Shows new referral rules for Dutch family physicians regarding patients with mental health problems

research question was: what is the potential for substitution of mental health care from specialized care and PCPs to family practices, and from specialized care to PCPs?

We investigated: (1) how many patients with and without psychiatric disorders were seen in the three mental health care settings before the reform, (2) how many patients with and without psychiatric disorders were referred by FPs and PCPs to primary and specialized care before the reform, and (3) how many patients with and without complex problems were treated by PCPs and in specialized care before the reform.

Methods

Data sources

In an observational, cross-sectional study, we extracted anonymized patient data from two national databases, to describe primary care, including family practices and primary care psychologists, and specialized mental health care in 2012.

Data on primary care were extracted from electronic health records of caregivers participating in the NIVEL Primary Care Database (NIVEL-PCD). All caregivers participating in the NIVEL-PCD, including FPs and PCPs, routinely record care they deliver to patients. Family practices participating in the NIVEL-PCD are representative of Dutch family practices [20], although group practices and practices in non-urban areas are somewhat overrepresented compared to national numbers [21]. The patient populations of the family practices are representative of the Dutch population according to sex and age. Only data from practices with the most complete records were used for this study ($n = 180$ practices; $n = 685{,}337$ patients). Not all FPs keep complete records of referrals. A smaller number of practices were included in the analyses on referrals ($n = 25$ practices; $n = 90{,}734$ patients). Practices with complete referral records did not differ from other practices regarding practice type, degree of urbanization, or practice size.

In 2012, 543 primary care psychologists were participating in the NIVEL PCD, providing care to 45,947 patients. The database covered 14.6% of all patients treated by primary care psychologists working in the Netherlands [22].

Data on specialized care were extracted from a national database for specialized care [23]. This database covers all caregivers, mostly psychiatrists and psychologists, working in Dutch specialized mental health care institutions, as well as solo operating entrepreneurs. Professionals working in specialized care are obliged by Dutch law to record all provided care that is paid for by health insurers in the national database. Therefore, virtually all Dutch patients treated in specialized mental health care were represented in this database.

Patient data

We extracted data on the number of seen or treated and referred patients and their diagnoses. To facilitate comparability between the three settings, all extracted numbers were converted to numbers of patients per 1,000 citizens based on the Dutch population number of 2012 [24].

FPs use the International Classification of Primary Care (ICPC) system to record diagnoses of patients within chapters of diseases during consultations. Within each ICPC chapter, a subdivision is made between symptoms (codes 01–29) and diseases or disorders (codes 70–99), although the Z chapter (social problems) is limited to symptom codes. Only patients with at least one consultation at the family practice with a diagnosis concerning psychological problems (P chapter) or social problems (Z chapter) were included in the study. We distinguished between patients with a psychiatric disorder (P70–P99) and patients without a psychiatric disorder (psychological symptoms, P01–P29, or social problems, Z01–Z29).

PCPs and caregivers in specialized care record a DSM-IV diagnosis for each patient during treatment. Diagnostic assessment usually takes place during an intake phase, when a wide range of diagnostic instruments may be used. The DSM-IV is a globally used classification system for psychiatric disorders, covering five axes [25]. Axis 1 represents the primary disorder or psychopathology of the patient. Axes 2 to 4 represent comorbid, underlying, or related problems. Caregivers use axis 2 to report personality disorders, axis 3 for somatic diseases, axis 4 for psychosocial problems, and axis 5 for the level of (dis)functioning of the patient. The latter was not included in this study, as it was not available for all patients in specialized care. We used the axis 1 diagnosis to determine if patients of PCPs or in specialized care had a psychiatric disorder or not. Patients had problems of higher complexity if they had comorbid problems on axis 2 (a personality disorder), axis 3 (somatic problems), or axis 4 (psychosocial problems).

Results

Patients with and without disorders in three settings

Figure 2 shows the number of patients with and without psychiatric disorders in each of the three major settings of Dutch mental health care. FPs saw 131.0 patients with psychological problems per 1,000 citizens, mostly patients without psychiatric disorders (71.3%). FP patients often had psychological symptoms such as anxious feelings, or social problems such as problems with their partner (Additional file 1: Table S1).

PCPs and caregivers in specialized care treated a smaller number of patients compared to FPs, 18.7 and 43.7 patients per 1,000 citizens, respectively. A considerable number of patients treated by primary care psychologists or in specialized care did not have

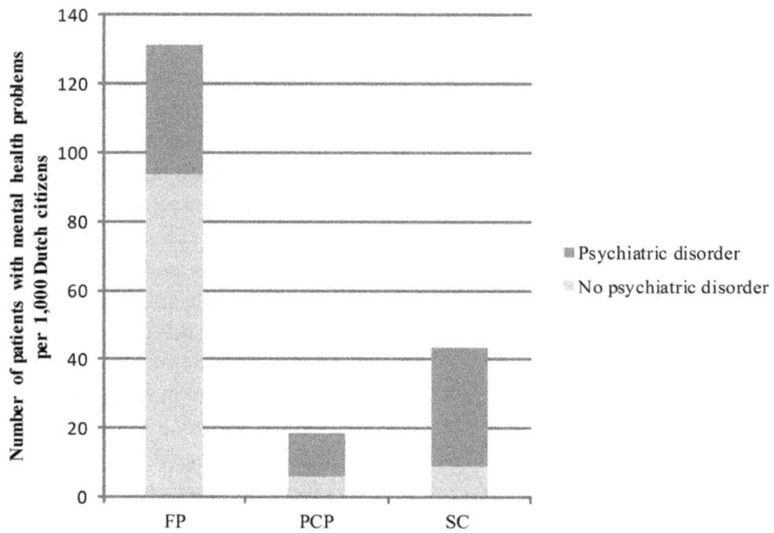

Fig. 2 Number of patients with and without a psychiatric disorder in three settings per 1,000 Dutch citizens in 2012. Shows how many patients with mental health problems were treated in 2012 by family physicians, primary care psychologists, and in specialized care in the Netherlands. Notes: FP = family practice, PCP = primary care psychologist, SC = specialized care

a psychiatric disorder, 32.8% and 20.8%, respectively. In total, 15.3 patients without a disorder per 1,000 citizens were treated by primary care psychologists or in specialized care. These patients were for example diagnosed with other worries or problems, adjustment problems, or had no diagnosis (Additional file 2: Table S2 and Additional file 3: Table S3).

Referrals

Figure 3 shows how many patients with and without psychiatric disorders were referred by FPs and PCPs to primary and specialized care (Additional file 4: Table S4 shows exact numbers). FPs in total referred 16.1 patients with psychological and social problems per 1,000 citizens to primary or specialized care, which is 12.3% of all the

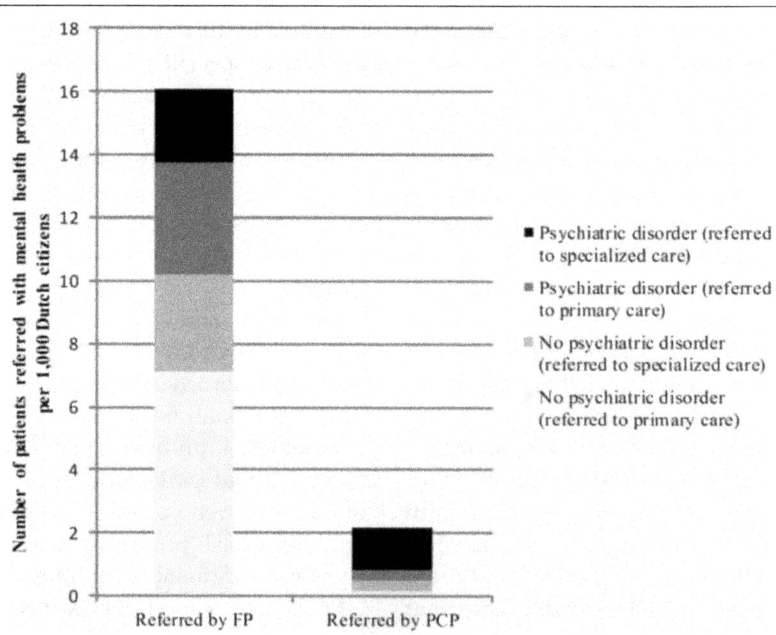

Fig. 3 Number of patients referred with and without psychiatric disorder per 1,000 Dutch citizens in 2012. Shows how many patients with mental health problems were referred in 2012 by family physicians and by primary care psychologists to primary and specialized care. Notes: FP = family physician. PCP = primary care psychologist. Primary care: (other) FP, (other) PCP, or social work

FP patients with psychological and social problems. Over half of the referred FP patients (63.2%) did not have a psychiatric disorder. PCPs in total referred 2.2 patients per 1,000 citizens to primary and specialized care, which is 11.7% of all patients they treated. Of the referred PCP patients, around one fifth (22.4%) did not have a psychiatric disorder.

Complexity of problems

Figure 4 shows that many patients treated by PCPs had comorbidity, mostly a psychiatric disorder combined with psychosocial problems (78.3%), or somatic problems (75.9%). Only one in every twenty PCP patients had a combination of a psychiatric disorder and a personality disorder (4.5%). Most patients treated in specialized care had comorbidity as well; most patients with a disorder also had psychosocial problems (90.8%). Fewer patients treated in specialized care had a psychiatric disorder combined with somatic problems (32.4%) or with a personality disorder (15.7%).

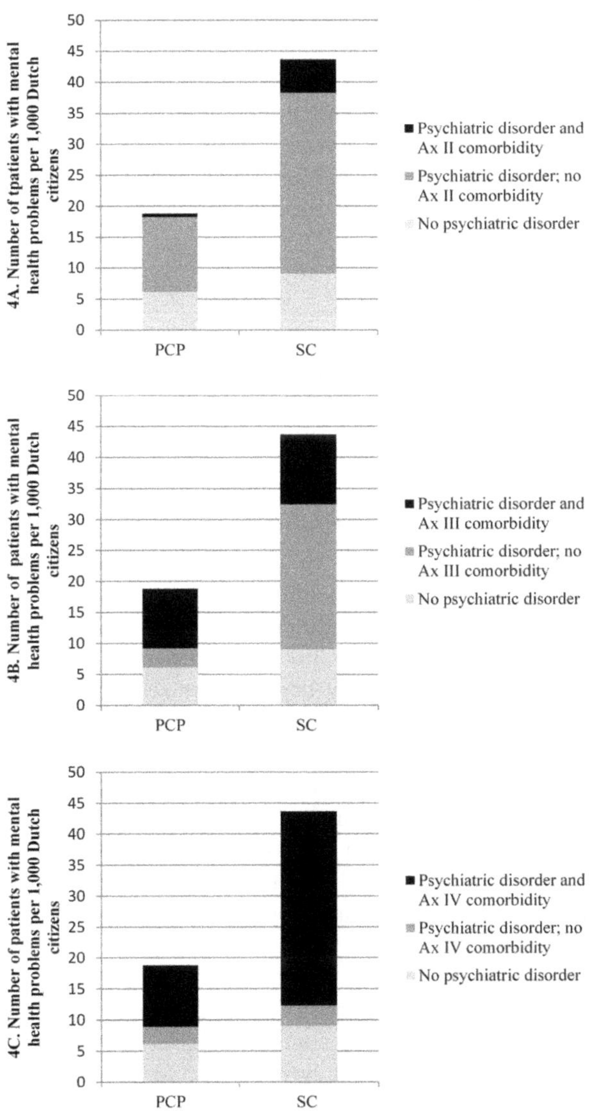

Fig. 4 Number of patients with and without comorbidity in two settings per 1,000 Dutch citizens in 2012. Shows how many patients with mental health problems treated in 2012 by primary care psychologists or in specialized care had comorbid problems. Notes: PCP = primary care psychologist. SC = specialized care

Discussion

Summary of findings

Prior to the recent reform of Dutch mental health care, a significant number of patients treated by PCPs (approximately one third) and in specialized care (approximately one fifth) did not have a diagnosed DSM-IV disorder. Over half of the patients with psychological and social problems referred by FPs to mental health professionals did not have a diagnosis of a psychiatric disorder. Most patients with a disorder in specialized care had complex problems, expressed by comorbidity on axis 4 of the DSM-IV (psychosocial problems). Comorbidity on axis 3 (somatic problems) or axis 2 (personality disorders) was less common.

Potential for substitution from PCPs and specialized care to family practice

The proportion of patients without a psychiatric disorder in mental health care observed in this study is in line with previous research [3–5]. If we evaluate this study as a baseline measure of the reform of the Dutch mental health care system, we expect that a part of the patients previously referred to and treated in mental health care from now on will receive treatment within family practices. Nurses with mental health expertise, who work in increasing numbers of family practices in the Netherlands, may be of crucial importance in the diagnostic assessment and treatment of those patients.

An apparent discrepancy was observed between the number of patients without a psychiatric disorder who were referred by FPs (over 60%) and the lower number of patients without a psychiatric disorder who were treated by PCPs and in specialized care (20.8% and 32.8%). It is highly plausible that (final) diagnostic assessment often takes place *after* referral, We have to consider the possibility that some of the patients might be falsely diagnosed after referral. Although the DSM-IV is highly useful, its limitations are widely debated, and it might stimulate overdiagnosis [26, 27]. Moreover, the Dutch health insurance only covers PCP and specialist treatment for patients with a DSM-IV disorder, which may encourage overdiagnosis even further. Remarkably, FPs now also face the risk of overdiagnosis, as the new referral criteria make a psychiatric disorder a necessity for every referral to mental health care.

Some of the patients recently treated by mental health care professionals or referred by GPs may not have had a diagnosed psychiatric disorder, but they may certainly have been in need of treatment. Previous research showed that approximately half of the patients in mental health care had no psychiatric disorder, but showed other important indicators of need for treatment, such as multiple subthreshold disorders, a recent stressor, psychosocial problems, or suicidal behavior [3, 4]. If we assume this is also true for the patients included in this study, the new referral criteria for FPs regarding psychiatric disorders could have an unwanted effect. Some patients, who are certainly in need of mental health care, but who do not meet formal criteria for a psychiatric disorder, may be deprived of appropriate treatment.

In either way, enabling and improving diagnostic assessment in family practices seems essential for substitution of mental health care. Good quality diagnostic assessment in family practice could facilitate the correct adoption of the new referral criteria. It could also improve the continuity of care from the patient's perspective. A screening instrument may be helpful, for example a symptom severity assessment [28]. MHNs could improve diagnostic assessment, both by performing it themselves or by indirectly improving FPs' knowledge and skills through collaboration.

Potential for substitution from specialized care to PCPs

We expect substitution towards PCPs to a lesser extent compared to substitution toward family practices, as most patients treated in specialized care with a disorder had at least comorbid psychosocial problems. However, it is debatable to what extent psychosocial problems genuinely represent a complicating factor, as they are often temporary and can be solved in a relatively straightforward way. Other comorbid diagnoses, such as personality disorders, were observed less frequently, but they are more likely to complicate treatment [29]. From this perspective, more potential for substitution from specialized care toward PCPs may exist than observed in this study.

Health care costs

Restraining costs was one the most important reasons for the recent Dutch mental health care reform. Our study indicates that, in the near future, at least some of the patients with mental health problems may be treated in (less expensive) primary care instead of in specialized care. This may result in a cost reduction. However, the recent Dutch reform might also have unintended cost effects. The accessibility of mental health care is likely to be improved, and some patients that might not have been treated at all before may now receive treatment in family practice. Moreover, it is unknown how many of the patients initially treated in family practice afterwards still need a referral to specialized care. Future research following patients through the different echelons of mental health care is needed to evaluate cost effects.

International relevance

The WHO states it is important to redirect funding towards community-based services, including the integration of mental health care into general health care settings [6]. Various health care system characteristics influence the role of the FP in mental health care [30, 31], for example the referral system, FP workload and mental health expertise, financial regulations, and patient expectations. These factors vary strongly between countries, and influence a possible shift of mental health care from specialized care to primary care. Potential for substitution is likely to exist in other countries besides the Netherlands, as was shown by the numbers of patients without a psychiatric disorder treated in mental health care [3, 4], and by the numerous international studies evaluating the integration of mental health care into primary care [7–12]. FPs in the UK [32] and Canada [33] are collaborating with professionals similar to mental health nurses, which might enable substitution.

Strengths and limitations

As this is a descriptive study, we cannot draw any conclusions on causality. A major strength of this study is that we were able to combine two national databases, thereby including a very large number of patients in primary care and virtually all patients in specialized care. This study can function as a baseline measure for the recent Dutch mental health care reform.

Caregivers working in different settings vary in their skills to recognize and diagnose mental health problems. Caregivers working in different settings use different classification systems (ICPC and DSM-IV), which may complicate comparability between the settings. Previous research has shown that GPs do not always recognize psychological problems, or that they may be aware of mental health problems but do not label patients with a specific psychological diagnosis [34]. Only about half of all persons with mental disorders had contact with their GP in the last six months [35]. The diagnoses of persons who do not seek help are not coded and were thus not included in this study.

Professionals working in mental health care sometimes postpone giving a diagnosis. This could mean some of the patients included in our study may have been diagnosed later on. However, data were extracted a considerable amount of time after treatment (2014 vs. 2012). We categorized patients without a diagnosis as patients without a disorder, as we assume that the complaints of many of these patients were not severe enough to have led to an official diagnosis of a disorder within a decent amount of time. PCPs had the possibility of explicitly choosing between "no axis 1 disorder" or "diagnosis postponed". The latter was only used for a one out of five patients without a diagnosis (Additional file 2: Table S2).

We were unfortunately not able to, besides the DSM-IV axis 2 to axis 4 comorbidity, include any other complicating factors, such as suicide risk. These factors were not routinely recorded by caregivers in any setting.

Conclusions

A recent reform of Dutch mental health care, including new FP referral criteria, will likely lead to a considerable increase in patients with psychological or social problems that have to be treated within family practices. Enabling and improving diagnostic assessment and treatment in family practices seems essential for substitution of mental health care.

Additional files

Additional file 1: Table S1. Number of patients seen for psychological or social problems at Dutch family practices per 1,000 citizens in 2012. Contains a table with the number of patients with mental health problems treated in 2012 in family practices, according to diagnosis.

Additional file 2: Table S2. Number of patients treated by primary care psychologists per 1,000 Dutch citizens in 2012. Contains a table with the number of patients with mental health problems treated in 2012 by primary care psychologists, according to diagnosis.

Additional file 3: Table S3. Number of patients treated in secondary care per 1,000 Dutch citizens in 2012. Contains a table with the number of patients with mental health problems treated in 2012 in specialized care, according to diagnosis.

Additional file 4: Table S4. Number of patients referred by FPs and PCPs per1,000 Dutch citizens in 2012. Contains a table with the number of patients with mental health problems referred in 2012 by family physicians and by primary care psychologists to primary and specialized care.

Abbreviations

FP: Family physician; ICPC: International Classification of Primary Care; MHN: Mental health nurse; NIVEL: Netherlands Institute for Health Services Research; NIVEL PCD: NIVEL Primary Care Database; PCP: Primary care psychologist; SC: Specialized care

Funding

This study was carried out with a grant of the Dutch Advisory Committee on Medical Manpower Planning (ACMMP). The funding body was involved in the design of the study, and not in the data collection, analyses, interpretation of data, and writing of the manuscript.

Authors' contributions

TM, DB, DHB, and PFV designed the study. TM and RB analyzed the data. TM wrote the first draft of the manuscript. All authors contributed to and approved the final manuscript.

Competing interests

The authors declare that they have no competing interests.

Consent for publication

Not applicable.

Author details

[1]Netherlands Institute of Health Services Research (NIVEL), PO Box 15683500 BN Utrecht, The Netherlands. [2]The Dutch Healthcare Authority, Utrecht, The Netherlands. [3]Tilburg University, Scientific Centre for Transformation in Care and Welfare (TRANZO), Tilburg, The Netherlands. [4]Department of General Practice, Groningen University, Groningen, The Netherlands.

References

1. Van Dijk CE, Verheij RA, Hansen J, et al. Primary care nurses: effects on secondary care referrals for diabetes. BMC Health Serv Res. 2010;10:230.
2. Van Hoof F, Knispel A, Meije D, Van Wijngaarden B, Vijselaar J. Trendrapportage GGZ 2010. [Trend report mental health care 2010]. Utrecht: Trimbos-instituut; 2010.
3. Bruffaerts R, Posada-Villa J, Al-Hamzawi AO, et al. Proportion of patients without mental disorders being treated in mental health services worldwide. Br J Psychiatry. 2015;206(2):101–9. doi:10.1192/bjp.bp.113.141424.
4. Druss BG, Wang PS, Sampson NA, et al. Understanding mental health treatment in persons without mental diagnoses: results from the National Comorbidity Survey Replication. Arch Gen Psychiatry. 2007;64(10):1196–203. doi:10.1001/archpsyc.64.10.1196.
5. Jorg F, Visser E, Ormel J, et al. Mental health care use in adolescents with and without mental disorders. Eur Child Adolesc Psychiatry. 2015. doi:10.1007/s00787-015-0754-9. Epub 2015 Aug 15.
6. WHO. Mental Health Action Plan 2013-2020. Geneva: WHO Publishing; 2013. [cited December 22 2015]. Available from: http://www.who.int/mental_health/publications/action_plan/en/
7. Cape J, Whittington C, Bower P. What is the role of consultation-liaison psychiatry in the management of depression in primary care? A systematic review and meta-analysis. Gen Hosp Psychiatry. 2010;32(3):246–54. doi:10.1016/j.genhosppsych.2010.02.003.
8. van der Feltz-Cornelis CM, Van Os TW, Van Marwijk HW, Leentjens AF. Effect of psychiatric consultation models in primary care. A systematic review and meta-analysis of randomized clinical trials. J Psychosom Res. 2010;68(6):521–33. doi:10.1016/j.jpsychores.2009.10.012.
9. Bower P, Knowles S, Coventry PA, Rowland N. Counselling for mental health and psychosocial problems in primary care. Cochrane Database Syst Rev. 2011;9:CD001025. doi:10.1002/14651858.CD001025.pub3.
10. Harkness EF, Bower PJ. On-site mental health workers delivering psychological therapy and psychosocial interventions to patients in primary care: effects on the professional practice of primary care providers. Cochrane Database Syst Rev. 2009;2009:CD000532. doi:10.1002/14651858.CD000532.pub2.
11. Green C, Richards DA, Hill JJ, Gask L, Lovell K, Chew-Graham C, Barkham M. Cost-effectiveness of collaborative care for depression in UK primary care: economic evaluation of a randomised controlled trial (CADET). PLoS One. 2014;9(8):e104225. doi:10.1371/journal.pone.0104225.
12. Jacob V, Chattopadhyay SK, Sipe TA, Thota AB, Byard GJ, Chapman DP & Community Preventive Services Task F. Economics of collaborative care for management of depressive disorders: a community guide systematic review. Am J Prev Med. 2012;42(5):539–49. doi:10.1016/j.amepre.2012.01.011.
13. Gilbody S, Bower P, Whitty P. Costs and consequences of enhanced primary care for depression: systematic review of randomised economic evaluations. Br J Psychiatry. 2006;189:297–308. doi:10.1192/bjp.bp.105.016006.
14. Griep EC, Noordman J, van Dulmen S. Practice nurses mental health provide space to patients to discuss unpleasant emotions. J Psychiatr Ment Health Nurs. 2015. doi:10.1111/jpm.12279. Epub 2015 Dec 28.
15. Van Boeijen CA, van Balkom AJ, van Oppen P, Blankenstein N, Cherpanath A, van Dyck R. Efficacy of self-help manuals for anxiety disorders in primary care: a systematic review. Fam Pract 2005. 2005;22(2):192–6. doi:10.1093/fampra/cmh708.
16. Cape J, Whittington C, Buszewicz M, Wallace P, Underwood L. Brief psychological therapies for anxiety and depression in primary care: meta-analysis and meta-regression. BMC Med. 2010;8:38. doi:10.1186/1741-7015-8-38.
17. Huibers MJ, Beurskens AJ, Bleijenberg G, van Schayck CP. Psychosocial interventions by general practitioners. Cochrane Database Syst Rev. 2007;3:CD003494. doi:10.1002/14651858.CD003494.pub2.
18. Kendrick T, Simons L, Mynors-Wallis L, et al. Cost-effectiveness of referral for generic care or problem-solving treatment from community mental health nurses, compared with usual general practitioner care for common mental disorders: Randomised controlled trial. Br J Psychiatry. 2006;189:50–9. doi:10.1192/bjp.bp.105.012435.

19. Van Orden M, Hoffman T, Haffmans J, Spinhoven P, Hoencamp E. Collaborative mental health care versus care as usual in a primary care setting: a randomized controlled trial. Psychiatr Serv 2009. 2009;60(1):74–9. doi:10.1176/appi.ps.60.1.74.
20. NIVEL Primary Care Database (NIVEL Zorgregistraties eerste lijn). Netherlands institute for health services research. 2015. [cited 2015 Dec 22] Available from: www.nivel.nl/en/dossier/nivel-primary-care-database. Accessed 22 Dec 2015.
21. Van Hassel DTP, Kasteleijn A, Kenens RJ. Cijfers uit de registratie van huisartsen: peiling 2013 [Numbers from the registrations of general practitioners: poll 2013]. Utrecht: NIVEL; 2014.
22. Magnée T, Verhaak P, Boxem R. Verschuivingen van de tweedelijns geestelijke gezondheidszorg naar de eerstelijn en gevolgen daarvan voor de benodigde beroepsbeoefenaren: 2009–2012. [Shifting from secondary mental health care to primary care and the consequences for needed professions: 2009-2012] Utrecht: NIVEL; 2014.
23. DBC-Informatiesysteem.nl [Internet]. Utrecht, the Netherlands: DBC-Onderhoud. [cited 2016 Jan 21] Available from: http://www.dbcinformatiesysteem.nl. Accessed 21 Jan 2016.
24. Statistics Netherlands (Centraal Bureau voor de Statistiek, CBS) [cited 2016 Jan 15] Available from: http://statline.cbs.nl/Statweb/publication/?DM=SLNL&PA=37296ned&D1=a&D2=0,10,20,30,40,50,62&HDR=G1&STB=T&VW=T. Accessed 15 Jan 2016.
25. American Psychiatric Association (APA). Diagnostic and statistical manual of mental disorders (4th ed., text rev.). Washington, DC: APA; 2000. doi:10.1176/appi.books.9780890423349.
26. Bolton D. Overdiagnosis problems in the DSM-IV and the new DSM-5: can they be resolved by the distress-impairment criterion? Can J Psychiatry. 2013;58(11):612–7. Retrieved from http://www.ncbi.nlm.nih.gov/pubmed/24246431.
27. Pierre JM. The borders of mental disorder in psychiatry and the DSM: past, present, and future. J Psychiatr Pract. 2010;16(6):375–86. doi:10.1097/01.pra.0000390756.37754.68.
28. Sinnema H, Franx G, Spijker J, et al. Delivering stepped care for depression in general practice: results of a survey amongst general practitioners in the Netherlands. Eur J Gen Pract. 2013;19(4):221–9. doi:10.3109/13814788.2013.780018.
29. Newton-Howes G, Tyrer P, Johnson T, et al. Influence of personality on the outcome of treatment in depression: systematic review and meta-analysis. J Pers Disord. 2014;28(4):577–93. doi:10.1521/pedi_2013_27_070.
30. Dezetter A, Briffault X, Bruffaerts R, De Graaf R, Alonso J, Konig HH, Kovess-Masfety V. Use of general practitioners versus mental health professionals in six European countries: the decisive role of the organization of mental health-care systems. Soc Psychiatry Psychiatr Epidemiol. 2013;48(1):137–49. doi:10.1007/s00127-012-0522-9.
31. Verhaak PF, van den Brink-Muinen A, Bensing JM, Gask L. Demand and supply for psychological help in general practice in different European countries: access to primary mental health care in six European countries. Eur J Public Health. 2004;14(2):134–40. Retrieved from http://www.ncbi.nlm.nih.gov/pubmed/15230497.
32. Gray R, Parr AM, Plummer S, Sandford T, Ritter S, Mundt-Leach R, Gournay K. A national survey of practice nurse involvement in mental health interventions. J Adv Nurs. 1999;30(4):901–6. Retrieved from http://www.ncbi.nlm.nih.gov/pubmed/10520103.
33. Joling KJ, van Marwijk HW, Piek E, van der Horst HE, Penninx BW, Verhaak P, van Hout HP. Do GPs' medical records demonstrate a good recognition of depression? A new perspective on case extraction. J Affect Disord. 2011; 133(3):522–7. doi:10.1016/j.jad.2011.05.001.
34. Kates N, McPherson-Doe C, George L. Integrating mental health services within primary care settings: the Hamilton Family Health Team. J Ambul Care Manage. 2011;34(2):174–82. doi:10.1097/JAC.0b013e31820f6435.
35. Verhaak PF, Prins MA, Spreeuwenberg P, Draisma S, van Balkom TJ, Bensing JM, Penninx BW. Receiving treatment for common mental disorders. Gen Hosp Psychiatry. 2009;31(1):46–55. doi:10.1016/j.genhosppsych.2008.09.011.
36. Dutch Civil Law, Article 7:458. [cited 2015 Dec 22] Available from http://www.dutchcivillaw.com/civilcodebook077.htm. Accessed 22 Dec 2015.

6

Challenges in supporting lay carers of patients at the end of life: results from focus group discussions with primary healthcare providers

Katja Krug*, René Alexander Ballhausen, Regine Bölter, Peter Engeser, Michel Wensing, Joachim Szecsenyi and Frank Peters-Klimm

Abstract

Background: Family caregivers (FCGs) of patients at the end of life (EoL) cared for at home receive support from professional and non-professional care providers. Healthcare providers in general practice play an important role as they coordinate care and establish contacts between the parties concerned. To identify potential intervention targets, this study deals with the challenges healthcare providers in general practice face in EoL care situations including patients, caregivers and networks.

Methods: Focus group discussions with general practice teams in Germany were conducted to identify barriers to and enablers of an optimal support for family caregivers. Focus group discussions were analysed using content analysis.

Results: Nineteen providers from 11 general practices took part in 4 focus group discussions. Participants identified challenges in communication with patients, caregivers and within the professional network. Communication with patients and caregivers focused on non-verbal messages, communicating at an appropriate time and perceiving patient and caregiver as a unit of care. Practice teams perceive themselves as an important part of the healthcare network, but also report difficulties in communication and cooperation with other healthcare providers.

Conclusion: Healthcare providers in general practice identified relational challenges in daily primary palliative care with potential implications for EoL care. Communication and collaboration with patients, caregivers and among healthcare providers give opportunities for improving palliative care with a focus on the patient-caregiver dyad. It is insufficient to demand a (professional) support network; existing structures need to be recognized and included into the care.

Keywords: Family caregivers, Focus group discussions, Primary care, Healthcare provider in general practice, End-of-life care, Palliative care

* Correspondence: katja.krug@med.uni-heidelberg.de
Department of General Practice and Health Services Research, University Hospital Heidelberg, Im Neuenheimer Feld 130.3, 69120 Heidelberg, Germany

Background

Most patients at the end of life (EoL) are at home and receive out-patient care in Germany. They face the challenge to organise their lives and optimize their quality of life [1]. Decisions on the place of EoL care are influenced by available social support networks (involving lay carers such as family members, friends, and neighbours), preferences of patients, and supply of professional healthcare providers [2]. Patients, whose families are involved in their care as family caregivers and whose families are able to cope with the palliative care situation, are less likely to receive hospital care at the EoL [3] and more likely to die at home [4]. Admission to hospitals during the last days of life [5, 6] are often due to family caregivers feeling overburdened and without adequate professional support [7].

Lay carers are mostly family caregivers, friends and neighbours. Spouses comprise the largest part of those who support and care (28%), followed by daughters (26%) and parents (14%) [8]. These caregivers often devote a large part of their time (on average 37 h per week) to the care of a single patient [8] which leads to social isolation and higher perceived caregiver burden [9]. Caregivers are also prone to physical impairments, i.e. sleep deprivation and weight loss [9]. Caregiving is not only physically demanding, lay carers often develop psychological symptoms, i.e. depression and anxiety [9, 10], they experience stress due to caregiving [11] and may need support themselves. A higher caregiver burden is associated with lower education and living together with the care recipient [9]. Lay carers may receive support from other lay carers as well as professional healthcare providers. Coordination of care across all care givers is regarded a high priority by patients [12].

In Germany, palliative care has been developed as part of the hospice movement, which cumulated in the foundation of the first palliative care unit in 1983 [13]. For outpatients with life-limiting advanced diseases and complex care needs, a national bill on specialized ambulatory palliative care (SAPV, §37b social security statutes book V) was introduced in 2007. Approximately 10% of outpatients were estimated to be in need of SAPV [14]. For palliative outpatients without complex care needs, general practitioners (GPs) are traditionally in the best position to provide palliative care, including EOL care. A specific qualification program for GPs in palliative care or structured palliative care, comparable to the Gold Standards Framework in the United Kingdom [15], does not exist nationwide. There are local initiatives available, i.e. a palliative care initiative in northern Baden (PAMINO [16]). They also provide a platform for networking among general practices.

Networks can be used to share experiences with colleagues, since in Germany, general practices are mainly single-handed with few staff (medical assistants) [17]. Medical assistants take over administrative tasks from physicians and are also increasingly involved in patient care, i.e. disease and care management and home visits [17]. The practice teams should not only take care of the medical problems of patients, but also give social and logistic support. With patients at the EoL, healthcare providers in general practice are confronted with a complex situation involving both patients and caregivers as well as other healthcare providers. This study aims to close the knowledge gap about the challenges healthcare providers in general practice recognize which are posed by patients, lay carers, and professional carers in the care situation at the EoL of a patient and how the providers deal with those challenges.

Methods

The study was part of the PalliPA project (Verbesserung der häuslichen Versorgung von Palliativpatienten durch Unterstützung pflegender Angehöriger – Improvement of palliative care at home by supporting family caregivers) and focused on one aspect of EoL care important throughout the care process: the role of general practice teams in supporting family caregivers of patients at the EoL [18]. The project was framed as an exploratory trial for a subsequent implementation study. Before an intervention was developed, implemented and evaluated, a concurrent observation of the care problem was necessary. A qualitative approach with focus group discussions was used to gather a wide range of ideas and opinions regarding challenges in EoL care situations from healthcare providers in general practice. Interviews allow participants to discuss a given topic from their personal point of view, whereas in focus group discussions participants can discuss among themselves which can result in an additional source of information [19]. The focus group discussions in this study were structured with a questioning guideline covering aspects of good palliative care, identification and support of lay carers (Table 1). The questioning guideline was pilot tested with 2 palliative care physicians before conducting the formal focus group discussions.

To take part in the focus group discussions, healthcare providers in general practice with a special interest in palliative care were approached. This was based on the premise that those practice team members would be more highly motivated to identify and develop a gold standard for palliative care in German general practice than a representative sample. This approach follows purposeful sampling with the aim of a homogeneous sample [20]. The approached recruitment sample consisted of healthcare providers in general practice from the federal state of Baden-Wuerttemberg. It was intended that participants were currently taking care of palliative patients.

Table 1 Questioning guideline (main questions for reported analysis)

What motivated you at first to engage in palliative medicine?
What facilitates or hampers successful palliative care from your point of view?
Thinking of your last palliative care patient:
When did the family caregivers (FCs) get involved?
What was triggering the approach to the FCs?
Who initiates the contact between practice and FCs?
In which situations do you contact FCs directly?
What role does the staff actually play regarding the contact to the FCs?
How do you know if FCs are burdened?
What do you as a practice team do to support FCs?
What offers of assistance do you give?
How do FCs react to offers of assistance?
Can you remember a situation where FCs were especially reluctant or demanding? How did you react?
Do you talk about the possibility to admit the patient to a hospital? In which situations?
What has to change to enable your practice to better support FCs?
What kind of support would you like to have?

Contact information for potential participants was sourced from the publicly available register of the Association of Statutory Health Insurance Physicians (Kassenärztliche Vereinigung) Baden-Wuerttemberg. All general practitioners with an additional qualification in palliative medicine were identified and invited to participate in the study. Invitations were mailed to 258 general practices with 275 general practitioners.

Four 90-min focus group discussions were part of 2 recruitment meetings where the study was introduced and some background information on lay carers provided (i.e. facts on how many people take care of a family member underlining the importance of the topic). For the purpose of getting a multi-faceted picture, focus group discussions were mixed (general practitioners (GPs) and medical assistants), but GP and assistants from one practice did not attend the same focus group discussion. The focus group discussions were moderated by one of 3 members of the research team, who all had extensive experience in conducting focus group discussions and had also been involved in developing the questioning guideline (2 medical doctors (PE, FPK) experienced in qualitative research, 1 social scientist (KK)); the moderating medical doctors were also working as GPs and had an additional qualification in palliative medicine. The focus group discussions took place in the Department of General Practice and Health Services Research; GPs interested in the study but not able to attend the focus group discussions were asked to take part in a telephone interview covering the same aspects as the focus group discussions. Before conducting focus group discussions and interviews, all participants provided written informed consent to participating in, audio-recording and analysis of the focus group discussions.

The structured focus group discussions and interviews were audio-recorded and transcribed verbatim. Transcripts were analysed with content analysis [21] using ATLAS.ti. Two researchers (RAB, KK) reviewed and coded the transcripts independently. First, codes were derived deductively on the basis of the questioning guideline (Table 1); additional topics were derived inductively from the transcripts. During the iterative coding process, the codes were regularly compared, discussed and adapted for further use in the analysis. Finally, consensus was reached with a third researcher (FPK). The whole research team discussed and interpreted the results. While the analysis was performed on the original German data, quotes are translated into English for reporting in this paper.

Results

Thirty-five practices responded to the invitation (14%), of which 22 declined participation. The most common reason given for not taking part was lack of time. Four focus group discussions were conducted with 19 participants from 11 practices (12 GPs, 7 medical assistants), two additional telephone interviews with GPs who were not able to participate in the focus group discussions. Participant characteristics are given in Table 2. Data saturation was reached after 3 focus group discussions; no new topics emerged in the last focus group discussion and in the telephone interviews.

In the perspective of the participants from general practices, 3 main categories with 8 subcategories emerged: challenges with the patients, challenges with the caregivers, and challenges within the professional network. An overview is given in Fig. 1.

Challenges with patients

The majority of the participants faced challenges in dealing with patients, especially when they encountered resistance or reactions they did not anticipate: (1) they needed to recognize and accept non-verbal forms of the patient's volition, (2) they needed to communicate according to the situation, and (3) they needed to realize their own attitudes regarding an "appropriate" death.

(1) Healthcare providers recognized patients who were not able to communicate verbally as a group where palliative care has to be accomplished in the best interest of the patient. Participants particularly stressed the point of interpreting patient's behaviour:

> *With dementia patients [...] if someone does not eat or drink anymore, that's also a form of volition. Then I*

Table 2 Description of participants

	Abbreviation	Details	Professional experience[a]
Focus group discussion 1	S1	practice of GP3	additional palliative care certificate since 2 years
	S2	practice of GP4	
	S3	practice of GP4	since 10 years in the practice
	GP1	with S5	since 22 years in the practice, qualification in palliative medicine since 1 year
	GP2	with S4	since 26 years in the practice, qualification in palliative medicine since 5 years, SAPV
Focus group discussion 2	S4	practice of GP2	since 9 years in the practice, additional palliative care certificate
	S5	practice of GP1	
	GP3	with S1	since 24 years in the practice, qualification in palliative medicine since 1 year
	GP4	with S2 and S3	general practitioner since 10 years, since 6 years in the practice
	GP5		since 27 years in the practice
Focus group discussion 3	GP6	with S7	since 13 years in the practice, qualification in palliative medicine since 7 years
	GP7	with S6	since 12 years in the practice, qualification in palliative medicine since 3 years, SAPV
	GP8		since 1 year in practice after neurosurgery for 14 years and general practice for 4 years
	GP9	same practice as GP11	qualification in palliative medicine since 2 years
Focus group discussion 4	S6	practice of GP7	since 1 year in the practice after completing training in another practice
	S7	practice of GP6	since 5 years in the practice after working in hospital
	GP10		since 10 years in the practice, qualification in palliative medicine since 5 years, care of palliative patients for at least 20 years
	GP11	same practice as GP9	qualification in palliative medicine since 3 years
	GP12		since at least 20 years in the practice, qualification in palliative medicine since 1 year
Telephone interview 1	GP13		
Telephone interview 2	GP14		since 3 years in the practice after geriatrics

[a]as deductible from focus group discussions and interviews, *S* Staff, *GP* General practitioner, *SAPV* Member of a specialized ambulatory palliative care team (Spezialisierte Ambulante Palliativversorgung)

would absolutely refrain from any infusion or PEG (percutaneous endoscopic gastrostomy tube) or subcutaneous or else. (GP3).

(2) Most of the practice team members acknowledged the need to prepare patients for the time to come and to organize support on time, but they also experienced patients declining help if they did not perceive it as urgent:

I sometimes notice that if you want to organise things ahead [...] but the patient is reasonably well, they decline. (GP6).

(3) The majority of participants did not explicitly formulate their attitudes towards an "appropriate" death, but described how their own opinion influenced care decisions:

For 2 years, I had an old lady, where I asked the relatives to get her into a nursing home, since the couple at home were both heavy alcoholics. And I thought it would be actually awful for this old lady if she had to die at home. (GP12).

Challenges with lay carers

In their contact with caregivers, participants reported a wide range of relations to caregivers: (1) not knowing the relatives of a patient, not knowing if a patient is also a caregiver, but also having a long and close relationship to the caregiver. Healthcare providers were also (2) challenged by either demanding or refusing family caregivers and found individual ways to cope in such situations.

(1) In Germany, there is no obligation to register with a GP (practice). Patients may freely choose their GP. Unless GPs document explicitly the social case history or patients report for themselves, GPs and their practice teams do not necessarily know if a patient has lay carers or is a caregiver to a family member themselves. If more than just one family member are patients in the practice, the social structures of the patients were better known to the healthcare providers:

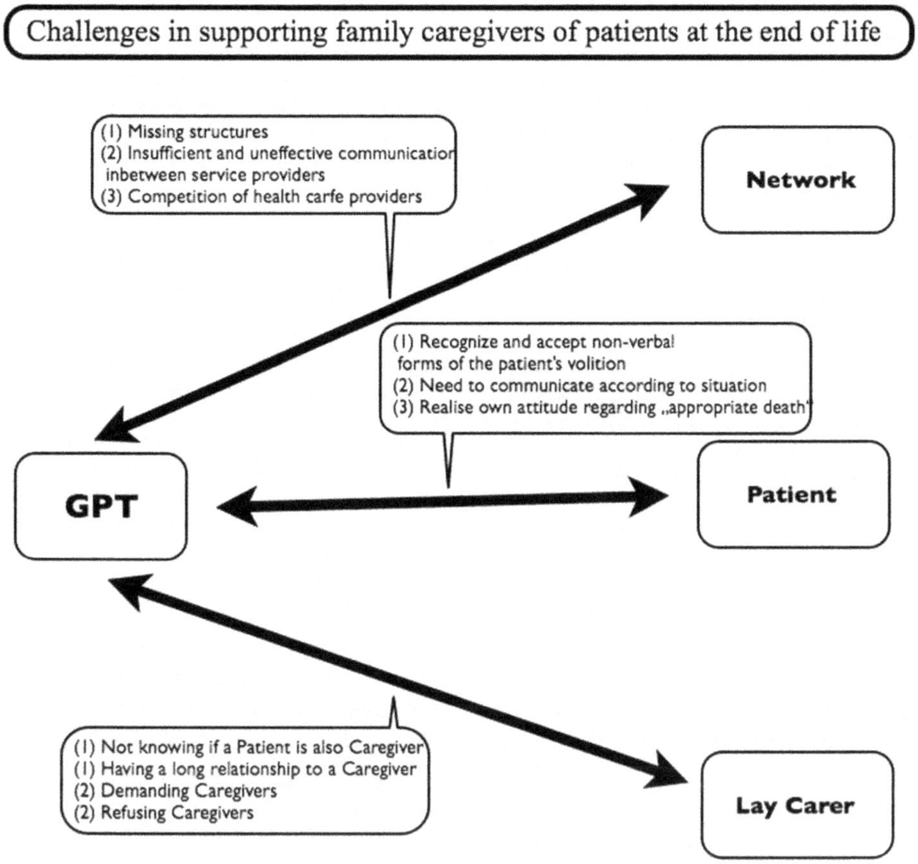

Fig. 1 Overview of challenges reported by members of general practice teams (GPT)

We definitely have people, where we don't know what's happening at home. (GP7).

Usually, they are patients we've known for years. We've known them since we've had the practice. And then we know the family structure, too. (GP9).

(2) Demands of family caregivers focused either on the care for the patient or on the caregivers themselves. For healthcare providers in general practice the request for support often came too late or was considered inappropriate:

Of course it happens that the relatives come in a state of absolute exhaustion and then dump everything on the table and say: Now it doesn't work anymore. And now you (the doctor) best do something immediately. (GP4).

Participants also described family caregivers, who were not responsible enough or taking sufficient action themselves from a practice' point of view:

Caregivers, who expect, that others ..., that [...] everything will be done, and who need to be nudged to become active by themselves. (GP14).

In some cases, demands of caregivers on patients were also brought up, especially when it came to decisions about further therapies closer to the EoL:

It goes both ways. There are relatives, who [struggle to accept the patient does not] want any therapy anymore, and then try to really convince the patient to do otherwise. (GP6).

Participants reported that caregivers (and patients) refused support sometimes rigorously, especially if they had the feeling of being able to cope:

A nursing home was not an option for them both. They didn't want to. The doctor advised to go to a nursing home. No. (S5).

Healthcare providers in general practice tried to give support at an early stage and to emphasize the caregiver's health. They also offered help for care aspects that were easier to accept for the family caregivers:

If you offer something in this (early) stage, it will be mostly rejected. [They say:] "No, I don't need that yet or it is okay or I can do it." [...] would be ideal, to get there at the right time. (GP4).

The participants perceived family caregivers as important supporters in the care of the patients. As such, they saw the necessity of treating patients and caregivers as a unit, with the caregivers' health influencing the trajectory of the patient's disease:

I try to address diplomatically that they are the most important persons and that their health is enormously important for the patient. Even if the caregiver is not one of my patients, it is the interest of the patient to have a healthy caregiver in all respects. Mentally, and physically. (...) That the quality of the care deteriorates if the exhaustion gets too much. (GP4).

Challenges within the professional network

To provide high-quality palliative care, healthcare providers in general practice need to work together with local professional support. They are involved in a multidisciplinary network which facilitates cooperation and involves nursing services, physiotherapy, spiritual care, volunteers and others.

At the same time, practice team members are faced with challenges within the network: (1) structures are missing, (2) the communication between cooperating partners does not involve all relevant information, and (3) partners who should cooperate in patient care are also competitors on the healthcare market.

(1) Although there is a widespread professional network, not all services are locally available. Especially inpatient structures are missing in some areas:

We don't have a hospice, we don't have a palliative care unit. (GP12).

(2) Relevant information is not shared between service providers on the interface of healthcare facilities; it is not given timely and unstated reasons for omission lead to unrequested interventions:

This gap between hospital and practice. Discharge on Friday afternoon, should get antibiotics and analgesics etc. I see the fax message maybe Saturday morning or Monday morning. (GP5).

An 88-year-old was discharged. I just had her admitted for transfusion, because she was anaemic again and again, and I almost knew there had to be a malignancy behind that. So I had her specifically admitted only for transfusion, and still they did a colonoscopy or tried to do it. Stenosing colorectal carcinoma, and now the clinic offered her an operation. (GP7).

(3) A big challenge perceived by some practice team members was the building of a cooperating network where the potential partners are also competitors for patient care:

The building of the team was difficult, since the nursing services are firstly competitors and sometimes quarrelling among themselves. But since we physicians took the initiative (...), we brought them all together using really a lot of diplomacy and tact. And so all of a sudden, the structure, the nursing services among themselves, has changed. (GP7).

Discussion

Healthcare providers in general practice are faced with a multitude of challenges in EoL care in communicating with patients, lay carers and other professional healthcare providers. From their point of view, practice team members have to deal with an appropriate communication with patients, interpreting patients' non-verbal messages and reacting accordingly. They need to identify lay carers and to find ways to deal with inappropriate demands and unnecessary refusals of support. They perceive themselves as an important part of the healthcare network, but also report difficulties in communication and cooperation with other healthcare providers.

To recognize the appropriate time to communicate with patients and to perceive patients' behaviour as a non-verbal expression of their wishes are essential communication skills in general practice. In EoL care, not only communication with patients but also with caregivers and within the professional network is of paramount importance. General practice teams need to be aware of the high potential of challenging situations as described in our study.

A systematic review showed that direct support of caregivers can reduce their psychological distress [22]. The interventions described comprise home visits by nurses of up to 1.5 h which are not feasible for German general practices. The topics important for family caregivers [23], on the other hand, are addressed in general practice, i.e. caregivers learn about symptom management, their health needs are discussed and they receive support provided by social networks and health services providers [24]. The results of the present study additionally stress the importance of communication with patients, caregivers and other health care providers to bring offers and demands of support together.

Another systematic review [25] summarized facilitators for a good patient-physician communication: the availability of the GP and the initiation of EoL issue discussions. Our participants additionally stressed the point of finding the right moment to initiate discussions with patients and caregivers to lead to effective results. Thus, communicating with and supporting the patient-caregiver *dyad* needs to be individually targeted [26]. Additionally, it underscores the importance of integrating early palliative care also in the primary care of diseases other than cancer [27].

Contrary to the situation in several other countries, such as the UK, general practices in Germany are not contractually required to identify (family) caregivers [28]. Still, the challenges for identification are comparable: family caregivers perceive themselves as relatives in the first place before considering themselves as carers [28]. As our participants reported, family caregivers have to be made aware of their need for support, even though they might refuse it. The healthcare providers perceived patients and caregivers as a unit of care and caregivers as potential "hidden patients" [29] and tried to support them to prevent caregiver collapse.

The perception of patients at the EoL and their caregivers leads to reflections on professional attitude which emerge not only in communication but also in the expression of practice team members' personal values and the evaluation of cooperation within the professional network.

While working with palliative patients and their family caregivers, healthcare providers in general practice are faced with their own assumptions of a "good" death, which goes further than the biomedical and psychosocial perspective [30] and might not concur with the views of patients and caregivers [31]. In our study, this topic was not explicitly addressed and thus, is not within the scope of this paper. In addition, to further analyse implicit assumptions of healthcare providers, another methodological approach would be needed.

The communication and cooperation with other healthcare providers needs to be optimized. The statements of the participants demonstrate that the communication has to be improved in both ways: from the practice to other service providers as well as from other service providers to the practice. All partners have to clarify their role and their expectations. This might also strengthen the communication with caregivers, who reported both unmet psychosocial needs and poor coordination of health-care services in a systematic review [32].

The results of our study show challenges of German healthcare providers in general practice, which were considered challenges in other European countries as well. In the UK, the Gold Standards Framework [33] addresses those topics and gives practice teams a guideline to deal with i.e. communication, coordination, and carer support. The assessment of burden in family caregivers poses a major challenge for general practitioners. Approaches for assessment have been described by Adelman et al. in a review [9], but to date in Germany no formal assessment strategies have been implemented. However, recent initiatives in the form of "burden relief programs for family caregivers", e.g. by the national elderly care insurance fund, have been introduced [34]. Nevertheless, awareness of such initiatives among general practitioners needs to be raised. Promotional information could be shared through GP networks. Recent evidence indicates German GPs actively utilize the German palliative care guidelines [35]. Information on burden relief programs for family caregivers could be included in this resource. Certainly there is room for improvement of palliative care in German primary care to be further improved on policymaking, practical and educational level [36]. Furthermore, our results are in agreement with other studies dealing with organizational challenges [37], the importance of communication and continuity in patient care as well as to the family caregivers [38, 39].

Strengths and weaknesses of the study

This study is part and the first step of a project to design and develop an intervention that may be implemented and evaluated in primary care to support lay carers. Focus group discussions were conducted with healthcare providers from general practices who were potential participants in the project [18]. They aimed at identifying facilitators and barriers of optimal palliative care in general practice, particularly on supporting lay caregivers. As a result of the focus group discussions, interventions were developed together with participants in the further project process [18].

The results are based on focus group discussions with a highly selective sample. We purposefully included primary healthcare providers with a special interest in palliative care. Thus, the participants were probably more familiar with the situation of family caregivers of patients at the EoL and could share the strategies they had developed to deal with the specific challenges occurring in such complex situations. We did not countercheck the impressions of the participating healthcare providers with the views of patients, lay carers, and other professional caregivers. Therefore, their views remain highly subjective and might be due to individual perceptions. In spite of this subjectivity, the topics were generally taken up by the participants of the focus group discussions. Reported experiences of general practice teams from our study are in part addressed in findings of studies examining the patient/caregiver end of the EoL care continuum. In particular, communication difficulties with general practitioners, inconsistencies and discontinuity of care have been reported [40].

Although it is a sample of health care providers, participants could vividly report on the challenges they are faced with in palliative care. However, due to the mixture of GPs and medical assistants in the focus group discussions, statements might be influenced by a possible social status gradient. We sought to minimize this potential bias by assigning members of the same practice team to different focus group discussions that took place in parallel. Additionally, the experienced moderators were conscious to invite reticent participants to share their thoughts and opinions. Nonetheless, there could be other challenges participants were not aware of and therefore did not report. Still, it could be assumed that the challenge for healthcare providers in general practice teams without a special interest in palliative care is even greater.

Conclusion

Healthcare providers in general practice identified many relational challenges in daily primary palliative care. Based on our findings, strategies to resolve these may concern the dimensions knowledge, professional attitude and skills which could be further supported and developed as part mixed interventions with educational and organisational elements. Our results indicate that it is insufficient to demand a support network; existing structures need to be recognized and included into the care in general practices. At the same time, motivations contrary to collaborative care due to a competitive healthcare market need to be considered. Additionally, healthcare providers in general practice should assess the relationship between patients and caregivers as a significant reason for accepting or denying support.

Abbreviations

EoL: End of life; FCGs: Family caregivers; GPs: General practitioners; PalliPA: Project Verbesserung der häuslichen Versorgung von Palliativpatienten durch Unterstützung pflegender Angehöriger (Improvement of palliative care at home by supporting family caregivers); PAMINO: Palliativmedizinische Initiative Nordbaden (palliative care initiative in northern Baden); PEG: Percutaneous endoscopic gastrostomy tube; SAPV: Spezialisierte ambulante Palliativversorgung (specialized ambulatory palliative care)

Acknowledgments

We sincerely thank Sarah Jane Berger (Dept. of General Practice and Health Services Research, University Hospital Heidelberg) for language editing.

Funding

The study was supported by the German Ministry for Education and Research (Bundesministerium für Bildung und Forschung, BMBF, Grant Number 01GX1046).

Authors' contributions

KK, RB, PE, JS, and FPK conceived and designed the study. KK, RAB, RB, PE, and FPK acquired the data. KK, RAB, and FPK analysed the data. RB, PE, JS, and MW additionally contributed to the interpretation of the data. KK and RAB drafted the manuscript. All authors revised the manuscript for important intellectual content and gave final approval of the version to be published.

Consent for publication

Not applicable.

Competing interests

The authors declare that they have no competing interests.

References

1. Gomes B, Higginson IJ. Factors influencing death at home in terminally ill patients with cancer: systematic review. BMJ. 2006;332(7540):515–21.
2. Murray MA, Fiset V, Young S, Kryworuchko J. Where the dying live: a systematic review of determinants of place of end-of-life cancer care. Oncol Nurs Forum. 2009;36(1):69–77.
3. Gott M, Frey R, Robinson J, Boyd M, O'Callaghan A, Richards N, Snow B. The nature of, and reasons for, 'inappropriate' hospitalisations among patients with palliative care needs: a qualitative exploration of the views of generalist palliative care providers. Palliat Med. 2013;27(8):747–56.
4. Kern M, Wessel H, Ostgathe E. Ambulante Palliativbetreuung - Einflussfaktoren auf eine stationäre Einweisung am Lebensende. Z Palliativmed. 2007;8(4):155–61.
5. Jordhoy MS, Fayers P, Saltnes T, Ahlner-Elmqvist M, Jannert M, Kaasa S. A palliative-care intervention and death at home: a cluster randomised trial. Lancet. 2000;356(9233):888–93.
6. Howat A, Veitch C, Cairns W. A retrospective review of place of death of palliative care patients in regional North Queensland. Palliat Med. 2007;21(1):41–7.
7. Tiernan E, O'Connor M, O'Siorain L, Kearney M. A prospective study of preferred versus actual place of death among patients referred to a palliative care home-care service. Ir Med J. 2002;95(8):232–5.
8. Döhner H, Kofahl C, Lüdecke D, Mnich E. The National Survey Report for Germany. In: EUROFAMCARE Services for Supporting Family Carers of Older Dependent People in Europe: Characteristics, Coverage and Usage; 2007.
9. Adelman RD, Tmanova LL, Delgado D, Dion S, Lachs MS. Caregiver burden: a clinical review. JAMA. 2014;311(10):1052–60.
10. Lavela SL, Ather N. Psychological health in older adult spousal caregivers of older adults. Chronic Illn. 2010;6(1):67–80.
11. Lund L, Ross L, Petersen MA, Groenvold M. Cancer caregiving tasks and consequences and their associations with caregiver status and the caregiver's relationship to the patient: a survey. BMC Cancer. 2014;14:541.
12. Han PK, Rayson D. The coordination of primary and oncology specialty care at the end of life. J Natl Cancer Inst Monogr. 2010;2010(40):31–7.
13. Cremer-Schaeffer P, Radbruch L. Palliative care in the light of legal and regulatory requirements in Germany. Bundesgesundheitsblatt Gesundheitsforschung Gesundheitsschutz. 2012;55(2):231–7.
14. Voltz R. Palliativmedizin: Eine Disziplin für den "ganzen Menschen". Dtsch Arztebl. 2008;105(1–2):A 20–2.
15. King N, Thomas K, Martin N, Bell D, Farrell S. Now nobody falls through the net': practitioners' perspectives on the gold standards framework for community palliative care. Palliat Med. 2005;19(8):619–27.
16. Engeser P, Reininghaus W, Zeise-Suess D, Wiesemann A. Palliativmedizin in Nordbaden (PAMINO-Projekt) Welche Einstellungen haben nordbadische Hausärzte zur Palliativmedizin. Z Allg Med. 2003;79:22.
17. Freund T, Everett C, Griffiths P, Hudon C, Naccarella L, Laurant M. Skill mix, roles and remuneration in the primary care workforce: who are the healthcare professionals in the primary care teams across the world? Int J Nurs Stud. 2015;52(3):727–43.
18. Hermann K, Boelter R, Engeser P, Szecsenyi J, Campbell SM, Peters-Klimm F. PalliPA: how can general practices support caregivers of patients at their end of life in a home-care setting? A study protocol. BMC Res Notes. 2012;5:233.
19. Powell RA, Single HM. Focus groups. International journal for quality in health care : journal of the International Society for Quality in Health Care / ISQua. 1996;8(5):499–504.
20. Palinkas LA, Horwitz SM, Green CA, Wisdom JP, Duan N, Hoagwood K. Purposeful sampling for qualitative data collection and analysis in mixed method implementation research. Admin Pol Ment Health. 2015;42(5):533–44.
21. Mayring P. Qualitative Inhaltsanalyse. In: Flick U, Ev K, Reinbek SI, editors. *Qualitative Forschung Ein Handbuch*. 5th ed. Reinbek: Rowohlt Taschenbuch; 2007.
22. Candy B, Jones L, Drake R, Leurent B, King M. Interventions for supporting informal caregivers of patients in the terminal phase of a disease. Cochrane Database Syst Rev. 2011;(6):CD007617.

23. Grande GE, Farquhar MC, Barclay SI, Todd CJ. Valued aspects of primary palliative care: content analysis of bereaved carers' descriptions. The British journal of general practice : the journal of the Royal College of General Practitioners. 2004;54(507):772–8.
24. Krug K, Bölter R, Ballhausen RA, Engeser P, Peters-Klimm F. Burden experienced by family caregivers of patients at the end of life: what do general practice teams offer? Gesundheitswesen (Bundesverband der Ärzte des Öffentlichen Gesundheitsdienstes (Germany)). 2016;78(S 01):e128–34.
25. Slort W, Schweitzer BP, Blankenstein AH, Abarshi EA, Riphagen II, Echteld MA, Aaronson NK, van der Horst H, Deliens L. Perceived barriers and facilitators for general practitioner-patient communication in palliative care: a systematic review. Palliat Med. 2011;25(6):613–29.
26. Guerriere D, Husain A, Zagorski B, Marshall D, Seow H, Brazil K, Kennedy J, Burns S, Brooks H, Coyte PC. Predictors of caregiver burden across the home-based palliative care trajectory in Ontario, Canada. Health Soc Care Community. 2016;24(4):428–38.
27. Thoonsen B, Vissers K, Verhagen S, Prins J, Bor H, van Weel C, Groot M, Engels Y. Training general practitioners in early identification and anticipatory palliative care planning: a randomized controlled trial. BMC Fam Pract. 2015;16(1):126.
28. Carduff E, Finucane A, Kendall M, Jarvis A, Harrison N, Greenacre J, Murray SA. Understanding the barriers to identifying carers of people with advanced illness in primary care: triangulating three data sources. BMC Fam Pract. 2014;15:48.
29. Kristjanson LJ, Aoun S. Palliative care for families: remembering the hidden patients. Can J Psychiatry. 2004;49(6):359–65.
30. Steinhauser KE, Clipp EC, McNeilly M, Christakis NA, McIntyre LM, Tulsky JA. In search of a good death: observations of patients, families, and providers. Ann Intern Med. 2000;132(10):825–32.
31. Escobar Pinzon LC, Claus M, Zepf KI, Letzel S, Fischbeck S, Weber M. Preference for place of death in Germany. J Palliat Med. 2011;14(10):1097–103.
32. Ventura AD, Burney S, Brooker J, Fletcher J, Ricciardelli L. Home-based palliative care: a systematic literature review of the self-reported unmet needs of patients and carers. Palliat Med. 2014;28(5):391–402.
33. Thomas K. Caring for the dying at home. Oxford: Radcliffe Publishing; 2003.
34. Hetzel C, Baumann R, Diekmann J, Frobose I. Description of a multidimensional health program for informal caregivers. Gesundheitswesen (Bundesverband der Arzte des Offentlichen Gesundheitsdienstes (Germany)). 2016;2018;80:S51-S6.
35. Schubert I, Heymans L, Fessler J. General practitioners' guideline for palliative care. A survey of guideline acceptance in quality circles of primary medical care. Medizinische Klinik (Munich, Germany : 1983). 2010;105(3):135–41.
36. Behmann M, Junger S, Radbruch L, Schneider N. Public health actions to improve palliative care in Germany: results of a three-round Delphi study. Health Policy. 2012;106(3):303–12.
37. Neergaard MA, Olesen F, Jensen AB, Sondergaard J. Shared care in basic level palliative home care: organizational and interpersonal challenges. J Palliat Med. 2010;13(9):1071–7.
38. Baile WF, Palmer JL, Bruera E, Parker PA. Assessment of palliative care cancer patients' most important concerns. Support Care Cancer. 2011;19(4):475–81.
39. Michiels E, Deschepper R, Van Der Kelen G, Bernheim JL, Mortier F, Vander Stichele R, Deliens L. The role of general practitioners in continuity of care at the end of life: a qualitative study of terminally ill patients and their next of kin. Palliat Med. 2007;21(5):409–15.
40. Krishnasamy M, Wells M, Wilkie E. Patients and carer experiences of care provision after a diagnosis of lung cancer in Scotland. Support Care Cancer. 2007;15(3):327–32.

7

Falls and long-term care: a report from the care by design observational cohort study

Emily J. Cameron[1], Susan K. Bowles[2,4], Emily Gard Marshall[3] and Melissa K. Andrew[4*]

Abstract

Background: Falls and the resulting complications are common among frail older adults. We aimed to explore risk factors and potential prevention strategies for falls in elderly residents of Long-Term Care Facilities (LTCF).

Methods: This was a cross sectional study design using data from the Care by Design (CBD) study, within Nova Scotia's Capital District Health Authority. This observational time series cohort study collected data before, during and after the implementation of CBD, a new model of coordinated primary care in LTCF. Here, we analyzed data collected after the implementation of CBD (September 1, 2011- February 28, 2012).

Results: Falls were frequent; 56.2% of our sample of 395 residents fell at least once. In univariate analyses, male gender ($p = 0.009$), dementia ($p = 0.005$), and use of Selective Serotonin Reuptake Inhibitors or Selective Serotonin-Norepinepherine Reuptake Inhibitors (SSRI/SNRI) ($p = 0.084$) showed statistically significant associations with having fallen. Benzodiazepine use appeared to be protective for falls ($p = 0.058$). In a fully adjusted multivariable linear regression model, dementia (β coefficient 0.96, 95% CI: 0.83,1.84; $p = 0.032$), visual impairment (β 0.84, 95% CI: 0. 13,1.56; $p = 0.021$), and use of any PIMs (β 0.34, 95% CI: 0.037,0.65; $p = 0.028$) were associated with increased risk of having fallen. Benzodiazepine use remained associated with reduced numbers of falls ($p = 0.009$), and SSRI/SNRI use was associated with increased numbers of falls ($p = 0.007$). Male gender was associated with increased falls in the model which excluded frailty ($p = 0.022$), though gender lost statistical significance once frailty was added to the model ($p = 0.06$).

Conclusions: In our sample of LTCF residents, falls were common. Cognitive impairment, male gender, visual impairment, PIM use and use of SSRI/SNRI medications were associated with increased risk of falls, while benzodiazepine use appeared to be associated with a decreased risk of having fallen. Falls remain an important problem among LTC residents. Screening for falls during patient encounters is recommended, along with further research to identify risk factors and target interventions.

Keywords: Falls, Long-term care, Nursing homes, Polypharmacy, Potentially inappropriate medication, Frail elderly, Primary health care

Background

Falls and the resulting complications among the elderly population are a common problem. Among older adults in Canada, ≥ 65 years old, 30% of those living in the community and 50% of residents living in care facilities will fall each year. The complications of falls may/have been found to lead to pain, functional impairment, disability and death in this population [1–3]. Due to the predicted increase in the proportion of elderly people in the population and known complications of falls in this population, it is important to assess the risk factors associated with falls. In assessing individual risk factors, it is important to screen for previous history of falls. One out of three older people fall each year, but less than half of those who fall actually tell their doctor [4]. Falling once doubles one's chances of falling again, and it also increases the patient's fear of falling [4, 5].

Prescribed medications have been shown to be an important contributor to falls. Medications such as benzodiazepines, neuroleptics, sedatives, and anti-hypertensive

* Correspondence: mandrew@dal.ca
[4]Department of Medicine (Geriatrics), Dalhousie University, Halifax, NS, Canada

drugs are some of the medications that are known to be associated with increased falls in elderly people [6]. As individuals age they may encounter more co-morbid conditions and higher numbers of medications than younger individuals (reference needed for increased comorbidity and meds). Hence, medications are one of the most important potentially modifiable risk factors for falls among the elderly. Nevertheless, data on the association between falls risk and number of medications taken by Long Term Care facility (LTCF) residents is limited.

Falls in older adults are not only due to extrinsic risk factors such as medications, but also due to intrinsic factors such as cognitive impairment, frailty, gender and age. Cognitive impairment and dementia are known to be associated with increased risk of falls; little is known about other intrinsic risk factors such as gender [7]. Frailty may also be a relevant predictor of falls; it is likely that as people become more frail their poor mobility may predispose to falls, though after a certain point they may have a lower risk of falls if they cease mobilizing [8]. The purpose of this study was to assess and quantify the risk factors associated with falls among older residents of LTCF in Nova Scotia, Canada.

Methods

Study design

This was a cross-sectional study using data from the Care by Design (CBD) study, within the Central Zone of the Nova Scotia Health Authority. CBD is a new model of coordinated primary care in LTCF that was implemented in 2009. Prior to CBD model, residents entering LTCF often kept their prior family physician or were responsible for finding a new one. As a result, residents of a single LTCF unit could have been cared for by several different physicians, leading to challenges in team cohesiveness and continuity of care, and lack of coordinated after hours coverage [9]. Key features of CBD included coordinated family physician coverage with a single family physician caring for all residents of a given LTCF floor or unit, regularly scheduled physician visits to the LTCF half a day per week to see residents who require care, clear 24/7 on call coverage, systematic Comprehensive Geriatric Assessment (CGA), and structured medication reviews. The CBD study was an observational time series cohort study which examined changes in healthcare and outcomes for LTCF residents as the new model of coordinated primary care was introduced. The CBD study thus collected data before and after the implementation of CBD. Data were collected from LTCF and, when a resident had an Emergency Health Services 911 call, from the EHS database and acute care Emergency department/hospital chart. For the purpose of our study, data collected during the post-CBD time period (September 1, 2011- February 28, 2012) were used [9]. We selected this time period as it occurred after the implementation of a Long-Term Care Comprehensive Geriatric Assessment tool (LTC – CGA), which provided rich information (e.g., more complete list of diagnoses and functional status) about residents' health (Additional file 1: Appendix) [10].

Sample

The sample comprised 395 LTCF residents. This included all of the residents who had an Emergency Health Services (EHS) 911 ambulance call, as well as a random sample of residents without an ambulance call because the overall CBD study had been designed to investigate the impact of the CBD model of care on Emergency Department transfers [11].

Measures

The number of falls was determined by chart review during a six-month timeframe. For the purposes of analyses using categorical variables, and to distinguish between non-fallers, infrequent fallers, and frequent fallers, falls were categorized as follows: no falls reported (N = 171), 1 fall (N = 106), 2-4 falls (N = 79), 5+ falls (N = 34). In regression analyses, the number of falls was treated as a continuous variable. Cognition was measured using both the Mini Mental State Examination (MMSE) score and the clinical diagnosis of dementia, which were both recorded on the LTC-CGA [12]. The LTC-CGA is completed by family physicians every 6 months and after any significant change in health status [10]. Medications were identified from most up to date medication list in the chart, and the research nurse data abstractors used clinical judgment to determine what medications the resident was currently prescribed. Polypharmacy was measured using drug counts and Potentially Inappropriate Medications (PIMs) were identified using the Beers list [13]. Frailty was measured by a clinical frailty scale adapted for use in LTC. Mildly frail individuals have limited dependence on others for instrumental activities of daily living. Moderately frail individuals are those who need help with both instrumental and non-instrumental activities. Severely frail people are completely dependent on other for the activities of daily living. Very severely frail people are completely dependent and are approaching the end of life. Terminally ill individuals have a life expectancy of less than 6 months, who are not otherwise evidently frail [14, 15]. Other risk factors for falls, such as visual impairment, patient transfer and mobility information was also abstracted from the LTC-CGA and/or chart notes [10, 14].

Analysis

Descriptive statistics included measures of central tendency means and Standard Deviation (SD) for normally distributed variables and medians with Inter Quartile

Rage (IQR) where distributions were skewed. Chi Square tests were used for comparison of categorical variables. Linear regression analyses were adjusted for relevant confounders (those with a priori importance such as age, sex, frailty, drug counts) and those drug classes with associations stronger than $p < 0.2$ in univariate analyses. Statistical analyses were done using Stata 8 and SPSS software packages.

Ethics

The study was approved by the Capital District Health Authority Research Ethics Committee and individual Research Ethics boards of participating LTCF, where these existed.

Results

Demographic information of the study participants is shown in Table 1. Residents were older (median age = 85 years) and predominantly female. Of the 285 individuals where sufficient data was collected to estimate frailty, approximately half (52%) were severely or very severely frail.

Of the 395 residents included in the analysis, 390 residents had falls data. The distribution of falls is shown in Fig. 1.

Table 1 Resident characteristics

Resident Characteristics	*N* = 395
Age (years)	Median (IQR)
Median age of residents	85 (77 – 90)
Sex	% (N)
% Female	68.1 (269)
Martial Status	% (N)
Married	16.7 (66)
Single	11.9 (47)
Divorced	8.6 (34)
Widowed	38.5 (152)
Unknown	24.3 (96)
Vision	% (N)
Impaired	39.1 (108)
Frailty	% (N)
Mild	7.6 (30)
Moderate	27.1 (107)
Severe	32.7 (129)
Very Severe	4.1 (16)
Terminally ill	0.8 (3)
Missing data	27.8 (110)
Cognition	%(N)
Dementia	64.1 (253)

Univariate analyses

Table 2 shows the results of univariate analysis. Male gender was a significant predictor of falls ($p = 0.009$). Further analysis of gender and falls category showed a greater percentage of men fell more often. Among the men in the study, 14.5% were reported to have fallen five or more times compared to 6.1% of women ($p = 0.04$).

There were more overall falls in residents with dementia than those without (63.35% vs. 41.84%); this difference was statistically significant ($\beta=0.85, p = 0.005$). For example, a group of 10 residents with dementia would experience 8 falls more than a group of 10 residents without dementia. Looking at the highest rate of falls, 10.8% of residents with dementia fell 5 or more times, compared with 6.1% of residents without dementia ($p = 0.001$).

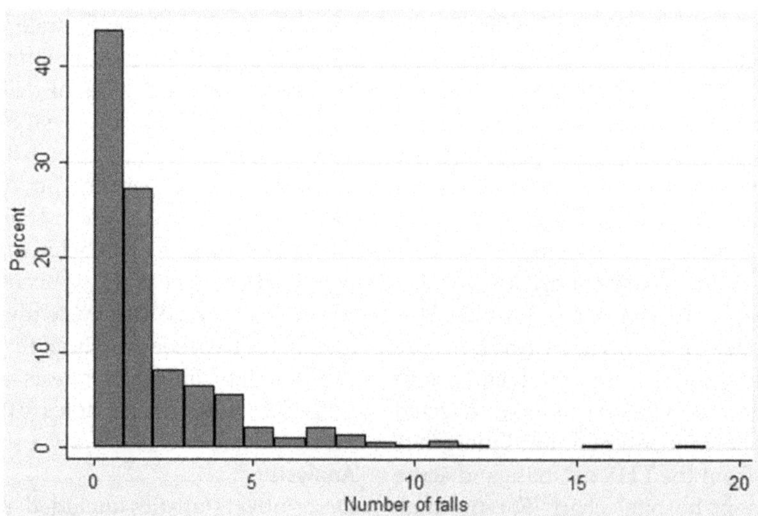

Fig. 1 Total number of Falls Reported per Resident

Table 2 Associations of individual variables with falls (univariate analyses)

Factor	β value (95% CI)	*P* value
Male Gender	−0.69 (−1.20, −0.17)	0.009
Dementia	0.85 (0.26, −1.43)	0.005
Increased Frailty	−0.16 (− 0.54- 0.21)	0.39
Benzodiazepines	−0.47 (− 0.96, 0.17)	0.058
SSRI	0.43 (−0.58, 0.91)	0.084

The number of residents taking each individual class of medication as well as the relationship between fall categories and medication by class is shown in Table 3. There was a trend towards residents taking benzodiazepines having fewer falls compared to those not taking benzodiazepines (p = 0.058), and use of SSRIs was associated with increased risk of falls (p = 0.084).

Further analysis was done to explore why benzodiazepine appeared to be protective for falls, particularly in relation to End of Life and mobility status. 54% of residents who were classified as end of life were on benzodiazepines, which equated to 26.8% of all benzodiazepine users being at end of life (p = 0.009). 47.5% of those taking benzodiazepines had independent transfers, while 32.8% were completely dependent for transfers (p = 0.036). 57.9% of residents on benzodiazepines were walking independently, while 34.2% were completely dependent with walking (p = 0.032).

In univariate analysis, frailty was not significantly associated with falls (p = 0.39). Table 4 shows associations between falls and frailty, classified using the frailty scale. There were no significant associations between frailty and gender (p = 0.21), frailty and falls categories (p = 0.95), or frailty and benzodiazepine use (p = 0.11).

Multivariate analyses

A linear regression model was performed, with the dependent variable being the number of falls adjusting for age, sex, dementia diagnosis, drug count, Potentially Inappropriate Medication (PIM) use, visual impairment, frailty, benzodiazepine and SSRI/SNRI use. As shown in Fig. 2, dementia (**β** 0.96, 95% CI: 0.83 – 1.84; P = 0.032), visual impairment (**β** 0.84, 95% CI: 0.13 – 1.56; p = 0.021), and use of any PIMs (**β** 0.34, 95% CI: 0.037-0.65; P = 0.028) were associated with increased risk of falls (Fig. 2). Consistent with our findings in the univariate analyses, benzodiazepine use remained associated with reduced numbers of falls (p = 0.009), and SSRI/SNRI use was associated with increased numbers of falls (p = 0.007). Age, drug count, and frailty were not significant predictors in this model. Gender was significantly associated with falls in the model which excluded frailty (p = 0.022), though it shifted from borderline statistical significance once frailty was added to the model (p = 0.06).

Discussion

Falls were frequent among the frail LTCF residents in our study, with 56.7% of residents having fallen at least once in the prior 6 months. We found that falls were associated with cognitive impairment, male gender, visual impairment and the use of certain medications. Potential Inappropriate Medication use (according to the Beers list) and SSRI/SNRI classes were associated with increased risk of falls, while benzodiazepines appeared to be associated with a decreased risk of falls.

Our results should be interpreted with caution. This was an observational study, and sampling of LTCF residents was not random; those with emergency ambulance calls were over-sampled. Data were abstracted from

Table 3 Medication class in relation to number of falls

Medication	N of residents taking each med. *N* = 395	0 (*N* = 171)	1 (*N* = 106)	2-4 (*N* = 79)	5+ (*N* = 34)	*P*-value
Typical antipsychotics	30	9 (30%)	9 (30%)	8 (27%)	4 (13.3%)	0.4
Atypical antipsychotics	156	66 (42.3%)	41 (26.3%)	33 (21.2%)	14 (9.0%)	0.96
SSRI/SNRI	219	97 (44.3%)	47 (21.5%)	51 (23.3%)	22 (10.0%)	0.03
Diuretic	193	85 (44.0%)	52 (26.9%)	36 (18.7%)	16 (8.3%)	0.94
Beta blocker	186	82 (44.1%)	48 (25.8%)	36 (19.4%)	17 (9.1%)	0.95
CCB	104	41 (39.4%)	29 (27.9%)	23 (22.2%)	8 (7.7%)	0.81
ARB	54	27 (50%)	11 (20.3%)	12 (20.45)	2 (3.7%)	0.31
Opioid	211	92 (43.65)	61 (28.9%)	41 (19.4%)	17 (8.1%)	0.83
Statin	149	68 (45.6%)	39 (26.2%)	30 (20.1%)	10 (6.7%)	0.72
Diabetic	106	45 (42.5%)	33 (31.1%)	20 (18.95)	7 (6.6%)	0.62
Bisphosphonate	64	28 (43.8%)	13 (20.3%)	17 (26.6%)	6 (9.4%)	0.41
Benzodiazepines	164	74 (45.1%)	53 (32.3%)	26 (15.9%)	10 (6.1%)	0.05

CCB Calcium Chanel Blocker, *ARB* Angiotensin Receptor Blocker, *SSRI/SNRI* Selective Serotonin Reuptake Inhibitors or Selective Serotonin-Norepinepherine Reuptake Inhibitors

Table 4 Frailty in relation to gender, benzodiazepine use and number of falls

	1- mild frailty	2 - moderate frailty	3 - severe frailty	4 – very severe frailty	5 – terminally ill	*P* value
Male Gender *N* = 92	11 (12%)	40 (43.4%)	33 (35.9%)	6 (6.5%)	2 (2.2%)	0.21
Female Gender *N* = 192	19 (10%)	67 (34.9%)	95 (49.5%)	10 (5.2%)	1 (0.5%)	0.21
Benzodiazepine Use *N* = 118	13 (11.0%)	42 (35.6%)	59 (50%)	2 (1.7%)	2 (1.7%)	0.11
0 Falls *N* = 113	14 (12.4%)	41 (36.3%)	50 (44.3%)	7 (6.2%)	1 (0.9%)	0.95
1 Fall *N* = 74	6 (8.1%)	27 (36.5%)	36 (48.6%)	4 (5.4%)	1 (1.4%)	0.95
2-4 Falls *N* = 70	5 (7.1%)	30 (42.9%)	31 (44.3%)	3 (4.3%)	1 (1.4%)	0.95
5+ Falls *N* = 27	5 (18.5%)	9 (33.3%)	11 (40.7%)	2 (7.4%)	0	0.95

LTCF charts, and thus we relied on documentation in the charts and on clinical reporting of measures like falls and dementia diagnoses. On the other hand, these results reflect the "real world" of clinical practice. Our study analyzed frailty and falls which is a relationship that has not previously been examined in Long Term Care populations to our knowledge.

Due to the retrospective nature of the study, despite the best efforts of the chart abstractors to glean the relevant data points from resident charts, some residents were missing data. For example, 110 individuals (27.8% of the sample) were missing frailty data because this had not been completed by their primary care teams. Based on prior experience in frailty studies, generally speaking frailty is more likely to be missing in the most vulnerable (who are also the most frail) [16]. Our findings may therefore be conservative, and this may also have contributed to our lack of finding of an association between frailty and falls.

Documentation and reporting of falls is a challenge. Our study did not use a standardized method of recording of falls, as the LTCF did not have a formal tool for recording falls. Falls were counted if they were documented in a resident's chart upon review of the preceding 6 months. It is possible that fall events would have been missed if they went undocumented (for example if the resident had not reported a fall to the care staff). Potential gaps in reporting of falls are not a problem unique to our study. Reporting differences by gender have been documented in the literature [17, 18]. This is potentially relevant to our study's finding of an association between male gender and increased fall numbers. The current literature supports that women fall more than men, but this may be due, at least in part, to gender differences in reporting. Stevens et al., examined gender differences in seeking care in the community-dwelling adults over the age of 65. They found that a significantly greater percentage of women than men sought medical care after a falls, talked with a healthcare provider about falls, talked with a provider to understand why they fell, and/or talked with a provider about fall prevention [17]. Since our study was conducted in LTCF, underreporting remains a possibility, though residents would presumably be more likely to come to staff attention when they fell. For this reason, our finding that men in our study had more documented falls appears all the more relevant. Taking our study findings in the context of the existing literature, more

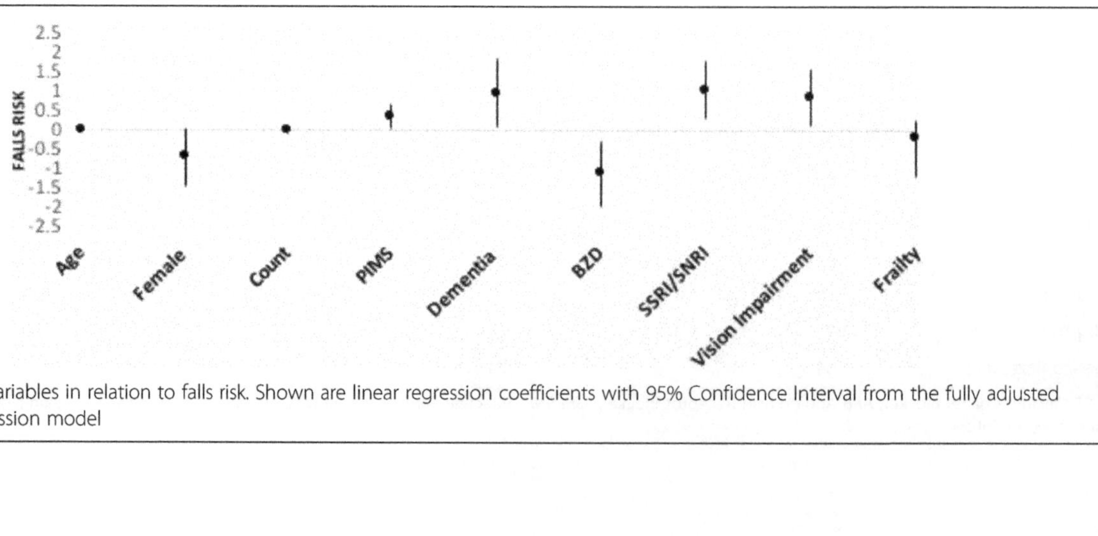

Fig. 2 Individual variables in relation to falls risk. Shown are linear regression coefficients with 95% Confidence Interval from the fully adjusted multivariable regression model

focused screening for falls among men may be warranted as a prevention strategy.

The relevance of medication use in relation to falls was another important finding in our study. Our study lacks information on medication doses and indications, which would be beneficial to the interpretation of our findings. In LTCF settings, mediations such as benzodiazepines, antidepressants and antipsychotics have been previously reported to be associated with increased risk of falls [6]. Our finding that SSRI/SNRI and PIMs were associated with increased risk of falls is thus in keeping with the current literature. However, our study found that benzodiazepines appeared to be protective for falls. We conducted further analysis to try and account for this surprising finding. We hypothesized that one potential explanation could be that benzodiazepines are more likely to be prescribed at end of life (when mobility might be restricted and falls risk thus attenuated). However, we found that the majority of benzodiazepine users were not classified as being at end-of life. Another explanation could be that those taking benzodiazepines were less mobile, and therefore less likely to fall, yet we found that over half (57.9%) of the residents on benzodiazepines were walking independently. A third explanation might be the increased education in appropriate prescribing of benzodiazepines among physicians. If residents at high risk of falls preferentially had benzodiazepines de-prescribed or not initiated, while those at lower risk of falls were left taking them, this could have led to an apparently inverse association. This is particularly interesting in our study as during the time period prior to our data collection, the CBD team implemented new prescribing guidelines and medication review protocols for the physicians caring for these patients. The focus was not specifically on benzodiazepines, but it still may have impacted the prescribing habits of the physicians.

Although not statistically significant, the frailty trends discovered in our study are interesting. We found that moderately and severely frail residents experienced more falls. These intermediate frailty categories were also were the highest benzodiazepine users. Moderate to severe frailty could be considered the most vulnerable group to experience falls, as they could be mobile but also dependent for most basic activities of daily living [14]. The extremes of frailty are likely to cancel each other out, with opposite influences. Very frail and terminally ill residents might tend to be bed bound (and thus at lower risk of falls) while those who with mild frailty would not be as likely to fall as they presumably have greater independence with mobility.

Generally speaking, women tend to be more frail than men [15]. Our lack of finding of an association between gender and frailty may reflect a placement bias. Less frail men may be more likely to be cared for at home by their surviving wives, moving to LTC only at with more advanced frailty. Women may have to move to LTC at lower levels of frailty if they have been widowed and have fewer options for care at home [19].

Our study also found visual impairment and impaired cognition to be correlated with increased risk of falls. The current literature lacks studies associating visual impairment and falls in residents of LTCF. Unfortunately, our study can only conclude visual impairment increased the risk of falls, but cannot comment of the specific degree or type of visual impairment, because we relied on a general clinical diagnosis of "visual impairment". However, visual impairment is something that is potentially modifiable, so it should not be overlooked as a risk factor for falls. On the other hand, dementia is a well-documented risk factor for falls [20]. Our study findings support the importance of dementia as a risk factor for falls in LTCF. Frequent cognitive screening and staging, and falls reduction interventions targeted to residents with dementia, may help to implement preventative measures.

Conclusions

Our study examined modifiable and non-modifiable risk factors for falls among LTCF residents. Keeping in mind the study limitations, we found that certain medications, impaired cognition, and visual impairment were associated with increased falls risk. This is consistent with the current literature and supports the need for screening and prevention of these risk factors. Screening for falls and associated risk factors should ideally occur during every patient encounter. Our finding that men fell more than women is a unique finding that requires more definitive research. Based on our findings, clinicians should consider asking men explicitly about falls as they may be less likely to be forthcoming. The finding that benzodiazepines were protective for falls may in fact reflect appropriate changing prescribing patterns of clinicians (e.g. benzodiazepines being stopped in those at risk for falls and started at end of life). Falls remain an important problem among LTC residents and further research is needed to inform clinical practice.

Abbreviations

ARB: Angiotensin Receptor Blocker; CBD: Care by Design; CCB: Calcium Chanel Blocker; CGA: Comprehensive Geriatric Assessment; CI: Confidence Interval; EHS: Emergency Health Services; IQR: Inter Quartile Rage; LTC: Long-Term Care; LTCF: Long-Term Care Facilities; MMSE: Mini Mental State Examination; PIM: Potentially Inappropriate Medication; SD: Standard Deviation; SSRI/SNRI: Selective Serotonin Reuptake Inhibitors or Selective Serotonin-Norepinepherine Reuptake Inhibitors

Acknowledgements

EJC was funded by the Dalhousie University Faculty of Medicine's "Research In Medicine" Program through a Department of Medicine University Internal Medicine Research Foundation Summer Studentship.

Funding
This study was funded by the Capital Health Research Fund and the Dalhousie University Department of Family Medicine. The funding organizations had no role in the design or implementation of the study protocol, or in preparation/analysis of the findings.

Authors' contributions
All authors contributed to developing the research questions and planning the analyses. EJC and MKA conducted the analyses. SKB and MKA classified the medications. All authors interpreted the analyses. EGM and MKA designed and conducted the overall Care By Design study and hold the data. EJC prepared the initial draft of the manuscript, and all authors provided revisions and approved the final version.

Competing interests
The authors declare that they have no competing interests.

Author details
[1]Faculty of Medicine, Dalhousie University, Halifax, NS, Canada. [2]Department of Pharmacy, Nova Scotia Health Authority-Central Zone, Halifax, NS, Canada. [3]Department of Family Medicine, Dalhousie University, Halifax, NS, Canada. [4]Department of Medicine (Geriatrics), Dalhousie University, Halifax, NS, Canada.

References
1. Gillespie L. Preventing falls in elderly people. BMJ. 2004;328:653–4.
2. Tinetti ME. Preventing falls in elderly persons. N Engl J Med. 2003;348:42–9.
3. Kannus P, Sievänen H, Palvanen M, Järvinen T, Parkkari J. Prevention of falls and consequent injuries in elderly people. Lancet. 2005;366:1885–93.
4. Important Facts about Falls | Home and Recreational Safety | CDC Injury Center. http://www.cdc.gov/homeandrecreationalsafety/falls/adultfalls.html. Accessed 16 Dec 2015.
5. Vellas BJ, Wayne SJ, Romero LJ, Baumgartner RN, Garry PJ. Fear of falling and restriction of mobility in elderly fallers. Age Ageing. 1997;26:189–93.
6. Woolcott JC, Richardson KJ, Wiens MO, Patel B, Marin J, Khan KM, Marra CA. Meta-analysis of the impact of 9 medication classes on falls in elderly persons. Arch Intern Med. 2009;169:1952–60.
7. Prevention I of M (US) D of HP and D, Berg RL, Cassells JS: Falls in older persons: risk factors and prevention. 1992.
8. Lannering C, Ernsth Bravell M, Midlöv P, Östgren C-J, Mölstad S. Factors related to falls, weight-loss and pressure ulcers–more insight in risk assessment among nursing home residents. J Clin Nurs. 2016;25:940–50.
9. Marshall EG, Boudreau MA, Jensen JL, Edgecombe N, Clarke B, Burge F, Archibald G, Taylor A, Andrew MK. A new long-term care facilities model in nova scotia, Canada: protocol for a mixed methods study of care by design. JMIR Res Protoc. 2013;2:e56.
10. Marshall EG, Clarke BS, Varatharasan N, Andrew MK. A long-term care-comprehensive geriatric assessment (LTC-CGA) tool: improving Care for Frail Older Adults? Can Geriatr J. 2015;18:2–10.
11. Marshall EG, Clarke B, Burge F, Varatharasan N, Archibald G, Andrew MK. Improving continuity of care reduces emergency department visits by long-term care residents. J Am Board Fam Med. 2016;29:201–8.
12. Folstein MF, Folstein SE, McHugh PR. "Mini-mental state". A practical method for grading the cognitive state of patients for the clinician. J Psychiatr Res. 1975;12:189–98.
13. Hajjar ER, Cafiero AC, Hanlon JT. Polypharmacy in elderly patients. Am J Geriatr Pharmacother. 2007;5:345–51.
14. Rockwood K, Abeysundera M, Mitnitiski A. How should we grade frailty in nursing home patients? J Am Med Dir Assoc. 2007;8:595–606.
15. Rockwood K, Song X, MacKnight C, Bergman H, Hogan DB, McDowell I, Mitnitski A. A global clinical measure of fitness and frailty in elderly people. Can Med Assoc J. 2005;173:489–95.
16. Andrew MK: Social vulnerability in old age. In: Brocklehurst's Textbook of Geriatric Medicine and Gerontology. Edited by Fillit HM, Rockwood K, Young J. Eighth edn. Philadelphia: Elsevier; 2016. p. 185-192.
17. Stevens JA, Ballesteros MF, Mack KA, Rudd RA, DeCaro E, Adler G. Gender differences in seeking care for falls in the aged Medicare population. Am J Prev Med. 2012;43:59–62.
18. Stevens JA, Sogolow ED. Gender differences for non-fatal unintentional fall related injuries among older adults. Inj Prev. 2005;11:115–9.
19. Andrew MK, Keefe JM. Social vulnerability from a social ecology perspective: a cohort study of older adults from the National Population Health Survey of Canada. BMC Geriatr. 2014;14:90.
20. Thurman DJ, Stevens JA, Rao JK. Practice parameter: assessing patients in a neurology practice for risk of falls (an evidence-based review): report of the quality standards Subcommittee of the American Academy of neurology. Neurology. 2008;70:473–9.

8

Training on domestic violence and child safeguarding in general practice: a mixed method evaluation of a pilot intervention

Natalia V. Lewis[1*], Cath Larkins[2], Nicky Stanley[2], Eszter Szilassy[1], William Turner[3], Jessica Drinkwater[4] and Gene S. Feder[1]

Abstract

Background: Children's exposure to domestic violence is a type of child maltreatment, yet many general practice clinicians remain uncertain of their child safeguarding responsibilities in the context of domestic violence. We developed an evidence-based pilot training on domestic violence and child safeguarding for general practice teams. The aim of this study was to test and evaluate its feasibility, acceptability and the direction of change in short-term outcome measures.

Methods: We used a mixed method design which included a pre-post questionnaire survey, qualitative analysis of free-text comments, training observations, and post-training interviews with trainers and participants. The questionnaire survey used a validated scale to measure participants' knowledge, confidence/ self-efficacy, and beliefs/ attitudes towards domestic violence and child safeguarding in the context of domestic violence.

Results: Eleven UK general practices were recruited (response rate 55%) and 88 clinicians attended the pilot training. Thirty-seven participants (42%) completed all pre-post questionnaires and nine were interviewed. All training sessions were observed. All six trainers were interviewed. General practice clinicians valued the training materials and teaching styles, opportunities for reflection and delivery by local trainers from both health and children's social services. The training elicited positive changes in total outcome score and knowledge and confidence/ self-efficacy sub scores which remained at 3-month follow up. However, the mean sub score of beliefs and attitudes did not change and the qualitative results were mixed. Two interviewees described changes in their clinical practice. Participants' suggestions for improving the training included incorporating more ethnic and class diversity in the material, using cases with multiple socio economic disadvantages, and addressing multi-agency collaboration in the context of changing and under-resourced services for children.

Conclusions: The pilot training for general practice on child safeguarding in the context of domestic violence was feasible and acceptable. It elicited positive changes in clinicians' knowledge and confidence/ self-esteem. The extent to which clinical behaviour changed is unclear, but there are indications of changes in practice by some clinicians. The pilot training requires further refinement and evaluation before implementation.

Keywords: General practice, Family practice, Domestic violence, Child safeguarding, Child protection, Pilot projects, Evaluation report, Pre-post-tests, Qualitative evaluation, Quantitative evaluation

* Correspondence: Nat.Lewis@bristol.ac.uk
[1]Centre for Academic Primary Care, School of Social and Community Medicine, University of Bristol, Canynge Hall, 39 Whatley Road, Bristol BS8 2PS, UK
Full list of author information is available at the end of the article

Background

Although the negative health impact of domestic violence and abuse (DVA) is well documented [1], training for health care professionals on how to identify and respond to patients experiencing DVA is virtually absent from undergraduate and postgraduate curricula [2, 3] and has a patchy presence within the continuing professional education [4–6]. A lack of special training is one of the multiple barriers prevailing clinicians from asking patients about DVA and adequately responding to disclosure [7–9]. DVA and child safeguarding (CS) are inter-related issues because (i) direct exposure to DVA has a negative impact on children's health and well-being to the extent that it can be considered maltreatment [10] and (ii) there is an overlap between direct child maltreatment and DVA [11–15]. The strong connection between DVA and child maltreatment is recognised in UK national guidance [16]. Health care professionals' key role in CS has been highlighted in recent policy developments [17, 18]. Opposite to DVA, training on CS for general practice is well established [16], but the link to DVA is rarely made [19]. General practitioners (GPs) are reported to remain uncertain of their CS responsibilities in the context of DVA [20]. Training to identify and manage DVA and, where appropriate, refer children affected by DVA to children's services is therefore required [21].

The pilot training evaluation reported here was a component of the RESPONDS study (*R*esearching *E*ducation to *S*trengthen *P*rimary care *on* *D*omestic Violence and *S*afeguarding) which integrated several evidence sources into the development of a training on DVA and CS for general practice [20, 22–26]. The aim of this study was to pilot the training and evaluate its acceptability, feasibility and the direction of change in short-term outcome measures. We hypothesised that the RESPONDS training would: (i) be acceptable to general practice clinicians and feasible to deliver; (ii) increase clinicians' knowledge on DVA and CS policy and procedures; (iii) increase clinicians' confidence and self-efficacy in supporting families exposed to DVA; (iv) improve clinicians' attitudes towards women and children exposed to DVA; (v) encourage reflection on clinicians' own practice regarding DVA and CS.

Methods

Design

We used a mixed method design [27–29] which included a pre-post questionnaire survey and qualitative analysis of free text comments from the survey, training observations, and post-training interviews. Based on previous research [30, 31], we expected low response rates from general practice staff and decided to use multiple data sources to obtain the maximum amount of data. Mixed methods enabled us to explore: (i) context for training and the experiences of trainers and participants (free text comments, observations, interviews); (ii) the extent to which learning is put into practice by participants (interviews, survey); (iii) the direction of changes in knowledge, confidence, attitudes and clinical behaviour (interviews, survey). Qualitative data helped contextualise and interpret the quantitative findings by enabling us to explore factors which may have facilitated or limited change in individual or collective practices [32].

We applied investigator triangulation, drawing on researchers from different academic disciplines, as well as methodological triangulation in order to 'cancel out' and double check any convergence, inconsistency, and contradiction that may arise within one paradigm. The aim of this was to increase confidence in the findings [27, 33]. Triangulation was both concurrent and sequential [34]. This enabled development from one element of the study to another [27]. Interim analysis of findings from the survey and the concurrent training observations informed the development of interview schedules for trainers and participants [35].

Study procedures

The Primary Care Research Network assisted with identification, sampling and recruitment of general practices for this study. We chose two geographical areas in south England and the Midlands, and drew a purposive sample of general practices of different size, location, ethnicity, socio-economic status, experience of previous DVA training, and provision of local DVA services. To increase practice response rate, we have followed strategies recommended for research in general practice [36]. Thus, each participating practice received a £500 incentive. All training participants received Continuing Professional Development (CPD) certificates stating that the RESPONDS session generated two hours of CPD in accordance with the current Royal College for General Practitioners (RCGP) Appraisal and Revalidation Guidance [37].

One week before the training (T1), practice administrators e-mailed all practice staff an invitation to the study and a link to an on-line SurveyMonkey questionnaire [38]. On the day of the training, researcher observing the session requested that all attendees complete the questionnaire if they had not already done so and provided a laptop for this task. Practice administrators emailed a second invitation and the survey link immediately after the training (T2). A third invitation was e-mailed three months post-training (T3). To increase response rate, weekly reminders were emailed at each time point. In order to match the pre- and post-training responses while protecting anonymity, the participants created a unique identification code which they used at the three time points. All the training sessions were observed. Telephone and face-to-face interviews were carried out with trainers at T2 and with training participants at T3.

After the training, we asked general practice teams to review their recording policies on DVA and CS. If they did not have recording policies, we requested to develop these in light of the received training. We asked practices to return the revised documentation to the research team within a month following the training.

The study was guided by two panels of professionals and service users who contributed to developing the interview schedule and analysis.

Intervention

The training aimed to fill gaps in knowledge and practice on the interface between DVA and CS revealed by the RESPONDS research [20, 22]. Development of the training is reported in detail elsewhere [26]. In brief, the training pack was developed collaboratively using clinical, academic, front line practitioner, service user and training expertise in DVA, CS and health. The RESPONDS training was focused on: (i) needs of children exposed to DVA emphasizing the safety of children and their non-abusive parents, (ii) management of adults and children living with DVA in the same family, (iii) the importance of consistent responses from general practice, DVA and children's social services. The content of the training addressed the following issues: (i) linking DVA and CS in practice; (ii) holding difficult conversations about DVA and speaking directly with children; (iii) responding to DVA disclosure; (iv) child protection referral process; (v) working with other professionals; (v) record keeping, safety and confidentiality.

An overarching feature of the RESPONDS training was to teach how to link DVA and CS in practice [39]. Multi-agency work with organisations who commission and provide services for children and families was emphasised throughout the training. The training focused on how clinicians can work with other professionals in supporting patients with experience of DVA while negotiating a child protection referral to ensure the safety of their children. Training provided information on how to seek advice and work with other health care professionals and third sector DVA agencies; it explained the role of children's social services, and described what general practice clinicians can expect following a child protection referral and what referral information is most helpful to provide. It also discussed the importance of inter-agency work in providing support for both threshold and sub-threshold children and their families. The training also taught how clinicians can provide support to perpetrators.

Each training session was delivered by two trainers, a health care professional and a local children's social work professional. To ensure fidelity to the model, all trainers attended the 'train the trainer event'. The training was delivered to individual general practice teams as a 2-h safeguarding level 3 [40] session during lunchtimes on each practice premises. Informed by the review of previous effective training in this field [22] as well as by the qualitative interviews and consultations with DVA experts and survivors [26], the teaching was interactive with an emphasis on discussion and reflection on practice. The session incorporated a film in which a female patient presented to a GP with depression and described her concerns about the behaviour of her teenage son. The GP asked the mother about DVA, spoke individually to the patient's son to elicit his experiences, and then discussed with the mother next steps, including making a referral to children's social service. The film was interspersed with short narratives from practicing GP and a social worker. These experts provided guidance on overcoming challenges faced in general practice when dealing with DVA and CS.

Quantitative measures and statistical analysis

The on-line questionnaire included a demographic section and validated outcome measure. The demographic section requested information about gender, age, job position and job experience. Participants were also asked whether they had a designated safeguarding role and whether they previously received DVA training. Ample free text space was provided at the end of the questionnaire to enable participants to comment on the training and to write down their contact details if they were interested in taking part in follow up interviews. Survey responses were downloaded from the Survey Monkey software [38] and imported into Stata [41] for subsequent analysis.

The validated outcome measure was the modified Domestic Abuse and Safeguarding Children Scale (M-DASC). An additional text file shows the M-DASC in detail [see Additional file 1]. The original DASC was developed for the evaluation of the inter-professional training in DVA and CS from a number of items used in previous research [42]. A group of six DVA and CS experts selected 10 items from the original DASC that were applicable to the general practice context and added 17 new items on identification and response to women and children exposed to DVA. The M-DASC consisted of 27 items with responses endorsed on a 1-5 scale (1 ='Strongly disagree' to 5 = 'Strongly agree'); possible range of total score was 1 to 135. Working through group discussion and consensus, the experts designated three M-DASC subscales: (1) knowledge of DVA and CS (16 items, possible range of scores 1-80), (2) confidence/

self-efficacy in responding to women and children exposed to DVA (14 items, range 1-70), and (3) beliefs/attitudes towards DVA (8 items, range 1-40). Some items appeared in more than one subscale [see Additional file 1]. We used total score and three subscale scores as continuous measures for the quantitative analysis.

To assess test-retest reliability of the M-DASC, a Pearson's product-moment correlation was used to measure the relationship between the two sets of repeated questions [43]. Internal consistency of the M-DASC was assessed with a Cronbach's alpha [44]. Frequencies were used to present categorical variables. We used the Fisher's exact test to compare two proportions for small samples [45].

We hypothesised that there would be positive changes in M-DASC measures taken post-training compared to the pre-training estimates, and used repeated-measures ANOVA to test the hypothesis [45]. The primary outcome was total M-DASC score; the secondary outcomes were three M-DASC sub scores. Time was a within-subject variable with three categories (T1, T2, T3). Between-subject covariates (gender, age, job position, job experience, previous DVA training) were pre-specified based on published research [46, 47]. We first ran a main analysis on a sample of participants who provided data at all three time points and then carried out a sensitivity analysis on a sample of participants who provided data at least twice (including at T1) . The results of the two analyses were then compared. We present a complete case analysis.

Test-retest reliability and internal consistency of the modified Domestic Abuse and Safeguarding Childrenscale

We assessed test-retest reliability of the M-DASC with 29 social work students at the University of Bristol. The students completed the questionnaire twice with a 2-week gap. Total scores and sub scores at both time points were highly correlated: (i) total score (r (27) = 0.79; $P < 0.001$); (ii) knowledge sub score (r (27) = 0.76; $P < 0.001$); (iii) confidence/self-efficacy sub score (r (27) = 0.74; $P < 0.001$); (iv) beliefs/ attitudes sub score (r (27) = 0.69; $P < 0.001$).

The Cronbach alpha (α) for the whole M-DASC had a very good level of internal consistency: 0.86 at the first time point and 0.91 at the second time point. [48]. Two subscales also demonstrated good levels of internal consistency at both time points (knowledge $\alpha = 0.82$ and 0.86 and confidence/ self-efficacy $\alpha = 0.79$ and 0.88, respectively). However, the beliefs/attitudes subscale had internal consistency below minimally acceptable level at the two time points ($\alpha = 0.22$ and 0.52, respectively).

Qualitative data and analysis

The qualitative element of the study had inductive and hypothetical logic. Working inductively from our earlier research [22, 42, 49] and existing literature [46, 50–52] we theorised that the process (delivery of and engagement with trusted training materials, group participation, and co-delivery by trainers from health and social care) would provide opportunities for reflection and that would subsequently lead to outcomes (increased knowledge of policy and procedures, increased confidence and self-efficacy, improved attitudes towards DVA and CS, and reflection on own role and practice). This informed our training observation guide [see Additional file 2] and interview schedule for trainers [see Additional file 3], which focused on documenting successes and challenges in the process and exploring initial outcomes (moments where training participants appeared to exhibit changes). We created an interview schedule for training participants [see Additional file 4] based on these observations, trainer interviews and the survey results at T2. This enabled us to explore concerns about factors which appeared to facilitate or limit the intervention delivery and where M-DASC measures indicated no change. Interviews were conducted by telephone or face-to-face, audio recorded, transcribed verbatim, and coded in NVivo [53].

The data were analysed using content analysis against our inductively theorised process and outcome measures (as above) to identify individual, local and system factors relevant to practices towards DVA and CS [27, 54]. From our previous research [42, 49] and literature [46, 50–52] we knew that gender, practice culture, and the availability of time and information about local resources were likely to be relevant to an individual's practice. We also speculated that individual pre-training attitudes and availability of support during the training were likely to be relevant to the direction of change in outcomes. Content was coded based on major themes identified in our previous research [26, 42, 49]. Each interview and free text comment was analysed systematically and coded according to the existing thematic coding structure. Additional codes were added where new themes emerged from the data and previous interviews and free-text comments were re-read and re coded with new codes if relevant.

Participants' quotes from survey free text comments are reported as 'Survey GPID', from observations as 'ObsID', from interviews with trainers and clinicians as 'TrID' and 'TGPID', respectively.

Results

Sample characteristics

Invitation letters and study information sheets were sent to 10 practices in the South and 10 practices in the Midlands. Overall, seven southern and five Midlands practices agreed to participate. However, one southern practice withdrew due to unexpected doctor capacity issue which resulted in 11/20 practices enrolled in the study (55% response rate). All southern practices had previous DVA training, although not all clinicians had been exposed to the training. The previous DVA training was received through IRIS – an evidence-based training, support and referral programme for general practice [4]. None of the Midland practices received previous DVA training.

Between May and July 2014, we delivered pilot training to 88 general practice clinicians. One pair of trainers worked with Midlands practices, the other two pairs worked with southern practices. The training team comprised of three health care professionals (named GP for safeguarding children, designated nurse for child protection, and liaison nurse from MARAC (Multi-Agency Risk Assessment Conference)) and three social workers (Early Help co-ordinator, children's social care senior practitioner, independent social worker). All the training sessions were observed by one of three researchers. All six (female) trainers were interviewed post-training (T2).

Overall, 25 training participants (21 in the South and four in the Midlands) expressed their interest in taking part in the follow up interviews (T3). However, four participants moved practice or went on maternity or long term sick leave, and seven did not reply to our email or phone invitations. In addition, five participants withdrew from follow up interviews due to increased workload. Consequently, we interviewed nine training participants (seven in the South and two in the Midlands; seven female, two male; two South Asian, seven white; all GPs; one aged 25-34; two aged 35-44; two aged 45-54; two aged 55-65; two safeguarding leads).

In total, 82/88 (93%) training participants completed the questionnaire at T1, 73/82 (60%) completed post-training survey at T2, and 42/82 (34%) completed 3-month follow up at T3. One questionnaire had all items missing and was excluded from analysis at this stage. After matching the questionnaires by ID, 37 participants had survey data at all three time points, 27 at two time points, and 18 at one time point. We coded those who completed all three questionnaires as 'completers' and those who did not provide data at all three time points as 'dropouts'. Data from survey completers who comprised 42% (37/88) of those trained were used in main statistical analysis. We then used 63/88 cases with at least two valid responses including T1 (72% of those trained) in a sensitivity analysis.

For 32 of the 42 variables used in this analysis, less than 10% of values were missing. Ages of the participants at T1 ranged between 25 and 64 years [Table 1]. All age groups were equally represented. Over three-quarters were GPs, followed by practice nurses and 'other professionals' (two practice managers, one health

Table 1 Comparison of survey completers and dropouts on socio-demographic and background characteristics

Variable	Categories	Total *n* = 82 *n* (%)	Dropouts *n* = 45 *n* (%)	Completers *n* = 37 *n* (%)	*P*
Gender	Female	55 (67)	27 (60)	28 (76)	0.16
	Male	27 (33)	18 (40)	9 (24)	
Age	<25-34	16 (20)	12 (27)	4 (11)	0.09
	35-44	23 (28)	13 (29)	10 (27)	
	45-54	25 (30)	9 (20)	16 (43)	
	55-64	18 (22)	11 (24)	7 (19)	
Job title	GP	63 (77)	34 (76)	29 (78)	0.52
	Nurse	14 (17)	8 (18)	6 (16)	
	Admin/ manager	2 (2)	2 (4)	0 (0)	
	Other	3 (4)	1 (2)	2 (5)	
Years of practice	0-9	20 (24)	15 (33)	5 (13)	0.08
	10-20	24 (29)	13 (29)	11 (30)	
	>21	38 (47)	17 (38)	21 (57)	
Safeguarding role	No	61 (79)	33 (79)	28 (80)	1.00
	Yes	16 (21)	9 (21)	7 (20)	
IRIS trained	No	47 (61)	38 (90)	9 (26)	<0.001
	Yes	30 (39)	4 (10)	26 (74)	
Geographic area	South	54 (66)	18 (40)	36 (97)	<0.001
	Midlands	28 (34)	27 (60)	1 (3)	

Note: Proportions are reported for available data. *IRIS* Identification and Referral to Improve Safety training, *SD* standard deviation, *P* p-value for the Fisher's exact test care assistant, one phlebotomist, one pharmacist). Nearly equal proportions of the participants had been practising for up to 20 years and for more than 20 years. About 20% of participants (16/77) had a designated safeguarding role. About 39% of respondents (30/77) received DVA training through IRIS [4]. When we compared survey completers and dropouts by their characteristics at T1, we found evidence of a selective dropout. Those participants who provided data at all three time points, and were thus included in the complete case analysis, were more likely to be IRIS-trained and to work in the South.

Qualitative evaluation of training acceptability and feasibility

Engaging and trustworthy training materials and delivery style

Participants opinions about training materials and delivery style were collected to evaluate the acceptability and feasibility of the training through exploring: (i) whether participants thought appropriate and trustworthy information was delivered (interviews); (ii) how they engaged with the video (interviews, observations); (iii) how well they thought the training had been delivered (interviews, observations); (iv) whether the training was compatible with participants' existing knowledge (survey, interviews, observations). We also assessed delivery style (observation, interviews) and trainers' experiences of delivering the training and engaging participants (observations, interviews).

Training participants considered that appropriate information was well presented and thoroughly delivered. Trainers were described as 'non-threatening' (TGP02) and the materials were compatible with participants' existing knowledge.

Training participants were observed to engage well with the video; it was 'realistic, very good' (TGP03) and 'very powerful' (TGP07) because it involved:

> *...seeing the GP actually talk to the child and all the different stages, and then discussing it, that was really useful, very different from just talking about it" (TGP07).*

Two respondents did not 'remember the video too well' (TGP02) or the child (TGP01) but saw the video as making them 'more alert' (TGP01) or provoking 'thoughts and ideas' (TGP02). One respondent who thought the video was unnatural and unrealistic saw the video as a prompt for team discussion on approaches that 'we all felt were more appropriate' (TGP09). In observations and trainer interviews, the suggested broad filter questions to patients experiencing DVA, were particularly valued with some saying 'I will definitely use that' (Obs04) or 'that's a good thing to ask' (Tr01). However occasional resistance to engagement was observed, particularly in three practices described by one trainer as 'old school' (Tr02). One GP responded to the mother in the video by saying 'well if she will nag' (Obs1).

Suggested improvements included videos that were more 'concise and punchy' (TGP07), 'multi-ethnic' (TGP02), 'class diverse' (TGP03) or 'a bit more complicated' (TGP08). Some participants felt that the training should address drug and alcohol use, parental non-consent and how to deal with 'an incredibly dysfunctional under-resourced market of referral services' (TGP05).

Opportunities for reflection

All interviewed participants concurred that there were 'enough' or 'definitely enough' opportunities for reflection, and seeing 'how my colleagues deal with it' (TGP01) was perceived as particularly useful. However we observed, and all interviewees agreed, that the extent to which training delivery enabled reflection on participants' own clinical cases depended on their experience. Two respondents suggested that this reflection case work could be a follow up training event. However, 10 of the 11 practices did not complete the post-training review of their recording policies on DVA and CS.

Group engagement

Group engagement was assessed through exploring how participants engaged in the group work (interviews, observations). The interviewees thought that most of their colleagues engaged in group discussions; it was 'authoritative but low key ... sort of join, join in and everybody felt very safe' (TGP04) and 'one of the best things' (TGP09). But in some practices, we observed a marked lack of engagement in group discussions, as on one occasion trainers felt 'we were just talking into an empty space' (Tr03) or groups were dominated by 'one [usually senior] doctor who would do a lot of the talking' (Tr01). The trainers agreed that talking a lot could mean they 'had a lot of questions and a lot to say' (Tr03), whereas 'not talking' did not mean 'not participating' (Tr02). One trainer suggested facilitating greater parity of engagement or participation through 'small groups, all at a similar [knowledge] level' (Tr02).

Provision of local multi-agency information

Each observed training session was delivered by health and social care frontline workers. Trainers reported the importance of multiagency delivery and this was echoed by participants:

> *"I think it's absolutely fantastic having professionals who are dealing with this day and day out" (TGP06).*

The 'social services input was that extra thing' (TGP08) that took training delivery beyond that delivered through IRIS which had no input from social worker. The RESPONDS training was 'able to defend that [social services] message rather than somebody who is just [a trainer]' (TGP05).

Quantitative analysis of training outcomes

In the questionnaire survey completed by the training participants at T1, M-DASC demonstrated a very good level of reliability of the whole scale (α = 0.91) and two subscales (knowledge subscale α = 0.85; confidence/self-efficacy subscale α = 0.88). However, the beliefs/attitudes subscale had reliability below minimally acceptable level (α = 0.51) [48].

The training elicited positive changes in total M-DASC score and two sub scores which remained at 3-month follow up [Table 2].

Compared with T1, the mean total M-DASC score increased by 11.7 units at T2 and stayed 10.8 units higher three months later (F (2, 108) = 19.83, $P < 0.001$). Compared with T1, the mean knowledge sub score increased by 8.6 units at T2 and remained 7.7 units higher at T3 (F (2, 108) = 24.02, $P < 0.001$). The confidence/self-esteem sub score was 6.7 and 6.3 units higher than at T1, respectively F (2, 108) = 16.72, $P < 0.001$).

The mean measure of beliefs and attitudes did not change either post-training (increase by 0.3 units) or at follow up (increase by 0.2 units) (F (2, 108) = 0.23, $P = 0.61$). It is worth noting that at the start of the training, scores on five out of eight items on this subscale [see M-DASC items 3, 5, 7, 9, 20 in Additional file 1] already indicated strong beliefs and positive attitudes towards DVA and CS which remained unchanged throughout the study (mean scores of 4 out of 5 possible).

We found some evidence that mean M-DASC score of GPs was higher compared to other general practice clinicians both at the start of the training and at 3-month follow up [Fig. 1]. At T1, mean M-DASC score of GPs was 87.7 (95% CI 85.0 to 90.4), compared to 73.0 of nurses (95% CI 67.0 to 79.0) and 70.0 of 'other practitioners' (95% CI 59.7 to 80.3). At T2, all professional groups improved their scores and the gap disappeared (97.9 vs. 90.2 and 87.5, respectively, all three 95% CIs overlap). At T3, although the total effect of the training remained, mean M-DASC score of GPs stayed higher (97.7, 95% CI 95.0 to 100.4) compared to nurses (88.8, 95% CI 82.9 to 94.8) or 'other professionals' (77.5, 95% CI 67.2 to 87.8).

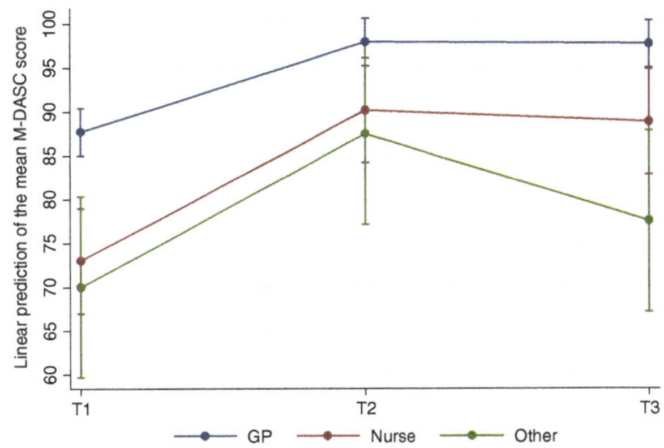

Fig. 1 Adjusted predictions of the effect of job position and RESPONDS training on total M-DASC score. Note. GP – general practitioners. Nurse – practice nurses. Other – other primary care practitioners. T1 – at the start of the RESPONDS training. T2 – immediately after the RESPONDS training. T3 – 3-month follow up. Line shows mean total M-DASC scores and 95% confidence intervals at three time points

Table 2 Modified Domestic Abuse and Safeguarding Children Scale (M-DASC) scores before and after training intervention ($n = 37$)

Scale/ subscale score	T1		T2		T3		P
	Mean	SD	Mean	SD	Mean	SD	
Total	84.4	10.6	96.1	7.1	95.2	8.7	<0.001
Knowledge	50.5	7.0	59.1	5.0	58.2	5.4	<0.001
Confidence/self-efficacy	42.8	6.3	49.5	4.5	49.1	5.8	<0.001
Beliefs/attitudes	24.5	1.8	24.8	1.9	24.7	2.0	0.61

Note: T1 – pre-training. T2 – immediately post-training. T3 – 3-month follow up. *SD* standard deviation, *P* *p*-value for the repeated-measures ANOVA test

We found some evidence of an interaction between previous IRIS training and the RESPONDS training, indicating that IRIS was associated with more sustainable M-DASC score between T2 and T3 (F (2, 58) = 3.81, $P = 0.05$) as seen from the plateau effect in Fig. 2 between T2 and T3. There was no difference in the M-DASC score by previous IRIS training either at T1 (mean difference between two categories 6.3, 95% CI -0.2 to 12.7; $P = 0.06$) or at T2 (mean difference 5.3, 95% CI -1.7 to 12.3; $P = 0.14$). However, at 3-month follow up, mean M-DASC score of IRIS trained respondents stayed 12.1 units higher compared to their non-IRIS trained colleagues whose mean score dropped (95% CI 4.7 to 19.6; $P = 0.02$).

Sensitivity analysis performed on a sample of participants who had valid responses at least at two time points including T1 ($n = 63$) produced results similar to the analysis of 37 study completers who had valid responses at all three time points.

Qualitative evaluation of training impact on individual and collective practices

Knowledge

Most qualitative interviews supported the survey finding of increased knowledge post-training. All eight interviewees described some new or 'refreshed' (TGP06)

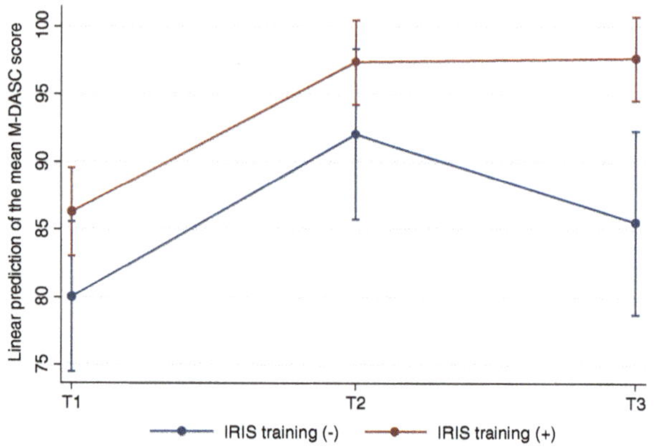

Fig. 2 Adjusted predictions of the effect of IRIS training and RESPONDS training on total M-DASC score. Note. IRIS – Identification and Response to Improve Safety – domestic violence training, support and referral programme for general practice. IRIS training (-) – participants without previous IRIS training. IRIS training (+) – participants with previous IRIS training. T1 – at the start of the RESPONDS training. T2 – immediately after the RESPONDS training. T3 – 3-month follow up. Line shows mean total M-DASC scores and 95% confidence intervals at three time points

knowledge. This included 'quite powerful learning about the impacts on children of domestic violence' (TGP04), and that 'people are actually very happy to just have the questions asked' (TGP03). Knowing 'the next steps' was seen to enable 'better conversation with the mother" (TGP06) and had led this GP to decide:

> *"The next time that I do [a referral], that's what I'm going to do...because if we're going to be all proactive, we want to make sure that we're involved in the loop" (TGP03).*

For IRIS-trained participants, learning about appropriate DVA recording was, '[not] anything we hadn't already heard' (TGP05). However it was striking that in three non-IRIS practices the content on the use of codes in record-keeping appeared to be new, especially for junior colleagues (Obs. 2, 4 & 5), and one of those practices went on to develop a new recording system (TGP02).

Current information about 'where to send them for help' (TGP01) (e.g., a website for young people, MARAC, the Early Help Scheme) was valued in both IRIS trained and non-IRIS practices. Even those who knew all the agencies mentioned nonetheless felt the training enabled them to 'know who to speak to' (TGP07) or it provided 'a lot more of a framework in my thinking' (TGP03) on how to access support. Understanding children's social services was particularly important. Respondents reported 'an understanding of where [the referral] goes' (TGP04). One GP had chosen to refer a DVA case to social services despite earlier negative experiences of no action following a referral. Another participant noted that in the future she would:

> *"more readily [make] a referral to Social Services for, you know, a sort of a supportive basis, than I would have done previously... [training was useful] in terms of perhaps lowering the threshold when I might talk to them" (TGP09).*

However, one survey respondent 'actually felt more muddled after this training' because 'there does seem to be an impressive array of disjointed services available.' (Survey GPb). One example of the increased knowledge of referral mechanisms was seen to emerge at the local level, as Trainer 2 noted that 'one of the practices had [subsequent to the training] made a referral, so something had obviously gone in'.

Confidence and self-efficacy

In line with the survey results, six interviewees explained that their 'general improved confidence' (TGP05) was 'sort of built up' (TN2) through being given information about role expectations,'owning the subject' (TGP04), and developing understanding of how to proceed in consultations:

> *"[The training] made me feel particularly confident about discussing this with children, you know, being able to ask them how it was affecting them ...being able to raise that with the mum .... It has changed my management a bit of a couple of patients I've seen since" (TGP07).*

However, confidence remained 'still not very high' where 'the child is ... indirectly affected [by DVA]'(TGP01), where the survey respondent had not had time to apply the learning in practice (Survey GPa) or because they had increased awareness of 'the reality of the limited service on offer by social services to support children if there is not consent.' (Survey GPc).

Beliefs and attitudes

In contrast to the survey result of no change in the mean measure of beliefs and attitudes, qualitative findings were rather mixed. Thus, participants in two sessions were observed (Obs 2 & 5) to make the link from DVA to CS when they had not done so before or ended up 'agreeing with the whole idea that you need to ...treat it as a safeguarding issue' (Tr05). However, Trainer 4 remained concerned that training participants in other sessions 'were still speaking of them as two separate issues'. Five interview respondents identified changes in their attitudes regarding the potential effects of children's exposure to DVA and the need to ask children about DVA, contrasting this to their previous approach:

> *"If I saw children with disturbed behaviour I tended not to think, you know, could it be due to difficulties at home? ... And I think that [training] completely changed my mind, so I actually always ask that now every time I see a child with behaviour problems" (TGP07).*

Although some training participants 'looked quite shocked that the GP in the video suggested talking to the child,' encouragement to talk to a child alone came through discussion with colleagues (Tr03).

For those who remained hesitant about talking to children, this was because they 'possibly would not look for the child' if the mother had not brought the child in (TGP01); they felt 'unclear [what] my role is in terms of actually bringing the child in for a separate consultation' (TGP05); or, were 'generally much happier to talk to children' but still reluctant 'to muddy the waters' by talking to a child directly in a specific case (TGP03).

In three training sessions, the researchers observed and trainers identified having 'not enough of a focus on making the link from DVA to children' (Tr04) or the need to feel 'a bit more confident in making such link' (Tr02). One GP with experience in a paediatric post and a safeguard lead explained that his attitudes towards abused women were already positive before the training.

Engagement in reflection on own clinical practice

Only one out of eleven practice carried out the follow up review of their DVA and CS recording policies. Engagement in reflective practice was not addressed by an M-DASC subscale and there is no evidence of change on the one statement most directly indicative of reflective practice 'I understand how my own experiences may influence my capacity and willingness to engage with issues of domestic violence and abuse' [see M-DASC item 3 in Additional file 1]. Changes in reflective practice were not mentioned by the training participants we interviewed. When asked directly, one participant said the practice was already 'quite keen on training and then encouraging reflective practice' (TGP02) and a second said that training had provided a rare opportunity for reflection.

Discussion

General practice clinicians and trainers found the RESPONDS training in DVA and CS acceptable and feasible. They valued the engaging and trustworthy materials and teaching styles, opportunities for reflection and delivery by trainers from local health and children's social services. The questionnaire survey showed that the training increased clinicians' knowledge and confidence/self-efficacy, but did not change their beliefs/attitudes towards DVA and CS. This could be because the participants' responses at the start of the training already showed that they understood women experiencing abuse and were positive about engaging with issues of DVA. Perhaps those practitioners who underwent previous DVA training were more familiar with these issues or their positive attitudes were unrelated to the DVA training.

Qualitative findings were also mixed. Some clinicians were more confident in knowing how to proceed in a consultation, and had greater awareness of relevant service provision and referral routes. Some participants reported increased willingness to engage directly with children and to discuss this with the non-abusive parent and this led to some changes in case management. Some participants from practices without previous DVA training learned about recording and were developing new systems. However, some participants reported no change in their clinical behaviour and some felt more confused after the training.

Participants' suggestions for improving the training included incorporating more ethnic and social class diversity in the material, using cases with multiple deprivation and socio economic disadvantages, and addressing multi-agency collaboration in the context of changing and under-resourced referral services.

Engaging primary care clinicians in face-to-face training proved challenging and the planned follow-up review of recording policies on DVA and CS was not carried out by most practices. Low follow up rates in the survey and interviews indicate the difficulty of engaging general practice clinicians beyond training. The fact that only 55% of approached practices took part in the RESPONDS training suggests that there is a systematic barrier to upskilling general practice clinicians. Echoing Sahin and colleagues [55], the most cited reasons for non-participation in the training and evaluation were clinicians' need to prioritise clinical care over research and lack of protected time.

The differential follow up rates between the southern IRIS trained practices and Midland's non-trained practices, to both the survey and interview requests, could indicate a possible positive effect of previous IRIS training on engaging primary care clinicians with this public health and clinical problem. The southern practices were more likely to take part in the evaluation, suggesting some of the arguments about putting time aside for this issue had been won. It could be that IRIS trained participants were more likely to engage because they were familiar with the topic and with the DVA clinical champion involved in the RESPONDS video. The extent to which the selective follow up rate was associated with practice characteristics (e.g., clinician-patient ratio) is not known as we did not collect such data. The low response to the follow up review of recording policies on DVA and CS by IRIS trained practices could be explained by the fact that they already had recording policies as a result of previous training which was highlighted in the qualitative evaluation. This demonstrates the variability of DVA management and support in general practice across the UK, and the challenges of producing national training material, with activities suitable to all levels of experience.

Our findings are partly consistent with the systematic review of educational interventions on responses to children exposed to DVA [22]. This showed that training interventions improved participants' self-reported knowledge, attitudes and clinical competence up to a year post intervention. Our results showed that those training participants who completed the study already had positive attitudes about DVA and CS at the start of the training. This could be explained by the IRIS training which most RESPONDS completers received in the past. Such previous DVA training and on-going practice support through IRIS programme could generate further interest and self-motivation among clinicians to further develop their knowledge, confidence/ self-esteem and skills and to participate in research about DVA.

This study found few examples of changes in clinical behaviour after the RESPONDS training. Interviews suggested behaviour change in some individuals such as increased willingness to ask about DVA and talk to children. However, other interviewees reported no change in their clinical behaviour. There are many possible explanations for this. For example, practitioners could be convinced, but did not have resources to change their own practice, or they could make changes but did not report back to the researchers. Another explanation might be the clinicians' negative previous experience liaising with children's social services. This demonstrates how changing clinical behaviour may require more time for reflection and reinforcement, perhaps longer training with booster sessions, as well as protected time and on-going support for implementation. The systematic review of DVA training interventions found evidence of the effectiveness of whole systems approaches; this might involve combining training for health care practitioners with wider system level interventions, such as increasing awareness of DVA, tools for victim identification, and improved access to support services [56].

Strengths and limitations

This study evaluated an evidence based pilot training on DVA and CS using a mixed method approach which provided insight into training feasibility, acceptability and short-term outcomes. The design included a reliable measure of outcomes, the M-DASC scale and pre/ post evaluation at three time points. Running the pilot in two sites allowed the identification of the value of previous DVA training and on-going support through the IRIS programme. The qualitative data provided possible explanations of why change did and did not occur, giving valuable guidance for future refinement of the RESPONDS training.

There are a number of shortcomings to this evaluation that limit its external validity. The first weakness is the absence of a control group, therefore we cannot be certain that changes in clinicians' outcomes were due to the RESPONDS training rather than other factors. The second limitation is a measurement bias. The questionnaire survey relied on self-report, which might be hindered by social desirability and memory biases with a potential to exaggerate the effect of the training. The M-DASC had limited validation before use in this study and demonstrated poor internal consistency on the beliefs/ attitudes sub scale. Training observations were taken by one of three researchers. The third limitation is a selective bias. Poor engagement of general practice clinicians resulted in small sample size for qualitative interviews. As a result of selective dropout, we ended up with the sample of survey completers biased towards clinicians who had previously received IRIS training and were safeguarding leads, although our follow up rates (60% at T2 and 34% at T3) were higher than those reported in similar studies [42, 57]. The selective bias is particularly problematic in assessing changes in beliefs and attitudes where it is possible that only those clinicians who had positive attitudes towards DVA and CS participated in the evaluation of the RESPONDS training.

Further research

Given the mixed results of the RESPONDS pilot, we propose further refinement and testing of the training. The further refinement could include an amendment of the teaching material with regards to diversity. Further evaluation should explore clinical impact such as changes in the rate of patient disclosure of past or current DVA, and potential harms in the form of parental anxiety, child fear or anxiety and inappropriate referral. Such evaluation requires a controlled study design, adequate sample size and long-term follow up.

As a stand-alone intervention the RESPONDS training could be implemented after refinement, but there remains uncertainty about its effectiveness in actually changing clinician behaviour, improving outcomes for families experiencing DVA and its potential for integration with other DVA training for general practice. Ultimately we do not think that RESPONDS should be a stand-alone training intervention, but should be integrated into other DVA interventions for general practices, combining it with training about the identification of and response to female and male patients with experience of DVA. For women patients, we already have IRIS – a training, support and referral programme. IRIS was tested in a cluster randomised trial and demonstrated clinical effectiveness [4], cost effectiveness [58] and acceptability to patients [59] and clinicians [60]. Following the success of the trial, IRIS has been implemented in >30 localities in England and Wales [61]. For male patients who have experienced or perpetrated DVA, we have a pilot study of HERMES, a training and support programme modelled on IRIS which showed that there was an increase in the identification and documentation of male patients following the pilot training [62].

As a result of the positive findings of the IRIS trial and promising results of the HERMES and RESPONDS pilots as well as responding to the needs of clinicians preferring the DVA training to be connected and have simpler referral routes, we aim to combine these three interventions into an integrated programme (IRIS+) and test its effectiveness in a cluster randomised controlled trial, powered to detect difference in identification and appropriate referral of men, women and children exposed to DVA. We will test whether the IRIS+ model, which builds on IRIS, but includes elements of the HERMES and RESPONDS is practical and whether it is equally effective at identifying female patients, as well as male patients experiencing/perpetrating DVA and their children [63].

Policy and practice implications

A priority for policy and guidance is training on DVA and CS that addresses positive practice aimed at ensuring the safety of children and their parents exposed to DVA, with content regarding appropriate management of adults and children living in the same family [21]. The development of the RESPONDS pilot training and some promising findings of this evaluation are important steps in addressing those priorities in the general practice.

Conclusions

The pilot RESPONDS training in DVA and CS for general practice was feasible and acceptable to both trainers and participants. It had a positive effect on clinicians' knowledge and confidence/ self-esteem. The extent to which beliefs/ attitudes and clinical behaviour changed is unclear. However there are indications of changes in practice for some individuals. The training package requires further refinement and further, more rigorous evaluation before implementation.

Additional files

Additional file 1: Modified Domestic Abuse and Safeguarding Children Scale items before and after training intervention ($n = 37$). Note. T1 – pre-training. T2 – immediately post-training. T3 – 3-month follow up. DVA – domestic violence and abuse. Reverse score items are 4, 5, 7, 8, 12. SD – standard deviation.

Additional file 2: Training observation framework.

Additional file 3: Training evaluation interview schedule – trainers.

Additional file 4: Training evaluation interview schedule – training participants.

Abbreviations

ANOVA: Analysis of variance; CS: Child safeguarding; DASC: Domestic Abuse and Safeguarding Children scale; DVA: Domestic violence and abuse; GPs: General practitioners; ID: Unique identification number; IRIS: Identification and Referral to Improve Safety; MARAC: Multi Agency Risk Assessment Conference; M-DASC: Modified Domestic Abuse and Safeguarding Children Scale; RESPONDS: *R*esearching *E*ducation to *S*trengthen *P*rimary care *on* *D*omestic violence and *S*afeguarding

Acknowledgements

We would like to thank the general practices across England that participated in this pilot training and evaluation. We would like to express our special gratitude and thanks to the RESPONDS trainers who delivered the pilot training and participated in its evaluation. We thank Professor John Carpenter, Research Associate Cindy Mann, and three external peer-reviewers for comments on an earlier version of this paper.

Funding

This study is an independent research commissioned and funded by the Department of Health Policy Research Programme (Bridging the Knowledge and Practice Gap between Domestic Violence and Child Safeguarding: Developing Policy and Training for General Practice, 115/0003). The funding body was not involved in the design of the study, data collection and analysis, interpretation of data and in writing the manuscript. The views expressed in this manuscript are those of the authors and not necessarily those of the Department of Health.

Authors' contributions

GSF, ES, NS and CL designed this evaluation study. JD helped design the intervention and evaluation. GSF (principal investigator) led the study. ES managed the study. ES, CL, NS collected and analysed qualitative data. CL wrote up the qualitative findings. WT and NVL validated the M-DASC. NVL carried out quantitative analysis and drafted the manuscript. All authors were involved in the interpretation of the data, edited the draft, read and approved the final manuscript.

Competing interests

The authors declare that they have no competing interests.

Consent for publication

Not applicable.

Author details

[1]Centre for Academic Primary Care, School of Social and Community Medicine, University of Bristol, Canynge Hall, 39 Whatley Road, Bristol BS8 2PS, UK. [2]School of Social Work, Care and Community, University of Central Lancashire, Harrington Building, Preston PR1 2HE, UK. [3]School for Policy Studies, University of Bristol, Social Science Complex, 8 Priory Road, Bristol BS8 1TZ, UK. [4]Leeds Institute of Health Sciences, Charles Thackrah Building, 101 Clarendon Road, Leeds LS2 9LJ, UK.

References

1. Feder G, Howarth E. The epidemiology of gender-based violence. In: Bewley S, Welch J, editors. ABC of domestic and sexual violence. Chichester: John Wiley; 2014.
2. Valpied J, Aprico K, Clewett J, Hegarty K: Are Future Doctors Taught to Respond to Intimate Partner Violence? A Study of Australian Medical Schools. J Interpers Violence. 2015. doi:10.1177/0886260515592616.

3. Kamimura A, Al-Obaydi S, Nguyen H, Trinh HN, Mo W, Doan P, Franchek-Roa K. Intimate partner violence education for medical students in the USA, Vietnam and China. Public Health. 2015;129(11):1452–8.
4. Feder G, Davies RA, Baird K, Dunne D, Eldridge S, Griffiths C, Gregory A, Howell A, Johnson M, Ramsay J, et al. Identification and Referral to Improve Safety (IRIS) of women experiencing domestic violence with a primary care training and support programme: a cluster randomised controlled trial. Lancet. 2011;378(9805):1788–95.
5. Lo Fo Wong S, Wester F, Mol SS, Lagro-Janssen TL. Increased awareness of intimate partner abuse after training: a randomised controlled trial. Br J Gen Pract. 2006;56(525):249–57.
6. Papadakaki M, Petridou E, Kogevinas M, Lionis C. Measuring the effectiveness of an intensive IPV training program offered to Greek general practitioners and residents of general practice. BMC Med Educ. 2013;13:46.
7. Beynon CE, Gutmanis IA, Tutty LM, Wathen CN, MacMillan HL. Why physicians and nurses ask (or don't) about partner violence: a qualitative analysis. BMC Public Health. 2012;12:473.
8. Ramsay J, Rutterford C, Gregory A, Dunne D, Eldridge S, Sharp D, Feder G. Domestic violence: knowledge, attitudes, and clinical practice of selected UK primary healthcare clinicians. Br J Gen Pract. 2012;62(602):e647–655.
9. Rose D, Trevillion K, Woodall A, Morgan C, Feder G, Howard L. Barriers and facilitators of disclosures of domestic violence by mental health service users: qualitative study. Br J Psychiatry. 2011;198(3):189–94.
10. McTavish JR, MacGregor JC, Wathen CN, MacMillan HL. Children's exposure to intimate partner violence: an overview. Int Rev Psychiatry. 2016;28:1–15.
11. Hester M. Making an impact: children and domestic violence: a reader. 2nd ed. Philadelphia: Jessica Kingsley Publishers; 2007.
12. Holt S, Buckley H, Whelan S. The impact of exposure to domestic violence on children and young people: a review of the literature. Child Abuse Negl. 2008;32(8):797–810.
13. Chang JJ, Theodore AD, Martin SL, Runyan DK. Psychological abuse between parents: associations with child maltreatment from a population-based sample. Child Abuse Negl. 2008;32(8):819–29.
14. Antle B, Barbee A, Sullivan D, Yankeelov P, Johnson L, Cunningham M. The relationship between domestic violence and child neglect. Brief Treat Crisis Interv. 2007;7(4):364–82.
15. Stanley N. Children Experiencing Domestic Violence: A Research Review. Dartington: Research in practice; 2011.
16. RCGP, NSPCC: Safeguarding Children and Young People: The RCGP/NSPCC Safeguarding Children Toolkit for General Practice. 2011: 223.
17. HM Government. Working together to safeguard children. A guide to inter-agency working to safeguard and promote the welfare of children. 2015. https://www.gov.uk/government/publications/working-together-tosafeguard-children–2. Accessed 28 Feb 2017.
18. Munro E: Department for Education. The Munro review of child protection: Final Report. A child-centred system. The Stationery Office Limited; 2011: 189.
19. Hester M. The three planet model: towards an understanding of contradictions in approaches to women and children's safety in contexts of domestic violence. Brit J Soc Work. 2011;41(5):837–53.
20. Szilassy E, Das J, Drinkwater J, Firth A, Hester M, Larkins C, Lewis N, Morrish J, Stanley N, Turner W, et al. Researching Education to Strengthen Primary care ON Domestic violence & Safeguarding (RESPONDS). Final Report for the Department of Health, Policy Research Programme Project. Bristol: University of Bristol; 2015.
21. NICE: Domestic violence and abuse: how health services, social care and the organisations they work with can respond effectively [NICE guideline]. 2014. http://www.nice.org.uk/Guidance/PH50. Accessed 1 Mar 2017.
22. Turner W, Broad J, Drinkwater J, Firth A, Hester M, Stanley N, Szilassy E, Feder G: Interventions to improve the response of professionals to children exposed to domestic violence and abuse: a systematic review. Child Abuse Rev. 2015. doi: 10.1002/car.2385.
23. Szilassy E, Drinkwater J, Hester M, Larkins C, Stanley N, Turner W, Feder G: Working Together, Working Apart: General Practice Professionals' Perspectives on Interagency Collaboration in Relation to Children Experiencing Domestic Violence. In: Humphreys C, Stanley N, editors. Domestic Violence and Protecting Children: New Thinking and Approaches. London: Jessica Kingsley Publishers; 2015: 214-31.
24. Larkins C, Drinkwater J, Hester M, Stanley N, Szilassy E, Feder G: General practice clinicians' perspectives on involving and supporting children and adult perpetrators in families experiencing domestic violence and abuse. Fam Pract. 2015;32(6):701-05.
25. Drinkwater J, Stanley N, Szilassy E, Larkins C, Hester M, Feder G: Juggling confidentiality and safety: a qualitative study of how general practice clinicians document domestic violence in families with children. BJGP 2017, bjgp17X689353. https://doi.org/10.3399/bjgp17X689353.
26. Szilassy E, Drinkwater J, Hester M, Larkins C, Stanley N, Turner W, Feder G: Making the links between domestic violence and child safeguarding: an evidence-based pilot training for general practice. Health Soc Care Commun. 2016, doi: 10.1111/hsc.12401
27. Greene JC. Mixed methods in social inquiry. 1st ed. San Francisco: Jossey-Bass; 2007.
28. Clarke A. Evidence-based evaluation in different professional domains. In: Shaw I, Greene JC, Mark MM, editors. Handbook of evaluation: policies, programs and practices. Thousand Oaks: Sage; 2006. p. 559–81.
29. Farquhar M, Preston N, Evans CJ, Grande G, Short V, Benalia H, Higginson IJ, Todd C, Morecare. Mixed methods research in the development and evaluation of complex interventions in palliative and end-of-life care: report on the MORECare consensus exercise. J Palliat Med. 2013;16(12):1550–60.
30. Williamson MK, Pirkis J, Pfaff JJ, Tyson O, Sim M, Kerse N, Lautenschlager NT, Stocks NP, Almeida OP. Recruiting and retaining GPs and patients in intervention studies: the DEPS-GP project as a case study. BMC Med Res Methodol. 2007;7:42.
31. Parkinson A, Jorm L, Douglas KA, Gee A, Sargent GM, Lujic S, McRae IS. Recruiting general practitioners for surveys: reflections on the difficulties and some lessons learned. Aust J Prim Health. 2015;21(2):254–8.
32. Brannen J. Mixing methods: The entry of qualitative and quantitative approaches into the research process. Int J Soc Res Methodol. 2005;8(3):173–84.
33. Denzin NK. The research act: a theoretical introduction to sociological methods. New Brunswick: NJ AldineTransaction; 2009.
34. Johnson RB, Onwuegbuzie AJ. Mixed methods research: a research paradigm whose time has come. Educ Res. 2004;33(7):14–26.
35. Miles MB, Huberman AM. Qualitative data analysis: an expanded sourcebook. 2nd ed. Thousand Oaks: Sage Publications; 1994.
36. Pit SW, Vo T, Pyakurel S. The effectiveness of recruitment strategies on general practitioner's survey response rates - a systematic review. BMC Med Res Methodol. 2014;14:76.
37. RCGP: The RCGP guide to the revalidation of general practitioners. Royal College of General Practitioners; 2014
38. SurveyMonkey Inc.: Survey Monkey. San Mateo,California, USA. https://www.surveymonkey.com/. Accessed 1 Mar 2017.
39. RESPONDS training pack. (2015). http://www.bristol.ac.uk/primaryhealthcare/researchthemes/responds/training-pack/. Accessed 1 Mar 2017.
40. RCPCH: Royal College of Paediatrics and Child Health. Safeguarding children and young people: roles and competences for health care staff. Intercollegiate document. 2014. 102.
41. StataCorp. Stata Statistical Software: Release 13. College Station: StataCorp LP; 2013.
42. Szilassy E, Carpenter J, Patsios D, Hackett S. Outcomes of short course interprofessional training in domestic violence and child protection. Violence Against Women. 2013;19(11):1370–83.
43. Krauss A, Chen P. Test-Retest Reliability. In: Lewis-Beck MS, Bryman A, Liao TF, editors. The Sage Encyclopedia of Social Science Research Methods. Thousand Oaks: Sage Publications; 2004. p. 1120–1.
44. Tavakol MRD, Tavakol M, Dennick R. Making sense of Cronbach's alpha. Int J Med Educ. 2011;2:53–5.
45. Acock A. A gentle introduction to Stata. 4th ed. US: Stata Press; 2014.
46. Elliott L, Nerney M, Jones T, Friedmann PD. Barriers to screening for domestic violence. J Gen Intern Med. 2002;17(2):112–6.
47. Saunders DG, Kindy Jr P. Predictors of physicians' responses to woman abuse: the role of gender, background, and brief training. J Gen Intern Med. 1993;8(11):606–9.
48. DeVellis RF. Scale development : theory and applications. 3rd ed. Thousand Oaks: Sage; 2012.

49. Carpenter J, Szilassy E, Patsios D, Hackett S. Outcomes of interagency training to safeguard children: final report to the Department for Children, Schools and Families and the Department of Health. Bristol: University of Bristol; 2010. p. 188.
50. Gabbay J, le May A. Evidence based guidelines or collectively constructed "mindlines?" Ethnographic study of knowledge management in primary care. BMJ. 2004;329(7473):1013.
51. Miller E, McCaw B, Humphreys BL, Mitchell C. Integrating intimate partner violence assessment and intervention into healthcare in the United States: a systems approach. J Womens Health (Larchmt). 2015;24(1):92–9.
52. Minsky-Kelly D, Hamberger LK, Pape DA, Wolff M. We've had training, now what? Qualitative analysis of barriers to domestic violence screening and referral in a health care setting. J Interpers Violence. 2005;20(10):1288–309.
53. Richards L. Handling qualitative data: a practical guide. London Thousand Oaks: SAGE Publications; 2005.
54. Franzosi RP: Content analysis, vol. 1. London: SAGE Publications Ltd; 2008.
55. Sahin D, Yaffe MJ, Sussman T, McCusker J. A mixed studies literature review of family physicians' participation in research. Fam Med. 2014;46(7):503–14.
56. Zaher E, Keogh K, Ratnapalan S. Effect of domestic violence training: systematic review of randomized controlled trials. Canadian Fam Physician Medecin de famille canadien. 2014;60(7):618–24. e340-617.
57. Saunders DG, Anderson D. Evaluation of a domestic violence training for child protection workers & supervisors: Initial results. Child Youth Serv Rev. 2000;22(5):373–95.
58. Devine A, Spencer A, Eldridge S, Norman R, Feder G. Cost-effectiveness of Identification and Referral to Improve Safety (IRIS), a domestic violence training and support programme for primary care: a modelling study based on a randomised controlled trial. BMJ Open. 2012;2:3.
59. Malpass A, Sales K, Johnson M, Howell A, Agnew-Davies R, Feder G. Women's experiences of referral to a domestic violence advocate in UK primary care settings: a service-user collaborative study. Br J Gen Pract. 2014;64(620):e151–158.
60. Yeung H, Chowdhury N, Malpass A, Feder GS. Responding to domestic violence in general practice: a qualitative study on perceptions and experiences. Int J Family Med. 2012;2012:960523.
61. UOB. IRIS. Identification & Referral to Improve Safety. Commissioning guidance. Bristol: University of Bristol; 2011.
62. Williamson E, Jones SK, Ferrari G, Debbonaire T, Feder G, Hester M: Health professionals responding to men for safety (HERMES): feasibility of a general practice training intervention to improve the response to male patients who have experienced or perpetrated domestic violence and abuse. Prim Health Care Res Dev. 2015;16(3):281-8.
63. REPROVIDE. (2016). http://www.bristol.ac.uk/primaryhealthcare/researchthemes/reprovide/. Accessed 1 Mar 2017.

9

What can family medicine providers learn about concussion non-disclosure from former collegiate athletes?

Elizabeth A. Beverly[1,2*], Todd R. Fredricks[1], Andrew Leubitz[1], Benjamin R. Oldach[1], Daniel Kana[1], Michael D. Grant[3], Jonathon Whipps[4] and Emily H. Guseman[1,2]

Abstract

Background: Despite the risks, concussion symptoms often go underreported by athletes, leading to delayed or forgone treatment and increased potential for concussion recurrence. One of the most serious long-term consequences of sports-related concussions is Chronic Traumatic Encephelopathy (CTE), a disorder associated with progressive neurological deterioration. The purpose of this study was to explore former collegiate athletes' understanding of concussions and motivations behind concussion non-disclosure in order to better assist family medicine providers in screening for and managing a history of concussions.

Methods: Informed by the theoretical framework Social Cognitive Theory, we conducted focus groups with former collegiate athletes using a field-tested discussion guide. Discussions were transcribed, coded, and analyzed via content and thematic analyses using NVivo 10 software.

Results: Thirty-two former collegiate athletes (24.5 ± 2.9 years old, 59.4% female, 87.5% white) participated in 7 focus groups. Three predominant themes emerged: 1) Concussions are Part of the Game: Participants believed that concussions were part of sports, and that by agreeing to play a sport they were accepting the inherent risk of concussions. Importantly, many were not familiar with concussion symptoms and what constituted a concussion; 2) Hiding Concussion Symptoms: Participants said they often hid concussion symptoms from coaches and trainers in order to avoid being taken out of or missing games. Participants were able to hide their concussions because most symptoms were indiscernible to others; and 3) Misconceptions about Concussions in Low Contact Sports: Several participants did not understand that concussions could occur in all sports including low contact or noncontact sports. The former athletes who participated in low contact sports and experienced concussions attributed their concussions to personal clumsiness rather than their sport.

Conclusions: Family medicine providers as well as coaches, athletic trainers, teachers, and parents/guardians should reinforce the message that concussions can occur in all sports and inform patients about the signs and symptoms of concussions. Further, providers should ask all patients if they engaged in high school or collegiate athletics; and if yes, to describe their hardest hit to their head in order to obtain a complete medical history.

Keywords: Concussions, Concussion non-disclosure, Chronic traumatic Encephelopathy, Sports, Qualitative methods, Family medicine

* Correspondence: beverle1@ohio.edu
[1]Department of Family Medicine, Ohio University Heritage College of Osteopathic Medicine, Athens, OH 45701, USA
[2]The Diabetes Institute, Ohio University, Athens, OH 45701, USA
Full list of author information is available at the end of the article

Background

Head injuries are prevalent in collision and high contact sports such as soccer, rugby, American football, mixed martial arts, boxing, judo, and karate as well as winter sports such as ice hockey, skiing, ice skating, and snowboarding [1]. Popular sports differ by country and therefore the sport associated with the highest number of head injuries often varies by country. For example, in Japan, judo is the leading cause of catastrophic head injury [1] whereas, in New Zealand, the leading cause of head injury was rugby [2]. In Australia, Australian Rules football, rugby league, and rugby union have the highest rates of heady injury compared to any other team sport in the world, with 3 to 10 concussions per 1000 playing hours [3–6]. Worldwide, the most common sports-related head injury is a concussion or mild traumatic brain injury (mTBI) [1]. The most serious sequela of sports-related concussions include acute subdural hematoma, acute epidural hematoma, cerebral contusion, traumatic cerebrovascular accidents, diffuse brain swelling, diffuse axonal injury, skull fractures, Chronic Traumatic Ecephelopathy (CTE) [1]. Chronic Traumatic Encephelopathy (CTE), a progressive disorder associated with repetitive head trauma [7–9], has received a great deal of attention from researchers and the media in the last several years.

In the United States (US), approximately 3.8 million sports-related concussions occur annually accounting for nearly 10% of all sports-related injuries [10–12]; whereas, approximately 300,000 sports-related head injuries occur in Europe per year [13]. Thirty percent of all sports-related concussions result in emergency department visits [14–16]. Of special interest is neuropathology among former players of American football, particularly those who played at the collegiate and professional levels. Recent reports from a convenience sample of deceased American football players indicates that CTE may be present in as many as 87% of former football players [17] and that age of first football exposure predicts neuropsychiatric impairment in adulthood [18]. Behavioral and mood symptoms among both mild and severe cases of CTE include impulsivity, depression, apathy, anxiety, hopelessness, explosivity, verbal and physical violence, suicidality, substance use, and post-traumatic stress disorder [17, 18]. Cognitive symptoms consist of memory loss, executive dysfunction, attention deficits, language and visuospatial problems, gait instability, and slowness of movement [17, 18]. Findings from a convenience sample of deceased American football players with CTE showed that the most common cause of primary death was neurodengerative [17]. Thus, the high rate of behavioral, mood, and cognitive symptoms as well as neurodegenerative disease observed in cases of CTE are of grave concern for athletes at risk for repetitive head trauma.

Despite the risks, concussion symptoms often go underreported by athletes, leading to delayed or forgone treatment and increased potential for concussion recurrence [19–21]. Signs and symptoms of concussions include but are not limited to: nausea, vomiting, headache, visual problems, loss of consciousness, cognitive impairments (e.g., difficulty concentrating, forgetfulness, confusion), sleep disturbances, and emotional changes (e.g., irritability, sadness, nervousness) [10, 22]. Although most concussion symptoms resolve within a week, symptoms may persist for months to years for some athletes [23, 24]. In recent years, symptom underreporting has driven the emergence of novel testing to develop an objective measure of concussive symptoms; however, symptom-based reporting still remains a key component of concussion evaluation among athletes [10]. Even if symptoms of a concussion are correctly identified and diagnosed, however, there is no consistent evidence-based precedent to determine when an athlete can safely return to play [25]. Despite increased awareness about symptom underreporting and the role symptom reporting plays in concussion evaluation, research that explores athletes' decision-making process to report or not report symptoms is limited.

Exploring athletes' understanding of concussions may be useful information for family medicine providers overseeing the primary care of children, adolescents, and young adults participating in sports. Further, understanding the motivations behind concussion non-disclosure may help family medicine providers communicate with current athletes by helping them navigate conversations via a specific line of questioning during a medical visit. Moreover, former athletes will continue to receive primary care from family medicine providers and providers will need to know their concussion history in order to evaluate the presence, severity, and prognosis of their concussion(s) in order to inform future management. Finally, providers will need to monitor their patients through the days, weeks, months, and years after a head injury and assess the degree of emotional difficulties as well as cognitive, memory, and executive functioning deficits over time. Therefore, the purpose of this qualitative study was to explore former collegiate athletes' understanding of concussions and motivations behind concussion non-disclosure. Our research question was: Why do athletes hide concussions from teammates, coaches, and trainers?

Methods

Research

This qualitative focus group study explored participants' understanding of concussions and motivations behind concussion non-disclosure among graduate and osteopathic medical students who formerly participated in undergraduate collegiate athletics. Focus groups are a qualitative technique in which data are collected through a semi-structured group interview of approximately five to twelve individuals [26]. The premise of focus group research is that attitudes, beliefs, perceptions, and expectations are not developed in isolation but rather through interaction with others [27, 28]. Thus, questions are asked in an interactive group setting where participants are free to talk with other group members. In this study, focus groups were selected to gain insight into athletes' experiences with concussions and concussion non-disclosure in a convenient sample of former collegiate athletes. We followed the consolidated criteria for reporting qualitative research (COREQ) [29].

Sample

Purposive sampling strategies [26] were employed to recruit English-speaking adults who played a collegiate sport (e.g., football, soccer, basketball, lacrosse, field hockey, baseball, softball, wrestling) at the Division I, II, or III level (Note: three participants competed on traveling club teams, in which they had to tryout in order to make the team), and were currently enrolled in a graduate or medical degree program at the University. In the US, collegiate sports are classified by divisions, such that Division I represents the highest level of athletic competition at the largest universities with partial to full athletic scholarships, Division II represents mid-level competition at mid-size universities with fewer financial resources compared to Division I school, and Division III represents lower-level competition at the smallest colleges; Divisions III schools are not allowed to offer athletic scholarships. Based on prior concussion reporting research [30–32], former collegiate athletes were selected to describe their experiences without pressure or fear of repercussions from coaches, trainers, and teammates for participating in the study. Prior diagnosis of a concussion was not required for participation as we were interested in former athletes' understanding of concussions and concussion non-disclosure. Participants were recruited via the University graduate and medical student email listservs containing approximately 5000 students. In the US, approximately 7% of male and female high school students transition to participate in collegiate athletics. Thus, of the 5000 University graduate and medical students, we estimated that 350 students participated in college sports. Potential participants were contacted via email by University owned and matained listservs distributed by the Principal Investigator (EAB) and word of mouth. The research team distributed the recruitment email on October 16, 2013; a reminder email was sent one week later. Students responded to the email to express an interest in participation. All students who expressed an interest to participate were included in the study.

The University Institutional Review Board approved the study protocol IRB number 13X181. All participants provided written informed consent prior to participation and received a $15.00 gift card as compensation for their time. Participants were explicitly informed that there were no "right" or "wrong" responses to the focus group questions, and that none of the information they provided would be used to evaluate their academic performance at the University or medical school in any way. Further, participants were told they could decline to participate at any time in the study process without explanation.

Theoretical framework

The semi-structured focus group discussion guide was based on Bandura's Social Cognitive Theory (SCT) [33]. Implementing a theoretical framework was essential to understanding factors that influence concussion non-disclosure. SCT may help describe how environmental influences affect an individual's reporting decisions about a concussion [33]. SCT represents the dynamic interaction of individual-level behavioral, personal, and environmental factors as demonstrated through a triadic causation reciprocal model [33]. Specifically, an athlete's environment may influence concussion reporting behavior by influencing how he/she perceives what will happen after reporting a concussion. As outlined by the tenets of SCT, the environment directly influences the athlete's behavior of reporting symptoms. For example, an athlete may witness a teammate reporting a concussion and receiving backlash from coaches and other teammates, therefore, influencing the likelihood of that athlete reporting a concussion. Today's media adds another dimension to the athlete's environment. Not only does the athlete have his/her own experience and teammates' experiences with concussions, but also their attitude and behavior may be influenced by high profile athletes' actions [34]. Thus, environmental factors may contribute to the stigma surrounding concussions and concussion reporting.

Data collection

The research team devised a semi-structured discussion guide using the SCT framework and field-tested it for flow and clarity of the questions with a group of five participants (see Table 1). Once the discussion guide was finalized, data collection commenced. Focus groups were segmented by gender to account for potential gender differences in concussion non-disclosure. Specifically, we separated female participants from male participants by focus groups to remove any undue influence in the discussion of sensitive information about the understanding of concussions and motivations behind concussion non-disclosure. This segmentation plan allowed researchers to use shared experiences as a springboard for deeper examination and discussion of related issues, thus promoting greater depth in understanding without the potential influence or constraint exerted by members of the

Table 1 Focus group discussion guide for study participants

1.	What is a concussion?
	Probe. What are the signs and symptoms of a concussion?
2.	Have you ever experienced a concussion? Please describe.
	Probe. Did a trainer/coach or physician diagnose you with a concussion?
	Probe. Did you diagnose yourself?
	Probe. What symptoms did you experience?
	Probe. Did you miss any practice time or games?
3.	Have you ever hit heads with an opponent or teammate while playing your sport? Please describe.
	Probe. How did you feel after it happened? How did you feel the next day?
	Probe. Did you miss any practice time or games?
	Probe. Did you think this could have been a concussion? Why or why not?
4.	If you have ever had a concussion, did you tell anyone at the time that it happened or did you hide it?
	Probe. Why did you hide it? Please explain
5.	Did any of your teammates every have a concussion and hide it from a coach or trainer?
	Probe: Why do you think they hid it? Please explain.
6.	Did you ever play your sport when you should not have because of a concussion or head injury? Please explain.
7.	What did the coach expect from you as a player if you had a concussion or head injury (diagnosed concussion or not diagnosed concussion?)
8.	How did you feel if a teammate did not play in a game because of a concussion or head injury?
9.	Did a coach/trainer ever tell you to play even if you had a concussion or head injury?
10.	Did a parent ever tell you to play even if you had a concussion or head injury?
11.	Did fear of getting a concussion affect how you played the game?
12.	Is there a stigma in your sport about concussions? If so, what is it?
	Probe. Do you think this differs by gender?
13.	What advice would you give current athletes playing your sport about concussions?
14.	What advice would you give coaches, physicians, and parents about concussions?

opposite gender. Focus groups continued until all interested students had participated.

Focus groups were conducted at University sites (conference rooms and study rooms). Trained moderators asked participants broad, open-ended questions about their understanding of concussions, personal and teammates' experiences with concussions, and concussion non-disclosure. A female moderator, an Assistant Profession in Family Medicine (EAB), conducted the women's focus groups and male moderators, three medical students and one Lecturer in Psychology (BRO, AL, DK, MDG), took turns conducting the men's groups. All moderators were trained by an expert in qualitative methods (EAB). When the medical students and Lecturer in Psychology (BRO, AL, DK, MDG) were not serving as the moderator, they served as co-moderators for the focus groups by writing notes to capture key points (i.e., written accounts of what happened during focus groups) as well as observations (e.g., participant nonverbal communication, expressions, behaviors) about the discussions. At the end of each focus group, moderators and co-moderators met to share impressions and observations. All focus group discussions were audio-recorded and transcribed verbatim; participants' names and identifiers were removed to protect their confidentiality. Participants also completed a brief demographic form and history of head injury questionnaire. Importantly, on the demographic form, participants were asked to name the sport they participated in during college. Sports were classified as collision sports or sports in which players collide as part of the game (e.g., rugby, American football), high contact sports or sports which require physical contact between players (e.g., soccer, lacrosse, basketball, water polo), and low contact sports or sports that have minimal or no means of touching other players (e.g., track and field, swimming).

Data analysis

The multidisciplinary research team, consisting of a health behaviorist/qualitative methodologist (EAB), three medical students (AL, BRO, DK), and a health psychologist (MDG), analyzed data using content and thematic analyses [27]. The research team included two professors (EAB, MDG) who teach at the university where the participants attended. In addition, the three medical students (AL, BRO, DK) were current students at the medical school and peers of some of the participants. Specifically, the research team summarized the discussion following each focus group. Next, team members (EAB, AL, BRO, DK, MDG) performed content analysis by independently marking and categorizing key words, phrases, and texts to identify codes [35, 36]. The research team applied descriptive coding to describe the data and analytic or theoretical coding to explain why what was occurring in the data might be happening [37]. Transcripts were reviewed to resolve discrepancies through group consensus (EAB, AL, BRO, DK, MDG). No negative or deviant cases were excluded from the analysis [38]. This process continued until saturation was reached; that is, until no new codes emerged. After all transcripts were coded and reviewed, one member of the research team (EAB) entered the coded transcripts in NVivo 10 software (QSR International, Victoria, Australia) to further organize and group codes. The team (EAB, AL, BRO, DK, MDG) then met to agree on final themes, or patterns, that linked substantial portions of the data across focus groups [39]. The research team (EAB, AL, BRO, DK, MDG) selected themes that characterized the participants' perceptions and experiences from data that occurred multiple times, both within and across transcripts. Each theme included words expressed by the participants to demonstrate that the concepts were grounded in the data. After the team coded and reviewed all transcripts, three clinician/researchers (TRF - family physician, EHG - clinical exercise physiologist, JW - clinical exercise physiologist) reviewed the codes and themes to achieve researcher corroboration [40].

Rigor

To support credibility (validity), we triangulated the investigators with experts from different disciplines (i.e., health behaviorist/qualitative methodologist, health psychology, medicine, exercise physiology); analyst triangulation provided a check on selective perceptions as well as a means to identify blind spots in the analysis. Further, five participants reviewed the findings to achieve participant corroboration [41]. Transferability (external validity) was supported via rich descriptions and verbatim quotations included in the data. To support dependability (reliability) of the data, a researcher not involved with the study conducted an external audit to examine both the process of the research study and to evaluate whether or not the findings, interpretations and conclusions were supported by the data [38]. Confirmability (objectivity) of the data was supported via tracking the decision-making process with an audit trail, which is a detailed description of the research steps conducted from the development of the project to the presentation of findings [42].

Results

Thirty-two former collegiate athletes (24.5 ± 2.9 years old, 59.4% female, 87.5% Non-Hispanic white, estimated response rate 9.1%; see Table 2) participated in 7 total focus groups (4 female focus groups and 3 male focus groups). Note, one of the male focus groups had 3 participants and another had 2 participants. These focus groups were supposed to have more male participants; however, several individuals did not attend leaving a small number of participants. We chose to move forward and conduct these focus groups with the small number of participants; the data collected were adequate and of high quality.

On average, participants competed in collegiate sports for 3.6 ± 0.8 years. A little over half of participants (*n* = 18; 56.3%) received an athletic scholarship while competing in their sport. Participants competed in the following sports: soccer (*n* = 4), track and field (*n* = 4), football (*n* = 3), tennis (*n* = 3), basketball (*n* = 3), field hockey (n = 3), baseball (*n* = 2), wrestling (*n* = 2), lacrosse (*n* = 2), rugby (*n* = 2), softball (*n* = 2), volleyball (*n* = 2), swimming (*n* = 2), ice hockey (*n* = 1), and golf (*n* = 1), with four participants competing in multiple sports.

Table 2 Demographic and Collegiate Sport Characteristics of Study Participants (*n* = 32)

Variable	n (%)
Age (years)	24.5 ± 2.9
Education (years)	17.3 ± 1.1
Enrolled in Master's degree program	15 (46.9)
Enrolled in Doctor of Philosophy program	3 (9.4)
Enrolled in Doctor of Osteopathic Medicine program	14 (43.8)
Gender	
Female (%)	19 (59.4)
Male (%)	13 (40.6)
Race (%)	
Non-Hispanic White	28 (87.5)
Asian	1 (3.1)
Black	1 (3.1)
Hispanic	1 (3.1)
Mixed Race	1 (3.1)
Competed in collegiate sport(s) (years)	3.6 ± 0.8
Division Level	
Division I (%)	14 (43.8)
Division II (%)	6 (18.8)
Division III (%)	9 (28.1)
Traveling Club Team (%)	3 (9.4)
Competed in collegiate sport with head gear (%)	12 (37.5)
Athletic Scholarship (%)	18 (56.3)
Training in concussion recognition with collegiate program (%)	12 (37.5)

A history of 48 head injuries were self-reported, with several participants reporting multiple concussions. Fifteen participants (46.9%) reported a concussion accompanied by a loss of consciousness and/or confusion, and of these, only ten (32.1%) reported that their concussion was medically diagnosed. None of the participants reported having early or late seizures accompanied with their concussions; however, two participants reported a concussion requiring an overnight hospital stay.

Focus group themes

Three predominant themes emerged from the focus group discussions: *Concussions are Part of the Game, Hiding Concussion Symptoms*, and *Misconceptions about Concussions in Low Contact Sports.* We included identifiers, indicating focus group number, gender, and ID, with quotations illustrating the themes.

Theme 1: Concussions are part of the game

Participants in all 7 focus groups recognized the frequency and seriousness of concussions. Interestingly, most participants believed that concussions were inherent in sports, particularly for collision sports and high contact sports like football, soccer, ice hockey, and rugby. They felt that by agreeing to play a sport, they were accepting the inherent risk of concussions, as evidenced by the following quotations:

> "I think that certain sports [there] are inherent risks that you're going to be hitting your head more, like hockey, football, soccer, and sports like that." (Focus Group 2, Female ID 6)

> "In general, I think at least like for my team in rugby, it's the mentality of buck up, whatever it is, and concussions are going to happen so just deal with it." (Focus Group 4, Female ID 16)

> "I think everyone would kind of agree with this, by agreeing to play a sport and be a part of the team you're kind of taking in those risks .... It comes with playing the sport." (Focus Group 5, Male ID 23)

> "It almost seems like part of the game. It's like yeah, you're playing football. You get hit. It hurts. You've got to be tough." (Focus Group 6, Male ID 30)

Nearly all participants expressed a desire to keep playing even if they witnessed or experienced a concussion themselves. Despite knowing the risks, participants cited passion and competitiveness as reasons for playing with a concussion. For example, one male participant and one female participant described their rationale for continuing to play if and when they had a concussion:

> "I would probably play myself if I had a concussion and it was a big game. Yeah, I wouldn't care. It's more about the competition than being safe. Even though there are high risks and I know what the risks are, I'd probably still play through it, and that's probably not a good idea." (Focus Group 7, Male ID 31)

> "I knew exactly what the risks were, especially when it happened my junior year because I was much farther into my education, but what I logicked [sic] out with myself was, I play tennis, there's not a lot of things I could contact again, and I mean if I die, I die doing something I love, worst-case scenario." (Focus Group 2, Female ID 9)

Importantly, some participants did not appear to fully understand what qualified as a concussion. Many referenced "seeing stars" or "black shiny stuff" at one point or another but continued to play through it. They rationalized this as head injuries were an expected part of playing sports:

> "It's [concussion] the sport. We don't think of it as a concussion. I don't want to say every time like I've seen stars from a head [hit] or that it happened hundreds of times in wrestling, but that to me isn't a concussion. That's just when you hit your head like at the house or something like that. I didn't lose consciousness or anything like that, just kind of got bumped a little bit. I mean, if that is a concussion, then [expletive]." (Focus Group 6, Male ID 29)

Theme 2: Hiding concussion symptoms

Participants in each focus group discussed hiding concussion symptoms in order to avoid being taken out of or missing games. Some participants withheld information from coaches and trainers while others misrepresented or fibbed about their concussions. The following series of quotations demonstrates the frequency of hiding concussion symptoms in the former collegiate athletes in the study:

> "I got to the point where, I mean I know it's wrong, but you're an athlete and you want to get back in there, so you flub some stuff." (Focus Group 2, Female ID 9)

> "I myself did this and other people; we just wouldn't tell people if we were injured until after the game." (Focus Group 4, Female ID 16)

> "I know I did that myself sometimes because I wanted to play. That's why you're there and you knew if you showed these symptoms that you'd get pulled, so you'd just sort of hide it or say nothing's wrong when they come up and talk to you." (Focus Group 5, Male ID 27)

> "I'd say we'd all experienced it at one point or another. And I remember actually one guy specifically saying like, 'Oh, did you see the black shiny stuff?' I was like yeah. He was like, 'Oh, okay.' And that was that. We just kept playing, but I never told coaches or trainers or anyone. I guess I thought that if I did, then they were going to make me come out of the game and stop playing. And I felt like I needed to be there and I was still able to do it well enough to be in there. So I was like, oh man, I don't want to come out because if I do, then I might have to miss the rest of the game. I was like well, I'll just tough it out and see what happens. Hopefully, I'll make it the rest of the game. I did so." (Focus Group 6, Male ID 30)

Participants also acknowledged that hiding concussion symptoms was possible in part because most symptoms were indiscernible to the outside observer. As articulated by these two participants:

> "It's one of those injuries where there aren't a lot of symptoms other than what's reported. For example, an ankle, there's bruising and swelling. You know, it's hurt. But I think pressure from coaches, pressure from other players, and people just want to play, I think that's a large part of [why] people play. Other people play through other injuries even when they're bad and they can get worse, but I think this is one of them that, because there's no physical sign, there's no bruising ... you don't even look bad." (Focus Group 7, Male ID 31)

> "You know it's serious, but at the same time, I feel fine. It's happened before, whatever. We're all pretty intelligent, but we still have those innate thoughts of 'Is it really that big of a deal?' It's hard to see the long, long road that I am going to lose memory quicker or something crazy like that. We can't put it all together in one big piece ... You probably should say something, but at the same time if you're not having the symptoms of throwing up and vomiting, you're not going to have the drive to really get pushed to say it [to a coach]." (Focus Group 6, Male ID 29)

Along these lines, several participants speculated that some athletes may hide concussion symptoms so as to not disappoint coaches and teammates. Participants explained that the invisibility of concussions called into question an athlete's toughness and dedication to the team. For example, these participants described circumstances in which a player's reputation may influence coaches' and teammates' impression of an athlete's concussion:

> "I think concussions are hard because a lot of what your teammates and coaches will think will probably reflect on what you've shown thus far in terms of how you respond to difficult situations or injuries. So if you're thought of as that tough kind of person, they're not going to doubt your concussion. But if maybe you're looked at as being softer, they're going be like, oh, this is just typical – this is what they do, they're fine. Because a concussion isn't something you can physically see, like a broken arm or something, so it's something that people can doubt." (Focus Group 3, Female ID 10)

> "Someone who's commonly hurt, you'd kind of like roll your eyes at them. But somebody who's never hurt, I think that they would be treated differently." (Focus Group 3, Female ID 17)

> "Well, it depends on the person. [Laughter from the group]. If the person faked a lot of stuff, but if the person worked hard and was a pretty tough individual, you'd think all right, he must be hurting there." (Focus Group 5, Male ID 20)

Theme 3: Misconceptions about concussions in low contact sports

While all participants were familiar with the incidence of concussions in sports, many did not understand that concussions could occur in any and all sports. Some participants felt that concussions were limited to only collision sports or high contact sports. Further, athletes in low contact sports or sports with minimal physical contact with other athletes (e.g., tennis, track and field, swimming) who experienced concussions, attributed their injuries to personal clumsiness rather than their sport. As demonstrated by these quotations:

> "I threw a shot put and it didn't go away, it went in my head because I didn't know what I was doing, yeah. But I'm clumsy." (Focus group 2, Female ID 7)

> "People are like, 'You play tennis and you had a concussion?' It's like, okay, I'm kind of clumsy, but yeah, it can happen ... I mean what are the odds." (Focus group 2, Female ID 9)

> "I think it's more about perspective, so you could look at it two ways. Football is more likely to get head injuries, so if someone had a concussion oh, okay, that makes sense. It was football. On the other hand, if it happens to someone in track, it's like oh, wow, really? Okay. I guess it's a fluke, but it's probably not as bad as someone who would get it in football just because of the high contact or high speed, high force, et cetera." (Focus group 7, Male ID 32)

Additionally, a few participants chose not report their head injuries to coaches and/or trainers because they felt it was embarrassing to have a concussion in a low contact sport. For example, this female participant described a head on collision with her teammate while swimming sprints in the same lane of the pool:

> "I ran into someone head-on and we were both like sprinting and I had a headache. No one told me I had a concussion, I didn't want to go to the trainer ... but I was really confused. I had a really bad headache the whole week and I just had trouble thinking and stuff ... That's why it's really embarrassing, because who does that?" (Focus group 3, Female ID 14)

Discussion

In this qualitative focus group study, we explored former collegiate athletes' understanding of concussions and their motivations behind concussion non-disclosure in sports. Our findings confirm a relatively high rate of concussions among former collegiate athletes, with a history of 48 total head injuries and 10 self-reported medically diagnosed concussions. Participants believed that concussions were part of sports, and that by agreeing to play a sport they were accepting the inherent risk of concussions. Of particular importance, many were not familiar with concussion symptoms and what constituted a concussion. These participants referenced symptoms of concussions (e.g., seeing stars) but continued to play through them. Participants also shared that they often hid concussion symptoms from coaches and trainers in order to avoid being taken out of or missing games. Participants explained that they were able to hide their concussions because most symptoms were invisible to coaches and trainers. Lastly, several participants did not understand that concussions could occur in all sports including low contact sports. The former athletes who participated in low contact sports and experienced concussions attributed their concussions to personal clumsiness rather than their sport. These findings highlight the importance of continued concussion awareness education among collegiate athletes, especially for athletes in low contact sports. Further, these findings draw attention to the importance of obtaining a detailed medical history so that family medical providers can integrate a history of concussions in current and future treatment plans.

Our research builds on earlier work exploring concussion non-disclosure among athletes. One study with high school athletes found that participants did not report concussions due to perceived lack of severity, not wanting to be removed from practice and/or a game, and not wanting to let down teammates and/or coaches [32]. Another study found that athletes did not report concussions because they lacked access to athletic trainers or other medical professionals, did not fully understanding the consequences of concussions, expressed a desire to play through the pain, and swore allegiance to the team [30]. Interestingly, a recent study found that US high school athletes with access to an athletic trainer had more knowledge about concussions; however, increased knowledge was not associated an increased likelihood to report suspected concussions [43]. A study with male collegiate football players' identified minimization of risk, misconceptions about the long-term effects of concussions, diagnostic uncertainty, pressure from coaches, and athletic and social identity as reasons for not reporting concussions [31]. Finally, a study evaluating the effect of mandated US high school concussion education showed that while the number of athletes reporting that they received concussion education increased, the number of athletes reporting that they sought medical attention did not increase [44]. Although our study only included former collegiate athletes, almost all collegiate athletes also participate in high school athletics, so our findings within this studied can be applied to high-school athletics as well. These same themes emerged in our focus groups, which suggest that high school and collegiate athletes lack a complete understanding of concussions including concussions are not a normal part of playing a game, what constitutes a concussion, and the long-term consequences of a concussion or repeated concussions. Providing access to athletic trainers, which is standard practice in collegiate sports in the US, may improve concussion knowledge [43]. In addition, efforts to develop and disseminate evidence-based concussion education programs are needed to increase knowledge of symptoms and improve self-reporting of concussions.

Worldwide, millions of students and young adults participate in sports. Given the high rate of sports-related concussions, family medicine providers should ask adolescents and young adults about prior experiences with head injuries at sport physicals. This is particularly important during the preparticipation sports evaluation [45]. In athletes with a history of concussions, providers should determine the number of concussions, how they occurred, whether or not they lost consciousness, how long the symptoms lasted, and how soon they went back to playing the sport [45]. Providers should explain to patients that they are asking these questions because it is important to have a complete history of head injuries, and that they are not trying to keep them from playing sports. If a patient appears hesitant, providers should reiterate that they will not interfere with them playing sports, and that they only want to know their complete history in order to provider better care for them in the future. In addition, providers should perform a complete neurologic exam on athletes with a history of concussions [45]. If an athlete shows signs and symptoms of a concussion or postconcussion syndrome, the athlete should not be cleared for participation until his/her symptoms have resolved [45].

For adult patients, family medicine providers should ask if they engaged in high school or collegiate athletics. If yes, providers should ask if they were ever hit so hard they saw stars, could not remember the next play, or were asked to sit on the bench for a few minutes. Another approach is to ask patients to describe their hardest hit to the head. Follow-up questions should include if they received medical help or were taken to the hospital. This line of questioning is important given many of the participants in this study were not familiar with what constituted a concussion, and family practitioners need this information in order to provide longitudinal care for their patients. Further, symptoms of chronic traumatic encephalopathy (CTE) typically occur eight to ten years after repetitive head trauma [17, 46–49]. Thus, providers need to probe patients about a history of head injuries before they present with behavioral, mood, and/or cognitive symptoms of CTE. Along these lines, family medicine providers need to be familiar with current principles of concussion diagnosis and management to prevent long-term consequences like CTE. However, recent research shows gaps in the knowledge of concussion diagnosis and management among primary care providers [50–53]. Thus, continued efforts are needed to train and educate current and future providers to improve the care of athletes with head injuries.

Limitations

Study limitations include the homogeneity of the study sample with regards to setting, sample size, race/ethnicity, and self-reported data. The study was conducted at one Midwestern university, with a small number of former collegiate athletes. Next, self-reported data were vulnerable to social desirability bias. To minimize bias, the researchers informed participants that their responses were confidential and could not be linked back to their personal identity. The researchers also emphasized the voluntary nature of participation and explicitly informed the participants that their responses had no bearing on their student status. Further, the study sample was predominantly white (87.5%); thus, future mixed method is needed to confirm the themes in a larger, more diverse athlete population. Lastly, the authors chose former collegiate athletes as participants in the study to enable them to speak openly about their experiences with concussions without fear of repercussion from coaches, trainers, or teammates. However, this choice may have resulted in different findings compared to a population of current athletes.

Conclusions

Recent research on CTE underscores the need for family medicine providers to address head injuries across the lifespan. Family medicine providers are uniquely positioned to address the risks associated with concussions at all levels of sport participation – before, during, and after. Family medicine providers have the most frequent opportunities to speak with athletes of all ages at well-patient visits, sick visits, sport physicals, etc. This can include youth athletes in low and high contact sports as well as athletes in recreational or intramural leagues. In office discussions should include routine questions about hard hits to the head and "seeing stars," not necessarily concussions given that many athletes have an incomplete understanding of concussions, and talk about the signs and symptoms of concussions. By not being affiliated with the team, family medicine practitioners can provide a non-biased third-party evaluation on concussion, perhaps improving concussion recognition and treatment in athletes across sports and ages. Future research is needed to create a simple questionnaire designed to measure patients' "bumps, dings, seeing of stars" in family practice to supplement the more sophisticated concussion screening tools. In addition, qualitative research with current high school and collegiate athletes is needed to inform a line of questioning for family medicine providers to encourage current athletes to disclose head injuries to providers.

Abbreviation

CTE: chronic traumatic encephalopathy

Acknowledgements

We thank the participants who shared their experiences and perceptions with us.

Funding

This work was supported by The Ohio University Heritage College of Osteopathic Medicine.

Authors' contributions

EAB, TRF, AL, BRO, DK, and MDG provided substantial contributions to conception and design of the study; EAB, AL, BRO, DK, and MDG acquired the data and conducted the qualitative data analysis; EAB, AL, BRO, DK, and MDG provided substantial contributions to the interpretation of data; EAB, TRF, JW, and EHG drafted the article; EAB, MDG, JW, and EHG revised the article critically for important intellectual content; and EAB, TRF, AL, BRO, DK, MDG, JW, and EHG have read and approved the final version of the manuscript to be published.

Competing interests

The authors declare that they have no competing interests.

Author details

[1]Department of Family Medicine, Ohio University Heritage College of Osteopathic Medicine, Athens, OH 45701, USA. [2]The Diabetes Institute, Ohio University, Athens, OH 45701, USA. [3]Department of Psychology, Ohio University, Athens, OH 45701, USA. [4]The Graduate College, Ohio University, Athens, OH 45701, USA.

References

1. Nagahiro S, Mizobuchi Y. Current topics in sports-related head injuries: a review. Neurol Med Chir. 2014;54:878–86.
2. King D, Gissane C, Brughelli M, Hume PA, Harawira J. Sport-related concussions in New Zealand: a review of 10 years of Accident Compensation Corporation moderate to severe claims and costs. J Sci Med Sport. 2014;17:250–5.
3. Makdissi M, McCrory P, Ugoni A, Darby D, Brukner P. A prospective study of postconcussive outcomes after return to play in Australian football. Am J Sports Med. 2009;37:877–83.
4. Makdissi M, Davis G, McCrory P. Updated guidelines for the management of sports-related concussion in general practice. Aust Fam Physician. 2014; 43:94–9.
5. Kemp SP, Hudson Z, Brooks JH, Fuller CW. The epidemiology of head injuries in English professional rugby union. Clin J Sport Med. 2008;18: 227–34.

6. Hinton-Bayre AD, Geffen G, Friis P. Presentation and mechanisms of concussion in professional rugby league football. J Sci Med Sport. 2004;7: 400–4.
7. McKee AC, Cairns NJ, Dickson DW, Folkerth RD, Keene CD, Litvan I, et al. The first NINDS/NIBIB consensus meeting to define neuropathological criteria for the diagnosis of chronic traumatic encephalopathy. Acta Neuropathol. 2016; 131:75–86.
8. Omalu BI, DeKosky ST, Minster RL, Kamboh MI, Hamilton RL, Wecht CH. Chronic traumatic encephalopathy in a National Football League player. Neurosurgery. 2005;57:128–34.
9. Omalu BI, DeKosky ST, Hamilton RL, Minster RL, Kamboh MI, Shakir AM, et al. Chronic traumatic encephalopathy in a national football league player: part II. Neurosurgery. 2006;59:1086–92.
10. Harmon KG, Drezner JA, Gammons M, Guskiewicz KM, Halstead M, Herring SA, et al. American medical Society for Sports Medicine position statement: concussion in sport. Br J Sports Med. 2013;47:15–26.
11. Gessel LM, Fields SK, Collins CL, Dick RW, Comstock RD. Concussions among United States high school and collegiate athletes. J Athl Train. 2007;42: 495–503.
12. Powell JW, Barber-Foss KD. Traumatic brain injury in high school athletes. JAMA. 1999;282:958–63.
13. Thurman DJ, Branche CM, Sniezek JE. The epidemiology of sports-related traumatic brain injuries in the United States: recent developments. J Head Trauma Rehabil. 1998;13:1–8.
14. Meehan WP 3rd, d'Hemecourt P, Comstock RD. High school concussions in the 2008-2009 academic year: mechanism, symptoms, and management. Am J Sports Med. 2010;38:2405–9.
15. CDC. Nonfatal traumatic brain injuries related to sports and recreation activities among persons aged ≤19 years--United States, 2001–2009. Morb Mortal Wkly Rep. 2011;60:1337–42.
16. Bakhos LL, Lockhart GR, Myers R, Linakis JG. Emergency department visits for concussion in young child athletes. Pediatr. 2010;126:e550–6.
17. Mez J, Daneshvar DH, Kiernan PT, Abdolmohammadi B, Alvarez VE, Huber BR, et al. Clinicopathological evaluation of chronic traumatic encephalopathy in players of American football. JAMA. 2017;318:360–70.
18. Alosco ML, Kasimis AB, Stamm JM, Chua AS, Baugh CM, Daneshvar DH, et al. Age of first exposure to American football and long-term neuropsychiatric and cognitive outcomes. Transl Psychiatry. 2017;7:e1236.
19. Kroshus E, Baugh CM, Daneshvar DH, Viswanath K. Understanding concussion reporting using a model based on the theory of planned behavior. J Adolesc Health. 2014;54:269–74.
20. McCrea M, Hammeke T, Olsen G, Leo P, Guskiewicz K. Unreported concussion in high school football players: implications for prevention. Clin J Sport Med. 2004;14:13–7.
21. Torres DM, Galetta KM, Phillips HW, Dziemianowicz EM, Wilson JA, Dorman ES, et al. Sports-related concussion: anonymous survey of a collegiate cohort. Neurol Clin Pract. 2013;3:279–87.
22. McCrory P, Meeuwisse W, Aubry M, Cantu B, Dvorak J, Echemendia R, et al. Consensus statement on concussion in sport - the 4th international conference on concussion in sport held in Zurich, November 2012. Phys Ther Sport. 2013;14:e1–e13.
23. Guskiewicz KM, McCrea M, Marshall SW, Cantu RC, Randolph C, Barr W, et al. Cumulative effects associated with recurrent concussion in collegiate football players: the NCAA concussion study. JAMA. 2003;290:2549–55.
24. McCrory P, Johnston K, Meeuwisse W, Aubry M, Cantu R, Dvorak J, et al. Summary and agreement statement of the 2nd international conference on concussion in sport, Prague 2004. Br J Sports Med. 2005;39:196–204.
25. Giza CC, Kutcher JS, Ashwal S, Barth J, Getchius TS, Gioia GA, et al. Summary of evidence-based guideline update: evaluation and management of concussion in sports: report of the guideline development Subcommittee of the American Academy of neurology. Neurology. 2013;80:2250–7.
26. Morse J, Field P. Qualitative research methods for health Profesionals. 2nd ed. Thousand Oaks: Sage Publications; 1995.
27. Krueger R, Casey M. Focus groups: a practical guide for applied research. 2nd ed. Thousand Oaks: Sage Publications, Inc; 2000.
28. Morgan D. Focus groups as qualitative research. Newbury Park: Sage; 1988.
29. Tong A, Sainsbury P, Craig J. Consolidated criteria for reporting qualitative research (COREQ): a 32-item checklist for interviews and focus groups. Int J Qual Health Care. 2007;19:349–57.
30. Sanderson J, Weathers M, Snedaker K, Gramlich K. "I was able to still do my job on the field and keep playing": an investigation of female and male athletes' experiences with (not) reporting concussions. Commun Sport. 2017;5:267–87.
31. Lininger MR, Wayment HA, Huffman AH, Craig DI, Irving LH. An exploratory study on concussion-reporting behaviors from collegiate student Athletes' perspectives. Athl Train Sports Health Care. 2017;9:71–80.
32. Register-Mihalik JK, Guskiewicz KM, McLeod TC, Linnan LA, Mueller FO, Marshall SW. Knowledge, attitude, and concussion-reporting behaviors among high school athletes: a preliminary study. J Athl Train. 2013;48:645–53.
33. Bandura A. Health promotion by social cognitive means. Health Educ Behav. 2004;31:143–64.
34. Anderson E, Kian EM. Examining media contestation of masculinity and head trauma in the National Football League. Men Masc. 2012;15:152–73.
35. Content Analysis KK. An introduction to its methodology. 2nd ed. Thousand Oaks: Sage Publications; 2004.
36. Pope C, Mays N. Qualitative research in health care. 2nd ed. London: BMJ Books; 2000.
37. Miles MB, Huberman AM. Qualitative data analysis: an expanded sourcebook. 2nd ed. Thousand Oaks: SAGE Publications, Inc.; 1994.
38. Lincoln Y, Guba E. Naturalistic inquiry. New York: Sage Publications; 1985.
39. Morse JM, Field P. Nursing research: the application of qualitative approaches. 2nd ed. London: Chapman and Hall; 1996.
40. Trochim W, Donnelly JP, Arora K. Research methods: the essential Knowledge Base. 2nd ed. Boston: Cengage Learning; 2016.
41. Denzin N. The research act: a theoretical introduction to sociological methods. 2nd ed. New York City: McGraw-Hill; 1978.
42. Russell CK, Gregory DM. Evaluation of qualitative research studies. Evid Based Nurs. 2003;6:36–40.
43. Wallace J, Covassin T, Nogle S, Gould D, Kovan J. Knowledge of concussion and reporting behaviors in high school athletes with or without access to an athletic trainer. J Athl Train. 2017;52:228–35.
44. Carroll-Alfano M. Mandated high school concussion education and collegiate Athletes' understanding of concussion. J Athl Train. 2017;52:689–97.
45. Mirabelli MH, Devine MJ, Singh J, Mendoza M. The Preparticipation sports evaluation. Am Fam Physician. 2015;92:371–6.
46. McKee AC, Cantu RC, Nowinski CJ, Hedley-Whyte ET, Gavett BE, Budson AE, et al. Chronic traumatic encephalopathy in athletes: progressive tauopathy after repetitive head injury. J Neuropathol Exp Neurol. 2009;68:709–35.
47. Robbins CA, Daneshvar DH, Picano JD, Gavett BE, Baugh CM, Riley DO, et al. Self-reported concussion history: impact of providing a definition of concussion. Open Access J Sports Med. 2014;5:99–103.
48. Stamm JM, Bourlas AP, Baugh CM, Fritts NG, Daneshvar DH, Martin BM, et al. Age of first exposure to football and later-life cognitive impairment in former NFL players. Neurology. 2015;84:1114–20.
49. Stamm JM, Koerte IK, Muehlmann M, Pasternak O, Bourlas AP, Baugh CM, et al. Age at first exposure to football is associated with altered Corpus callosum white matter microstructure in former professional football players. J Neurotrauma. 2015;32:1768–76.
50. Zonfrillo MR, Master CL, Grady MF, Winston FK, Callahan JM, Arbogast KB. Pediatric providers' self-reported knowledge, practices, and attitudes about concussion. Pediatrics. 2012;130:1120–5.
51. Mann A, Tator CH, Carson JD. Concussion diagnosis and management: knowledge and attitudes of family medicine residents. Can Fam Physician. 2017;63:460–6.
52. Ryu WH, Feinstein A, Colantonio A, Streiner DL, Dawson DR. Early identification and incidence of mild TBI in Ontario. Can J Neurol Sci. 2009; 36:429–35.
53. Zemek R, Eady K, Moreau K, Farion KJ, Solomon B, Weiser M, et al. Knowledge of paediatric concussion among front-line primary care providers. Paediatr Child Health. 2014;19:475–80.

10

Implementing new care models: learning from the Greater Manchester demonstrator pilot experience

Rebecca Elvey[1*], Simon Bailey[1], Kath Checkland[1], Anne McBride[1], Stephen Parkin[2], Katy Rothwell[3] and Damian Hodgson[1]

Abstract

Background: Current health policy focuses on improving accessibility, increasing integration and shifting resources from hospitals to community and primary care. Initiatives aimed at achieving these policy aims have supported the implementation of various 'new models of care', including general practice offering 'additional availability' appointments during evenings and at weekends. In Greater Manchester, six 'demonstrator sites' were funded: four sites delivered additional availability appointments, other services included case management and rapid response. The aim of this paper is to explore the factors influencing the implementation of services within a programme designed to improve access to primary care. The paper consists of a qualitative process evaluation undertaken within provider organisations, including general practices, hospitals and care homes.

Methods: Semi-structured interviews, with the data subjected to thematic analysis.

Results: Ninety-one people participated in interviews. Six key factors were identified as important for the establishment and running of the demonstrators: information technology; information governance; workforce and organisational development; communications and engagement; supporting infrastructure; federations and alliances. These factors brought to light challenges in the attempt to provide new or modify existing services. Underpinning all factors was the issue of trust; there was consensus amongst our participants that trusting relationships, particularly between general practices, were vital for collaboration. It was also crucial that general practices trusted in the integrity of anyone external who was to work with the practice, particularly if they were to access data on the practice computer system. A dialogical approach was required, which enabled staff to see themselves as active rather than passive participants.

Conclusions: The research highlights various challenges presented by the context within which extended access is implemented. Trust was the fundamental underlying issue; there was consensus amongst participants that trusting relationships were vital for effective collaboration in primary care.

Keywords: General practice, Qualitative research, Primary health care, Health services evaluation, Organizational innovation, Access to health care

* Correspondence: rebecca.elvey@manchester.ac.uk
[1]The University of Manchester, Oxford Road, Manchester M13 9PL, UK
Full list of author information is available at the end of the article

Background

Demographic shifts, changes in economic conditions and increased demand on services have brought new urgency to the question of how best to organise health care services. In meeting these challenges, United Kingdom (UK) health policy since the year 2000 has consistently emphasised improving accessibility [1], increasing integration [1, 2] and shifting resources from hospital to community and primary care [3]. Resources have been provided for several initiatives aimed at increasing integrated working practices at the organisational and service levels of health and social care [4–7]. The latest government vision is of an' integrated,' accessible' health service, with primary care playing a key role in developing 'locally led,' 'innovative' services or 'new care models' [8]. Several initiatives, including the Vanguard programme [9] and the Prime Minister's GP Access fund [10] have been funded and through these, sites are providing services using various care models [10] including GP practices offering 'additional availability' appointments during evenings and at weekends.

In Greater Manchester, the local health and social care strategy set out ambitions to transform primary care, focussing particularly on providing accessible and responsive services [11], and also redesigning and integrating primary and secondary care [12]. In June 2013, the National Health Service (NHS) England Local Area Team invited general practices and clinical commissioning groups (CCGs) in Greater Manchester to submit proposals for a 'demonstrator pilot' programme (the demonstrators), informed by the Greater Manchester primary care strategy [13]. The specifications were that they must: support a defined community of at least 30,000 people; support the delivery of integrated services across primary, community and social care; consider the use of innovative or enhanced technology; and extend access to primary care. The aim of the programme was to identify issues and test solutions in practice to inform the Greater Manchester primary care strategy going forward. Eighteen applications were received and six 'demonstrator sites' were funded: four sites provided additional availability of appointments in general practice, other services included case management and rapid response. Although the short timeline for submission of proposals encouraged applicants to make use of existing relationships, many proposals included plans to forge new collaborations between general practices in an area, often with the encouragement and support of the relevant CCG. Table 1 summarises the services provided.

Given the rapidity and scale at which new models of service are spreading, evidence about early adopters, such as those in Greater Manchester, is important. There is a growing body of literature about the adoption of health service innovations more generally [14–17], but a relative paucity of high quality research focusing upon the implementation of organisational change in primary care [18]. Furthermore, whilst the importance of context and inter-group relations in supporting or preventing organisational change is well known [19, 20], the primary care context is less well understood [21, 22].

We conducted a process evaluation of the Greater Manchester primary care 'demonstrator pilot' programme, designed to identify key learning points from the implementation process to inform future service innovations of this kind. The overall study findings, including a quantitative evaluation, are reported elsewhere [23, 24]. The aim of this paper is to explore in depth the factors influencing the implementation of services within the demonstrator sites, in particular the context in which the services developed and the experiences of people involved with providing them.

Methods

The qualitative process evaluation used semi-structured interviews. The sampling strategy was purposive in that it was driven by the characteristics of the case study sites and designed to capture a range of views from people working at strategic and operational levels, within the main provider organisations – general practices – and other organisations involved, including hospitals and care homes. This resulted in an evolving list of potential interviewees, as early interviews provided detail on others involved in project delivery, who were then targeted for interview. Potential participants were contacted by email and/or telephone and were supplied with information about the purpose and aims of the study; participants were encouraged to ask questions about the study and the research team prior to interviews. The interviews were conducted in three stages: firstly, interviews with 'key informants,' typically site strategic leads; second, interviews with a range of people working in various roles at different levels; third, a set of six 'round up' interviews close to the end of the demonstrator period, with site strategic leads and a clinician with a key role, designed to gain a retrospective account of each demonstrator.

Semi-structured interview topic guides were devised, which included open-ended questions about the project, its aims and the context in which it had developed, the participants' own role, experiences of working in the pilot and views about what was working well, what was not working well and possible reasons why. The interviews were audio recorded, with participants' written consent and transcribed verbatim. Field notes were made during and after interviews. The software package NVivo10 was used to store and manage the data.

SB, RE and DH carried out the interviews between January 2013 and October 2014. All interviewees were experienced and trained in qualitative research to PhD

Table 1 TIDieR Checklist description of the demonstrator pilot sites

Item number	Item
1	BRIEF NAME Site A: Pro-active case management for care home residents
2	WHY High ambulance and GP callouts to care homes; too many non-elective admissions to hospital; Care home residents having long lengths of stay in hospital; lack of access to clinical (GP) records from care homes. Goals: to improve access to clinical care outside hospital, specifically reducing GP and ambulance call-outs, hospital attendances and admissions, to facilitate integrated records and allow direct patient access to these.
3	WHAT Pro-active case management for adult residents, most aged 65+, of five care homes, registered with one of three general practices in one CCG area. Risk-stratifying care home residents and providing enhanced care planning, including end of life and crisis planning, using risk stratification.
4	Procedure: Care home residents were risk stratified, using the model previously employed in Greater Lever. For each, the case manager, carried out an initial, face-to-face holistic assessment and put a care plan in place, which was recorded on the GP system using a template. At the start of the demonstrator the case manager had access to general practice records via a computer in her office, partway through the demonstrator, she acquired direct read-write access to the records via a laptop. After the initial assessment, the case manager would manage patients using a video conferencing facility. Materials: General practices involved used EMIS[a], Vision[a] and TPP[a], laptop provided to the case manager.
5	WHO The service was provided by an advanced nurse practitioner (ANP) who worked during the demonstrator as a case manager (seconded from an acute trust), with input from care home carers and managers, GPs, practice managers and other administrative staff, a CCG pharmacist and members of the local Mental Health Trust's dementia team. CCG and CSU project managers and the integrated care lead (from the local Foundation Trust) also contributed.
6	HOW An initial face to face assessment, followed by case management of patients using a video conferencing facility, with the ANP 'ringing in' to run through the residents on her caseload with care home staff, hearing about any changes and performing consultations with patients, where necessary.
7	WHERE The assessments and consultations took place in care homes, additional work was undertaken in general practices.
8	WHEN AND HOW MUCH Each care home resident had one initial assessment and then consultations were performed as required.
9	TAILORING Individual assessments were undertaken and care plans produced for each care home resident receiving case management.
10	MODIFICATIONS In practice, the video conferencing technology was not used for both technical and organisational reasons. Rather, the care home staff contacted the ANP by telephone, to discuss residents or to ask her to visit the home. Notably, when at a home, the ANP was often asked, by care home staff, to respond to acute problems for residents that were not on her caseload.
Item number	Item
1	BRIEF NAME Site B: Additional availability appointments
2	WHY Difficulty for patients in obtaining timely and convenient access to general practice; too many emergency hospital admissions. Goals: To improve access to care, specifically providing quicker and more convenient access to routine primary care, reducing attendances at A&E.
3	WHAT Additional availability appointments for registered patients of five practices in a township plus one other three miles away, (c. 33,000)
4	Procedure: Additional availability appointments were provided by two GPs, working 6.30 pm to 8 pm Monday to Friday and 8 am to 6 pm at weekends. Three of the practices involved were housed within a purpose - built primary care centre; two of these practices and the practice located outside Radcliffe were owned by the same GP partner. Most appointments were pre-booked, with six kept as emergency appointments for allocation after 6 pm. From 6 pm the practice phone lines diverted to A Healthier Radcliffe. Materials: The appointment booking system was hosted at one practice and the other five logged into this to book appointments. All six practices used Vision with access to the full record, allowed through a data sharing agreement on a read-write basis. GPs used a smartcard to log into each practice system.
5	WHO Two GPs and receptionists.
6	HOW Face to face appointments.
7	WHERE GP practices.
8	WHEN AND HOW MUCH Patients booked appointments as required. Each appointment was 10 min in length, 18 appointments per day were provided Monday –Friday and 12 per day Saturday and Sunday.
9	TAILORING N/A
10	MODIFICATIONS N/A
Item number	Item
1	BRIEF NAME Site C: Additional availability appointments; responsiveness appointments; homelessness service; extension of specialist advice lines
2	WHY Some patients being unable to access timely GP appointments; patients with long term conditions not having timely access to a healthcare professional; insufficient healthcare provision for homeless people. Goals: To improve access to care, specifically reducing A&E attendances, by providing urgent same day (responsiveness) and additional availability appointments in general practice. To improve specialist primary care services and reduce secondary care planned activity, by shifting specialist service provision from secondary to primary care.
3	WHAT 1. Additional availability appointments (33/35 practices). Procedure: Additional availability appointments were provided at four 'host' practices. The additional availability appointments were provided by 1 GP at each site, between 6 pm and 8 pm Monday to Friday, and 9 am to 11 am at weekends. The participating practices across the CCG area and A&E at the local acute trust booked appointments at the host practice, which were available on a quota basis, until 1 pm and then made available on a first come first served basis. Materials: Practices logged into the host practice's system. All practices ran EMIS, either EMIS web or as streaming practices with access to the full record, allowed through a data sharing agreement, on a read-only basis.
4	2. Responsiveness appointments (31/35 practices); Procedure: Practices fitted the responsiveness appointments within the regular working hours of the practice. For example, one practice allocated four telephone triage slots and four

Table 1 TIDieR Checklist description of the demonstrator pilot sites *(Continued)*

Item number	Item
	appointments to the on – call doctor and two appointments each to all other doctors (the number of doctors in the practice varied). Materials: a macro was put onto each practice system and used to log the outcome of appointment. 3. Homelessness service (1 practice); Procedure: provided under a Locally Enhanced Service arrangement, run at a practice with a large local homeless population (often transient). A health questionnaire for patients was completed, to ascertain health needs and then the patient was signposted to various services (clinics for dressings, immunisations, substance misuse services), several of which operated from the same premises as the practice. 4. Extension of specialist advice lines; Procedure: The 'specialist advice lines' were a facility for GPs to get advice from hospital consultants. The service was pre-existing and the additional specialities were added as part of the demonstrator. Materials: Advice lines operated through a dedicated email address for GPs to use.
5	WHO The additional availability appointments were provided by 1 GP at each site, supported by two reception staff, Lead organisation was a GP federation; some additional availability appointments were staffed by locum GPs; the A&E department could refer into the additional availability appointments, local voluntary services could refer into the homelessness service. Hospital consultants staffed the advice lines.
6	HOW Appointments took place face to face and via the telephone.
7	WHERE GP practices.
8	WHEN AND HOW MUCH Patients booked appointments as required. Each additional availability appointment was 10 min in length, 12 appointments per day were provided Monday-Sunday.
9	TAILORING N/A
10	MODIFICATIONS Some changes to the original timings and booking arrangements were made. The weekday additional availability appointments were originally offered entirely on a quota basis and the weekend appointments continued until 12 pm. It appeared some GPs ended up seeing the patient again in normal surgery hours after the additional availability appointment, because they were unsure about what had happened at the appointment. Some practices did not participate in providing the responsiveness appointments; Reasons for non - participation included a lack of capacity in the practice for responsiveness, concerns around IG for one practice and proximity, and being situated on the CCG geographical border.
Item number	Item
1	BRIEF NAME Site D: Additional availability appointments; GP-led care planning; multi-skilled care worker led care planning; hospital navigator service
2	WHY Too much demand on general practice; 'inappropriate' use of A&E for problems that could be handled in general practice; A&E used by frail elderly that resulted in avoidable admissions; increase in A&E attendances from 1 pm onwards (when practices are open). Goals: To develop integrated care in line with the CCG strategy. To improve access to care, specifically access to general practice, reduced A&E attendances and hospital admissions. To improve care of the frail elderly through care planning. To develop the IT infrastructure, specifically to allow hub clinicians to access patients' records, allow practices and patients to book appointments at the hub (a GP practice), and let practices know when their patients are in hospital.

Table 1 TIDieR Checklist description of the demonstrator pilot sites *(Continued)*

Item number	Item
3	WHAT 1. Additional availability appointments for patients registered with GPs in one locality. Procedure: A hub was set up to provide additional GP and nurse appointments, with three nurse clinics and three GP sessions each day. GPs provided additional appointments 4 pm to 9 pm on weekdays and 10 am to 8 pm at weekends. Practices ran the appointment bookings until 6 pm, after which time patients could phone and book directly. The acute trust provided a late-night path lab collection. Materials: Four practices used EMIS, two used Vision. Host practice accessed summary care record on Adastra* on a read-only basis. 2. Care planning Procedure: GPs produced care plans for their frailest elderly patients. The multi-skilled care worker visited patients aged 85 and over at home to identify and assess their needs and produce a care plan.
4	3. Navigator service Procedure: The navigator kept track of presentations to one local A&E department, focussing particularly on those aged 65 and over, so tended to see patients with confusion, falls, and long term conditions, particularly multiple sclerosis and chronic obstructive pulmonary disease. She assessed each patient (each patient was also assessed by the medical team and had tests done as appropriate). Where patients were medically fit and did not need to be admitted, the navigator took responsibility for ensuring that the relevant support was in place, either in the form of a placement, if they were not safe to return home, or home support services (e.g. from team providing crisis response).
5	WHO The project lead was a GP. Local out of hours provider (supplied GPs and receptionists for additional availability appointments); the navigator was an occupational therapist based at a local general hospital, the multi-skilled care worker was based at a foundation trust.
6	HOW See 'procedure' for a description of how each component operated.
7	WHERE Additional availability appointments took place in person, at GP practices, care planning took places in GP practices and at patients' homes, the navigator service operated in hospital.
8	WHEN AND HOW MUCH Patients booked appointments as required. Each additional availability appointment was 15 min in length, 28 appointments per day were provided Monday-Friday, 51 on Saturday and 24 on Sunday.
9	TAILORING Care plans were prepared for individual patients. The navigator service arranged tailored care packages for patients.
10	MODIFICATIONS The additional availability GP appointments were typically booked, but the nursing ones were less popular and were replaced with GP appointments after six weeks. Issues arose as practices which had been allocated appointments were unwilling to give up their allocated slots to other practices which had filled theirs.
Item number	Item
1	BRIEF NAME Site E: Additional availability appointments; mental health crisis clinics.
2	WHY Too much demand on general practice; lack of an accessible mental health service locally. Goals: To improve access to care, specifically providing quicker and more convenient access to routine primary care, reducing attendances at A&E and increasing access to mental health services, by extending access to routine primary care and providing additional mental health services in the community. To make better use of local resources and support the local population to do this, specifically to reduce attendances at A&E, reduce hospital admissions and facilitate quicker discharge from hospital, by providing signposting and education to local services

Table 1 TIDieR Checklist description of the demonstrator pilot sites *(Continued)*

Item number	Item
	in the community, improving patient pathways and supporting collaboration between professionals in different agencies.
3	WHAT 1. Additional availability appointments for patients registered with GPs in one locality. Procedure: The general practice additional availability appointments ran from the lead practice. A purposely developed Care Diary was used by GPs, the local out of hours provider and A&E staff to book patients into the additional availability appointments. Patients were triaged at A&E and, if the ailment could be managed in the community, they could be booked into a GP or nurse appointment by staff at A&E using the Care Diary. Materials: six practices used EMIS, two used Vision. EMIS practices were able to share records on a read-only basis, Vision practices were not able to access records. Since Dec 2014 all practices have been EMIS web allowing all to share records on a read-only basis.
4	2. Mental health crisis clinics for patients registered with GPs in one locality. Procedure: The clinics were organised by a trained counsellor, who co-ordinated the service and provided appointments, plus other counsellors (and trainees) who also worked at another local general practice. Appointments were provided between 6.30 pm and 9.30 pm, Monday to Friday.
5	WHO The project lead was a GP. The additional availability appointments were provided to registered patients, at the lead practice, by GPs, supported by receptionists, all supplied by the local Out of Hours provider. The mental health appointments were provided by trained counsellors and counselling students. The demonstrator appointed a dedicated project manager partway through. CSU and EMIS also contributed to the project.
6	HOW See 'procedure' for a description of how each component operated.
7	WHERE In person, at GP practices,
8	WHEN AND HOW MUCH Patients booked appointments as required. The additional availability appointments were each 10 min in length and 18 appointments were provided per day, Monday-Sunday. The mental health appointments were each one hour in length and three per day were provided, Monday- Friday.
9	TAILORING
10	MODIFICATIONS The additional availability GP appointments were typically booked, but the nursing ones were less popular. Issues arose as practices which had been allocated appointments were unwilling to give up their allocated slots to other practices which had filled theirs. Some local GP practices did not refer patients to the mental health appointments, the lead GP was aware of this but the reasons for non-engagement are not known.

Item number	Item
1	BRIEF NAME Site F: Rapid response step-up service; complex care service; enhanced end of life service; carer needs assessment service; mental health liaison, care homes; end of life training, care homes and locality.
2	WHY Too many non-elective hospital admissions; too many patients dying in hospital; district nurses were under pressure and did not have enough time to provide the right end of life care and support to patients and carers. Goals: To proactively identify and manage people with complex needs via a core integrated team that can draw on specialist support when necessary. To support people with heart failure by extending telehealth services. Support for people to be maintained in their own home or care home where this is their preferred place prior to and including death. A reduction in unplanned, avoidable non-elective activity prior to and including death.

Table 1 TIDieR Checklist description of the demonstrator pilot sites *(Continued)*

Item number	Item
3	WHAT Overall: The demonstrator was part of the restructuring across health and social care, through the development of an 'integrated hub' in each CCG locality. The demonstrator took place in one locality, where the first hub had been established. The hub premises accommodated social workers and third sector staff. Stockport had shared patient information via the Stockport Health record which enabled GPs, secondary care and Out of Hours services to access each other's systems. An extension of the Stockport Health Record, to include health and social care data and integrated care plans, was planned to support the implementation of the Stockport One Integrated Care Team and was further developed within the demonstrator community demonstrator to ensure that the whole range of services within the hub had appropriate access to information. In terms of specific systems operating locally, social care used CareFirst, district nurses used DominiC, the REaCH service used Staffplan, and domiciliary workers users used CM2000 (to log each visit).
4	1. Rapid response step-up service provided to people aged 18 and over. Procedure: GPs referred into the service via a dedicated number at a contact centre when they felt a patient did not need to go to hospital, but needed support putting rapidly in place. Once the GP had made the referral, the patient received a response within 2 h from a team comprising a district nurse and a social worker. The patient could be maintained in their own home or go into a step-up bed. This service ran from 9 am to 5 pm and the intermediate care service provided an Out of Hours service. Materials: six practices used EMIS, two used Vision. EMIS practices were able to share records on a read-only basis, Vision practices were not able to access records. Since Dec 2014 all practices have been EMIS web allowing all to share records on a read-only basis. 2. Complex care service Procedure: the population was risk stratified. Multidisciplinary teams (MDTs), involving a GP and a practice nurse, worked to agree an integrated pathway and model of care for individual patients. The work undertaken followed the same basis as the GP care plans which had already been developed, but allowed other healthcare professionals to contribute to these. The task of coordinating the care plan was undertaken by various professionals (GPs, district nurses, social workers) and also voluntary sector workers. The multidisciplinary group (MDG) was a wider network of professionals which operated at a more strategic level, looking across the locality and identifying, for example, high rates of chronic obstructive pulmonary disease and considering what action should be taken, rather than necessarily focussing only on patients within the high risk stratification. Materials: the People at Risk of Readmission tool was used for risk stratification 3. End of life care service Procedure: The end of life care service was newly designed service that focussed on integrating health and social care. This is a jointly delivered service between district nursing (health) and assistant practitioners (social care) in the community. The service delivers end of life care to people in the last weeks and days of life undertaking joint assessments, care planning and visiting the person in their home to deliver interventions that meet the needs of the patient and their carers or family. The health and wellbeing service was planned as an extension of the existing service, into a different area. The end of life training consisted of delivering a module to care home staff. The dementia-focussed training consisted of several one-hour training sessions delivered to care home staff. Materials: End of life training based on the Six Steps programme and providing follow up telephone support. 4. The mental health liaison in-reach service involved working with three care homes to provide advice and support, particularly care planning.
5	WHO The demonstrator was part of a programme of work developed by the CCG and local authority, a hub was established and a hub co-ordinator was employed; the local Foundation Trust, Community mental health trust and local authority reablement service were involved; Project managers and general practice staff contributed. The MDT and MDGs were comprised of GPs,

Table 1 TIDieR Checklist description of the demonstrator pilot sites *(Continued)*

Item number	Item
	district nurses, social workers, primary care pharmacist and third sector staff. The end of life service was provided by assistant practitioners (domiciliary workers) from the REaCH service. The end of life training for care homes was provided by end of life facilitators. The health and wellbeing service was led by project managers, liaising with general practice staff. The carer assessments were carried out in general practice, with input from GPs and administrative staff. The mental health liaison in-reach service was provided by a community psychiatric nurse and a support worker.
6	HOW All services were provided in person.
7	WHERE At GP practices, in patients' homes, in step-up facilities, care homes.
8	WHEN AND HOW MUCH Services were provided to patients as required.
9	TAILORING
10	MODIFICATIONS The aim was for district nurses to be co-located at the hub but this was not possible within the timeframes associated with the demonstrator. In practice, social workers were 'paperless' whilst district nurses used paper records.

[a]computer systems used in general practices and/or the companies that supply these systems

level. Most interviews were conducted in person at the participants' place of work and four were conducted via telephone. The majority of interviews were individual, with a few conducted in pairs or trios. The interviews lasted between 15 min and 2 h, most being around 1 h long.

Data analysis followed ta thematic approach. Categories were generated through reading the transcripts, with some themes following the research questions, whilst others were derived from the data themselves [25]. Team members read the transcripts and discussed emerging themes. Initial open coding was refined by consensus within the team as a whole, with the agreed coding framework applied to the complete dataset by SP, SB and RE. The process of coding and organising the data was iterative, with the framework being revised and refined as further coding was undertaken and categories and themes grouped together. Feedback on emerging findings was provided by the evaluation team at a series of 'action learning sets' that were accessible to all involved with the sites; these were supplemented by the dissemination of interim reports, in addition to the final report.

Results

Ninety-one people participated in interviews (Table 2). Iterative analysis identified six influencing factors: information technology; information governance; workforce and organisational development; communications and engagement; supporting infrastructure; and federations and alliances. We explore each of these in turn and show the range of views expressed.

Information technology

Innovative use of information technology (IT) was a prerequisite for obtaining funding, but all sites experienced IT challenges, often of unexpected complexity. Several participants described learning from initial 'teething problems'. Thus one pilot lead, acknowledging that technical problems were frustrating, emphasised that they were not insurmountable:

> *We've got a couple of different solutions, some a bit more clunky than others, but there are solutions there...So I think the technology I'm sure can be pretty easily worked out in a place like (name) anyway. (GP site lead)*

However, at some sites the technical IT problems were far from 'easy' to solve, delaying the initiation of services, reducing efficiency and even preventing some service components being initiated at all. Technical problems affected both hardware and software: system failures; difficulties getting remote access to systems or records from mobile devices; and obstructions to equipment installation were all described. Whilst the precise problems varied between sites, there was a common recognition of initial over-optimism about what IT could deliver and subsequent complications, preventing the implementation of some elements of services:

> *EMIS had a configure switch where you can just turn up and log into (it). That didn't work. There were a couple of things we had to do to test it. Once we realised that (it) wasn't working, we had to stop. (Project manager)*

The interoperability of practice systems presented key challenges. Practices trying to work together to provide additional appointments had expected to be able to access one another's patient records. Whilst problems might be expected between practices using different computer systems, even those using the same system experienced setbacks. Further work was necessary to standardise the way the system was used, to gain agreement on this and to train staff. Participants expressed frustration with the interim workarounds developed, which were often lengthy and complex without delivering the expected operability:

> *But the Vision 360, although there's a bit of light at the end of the tunnel, is not the all singing and all dancing as we thought it might be...it's so long winded to get from A to B. (Project manager)*

Beneath this lay more challenging issues of inter-organisational working and relationships, with some interviewees distinguishing between the technical IT solutions and the more difficult integrative work required:

> *The IT integration…is not that bad. That's just complicated easy stuff…It's the simple hard stuff. And it's the relational stuff, it's trusting somebody outside to come in, that you've got really no control over…Who is it? What are they doing? What training? You know… So that integration stuff is, I think a learning that we need to take forward from this…you've got to have the GPs on board to allow people to come in and do this… (GP site lead)*

All of the demonstrator areas eventually achieved the expected 'innovative use of IT,' but it was often more difficult than anticipated and participants were disappointed at not being able to depend on the computer systems to work in the ways they had expected. Workarounds were developed, but more sustainable solutions required extended engagement with suppliers and practices. For practices, having trust in anyone who would have access to their systems was crucial.

Information governance

Whilst linked to IT, information governance (IG) appeared in these narratives as a separate, complex issue. Respondents described unanticipated problems relating to inflexible governance procedures and disparity in governance protocols between organisations. These were described as 'hurdles' and 'organisational hoops.' Cultural differences were found between different types of organisation and between healthcare sectors. The quotes below reflect embedded perceptions of approaches to information governance in primary and secondary care respectively, with direct implications for implementation processes:

> *…the information governance at the hospital is much tighter than it is in general practice and so what we think is reasonable data to see, the hospital are not altogether happy. So they tend to insert much more stringent criteria than we do. (GP site lead)*

> *We're a big organisation, we have very stringent governance procedures…what the demonstrator's done is put us working with small, independent businesses, and I guess there's a flexibility [for general practices]… I think they've been a bit frustrated in dealing with a fairly bureaucratic system… [Proposed interventions] had lots of IG issues in them…there were processes to go through. We couldn't just say 'yeah, fine, we can do that tomorrow'… (Hospital manager)*

A dialogical approach was therefore required in the demonstrator sites to reconcile these perspectives to allow effective collaboration to take place between different organisations, particularly between primary and secondary care.

The human issues of trust and relationships had important implications for IG. The following quote illustrates the need to gain the trust of practices, which here seem to be portrayed as protective or cautious, in order for people outside the practice to access data:

> *We've got to earn the trust of the GP practices. First of all, to allow read only access. So that's been a big barrier to break down, because the practice managers were not keen to allow, even, read only access, and to allow people to actually enter data onto it, that's a step too far at the moment. (Manager)*

Whilst the provision of honorary contracts offered partial solutions to IG issues, more fundamental solutions involved open and early dialogue.?>

Workforce and organisational development

Several respondents in each of the four sites extending GP opening hours mentioned the challenge of GP capacity, raising issues such as skill shortages, concerns about work-life balance and sustainability:

> *…one of the main problems I think is getting the clinical cover … they may be able to do it for so long but it's not sustainable on a long term basis (Site lead)*

These pilots aimed to provide additional *routine* appointments, rather than conventional out of hours care. Thus, alongside routine GP appointments, nurse appointments were also offered. However, there was no standard practice nurse training or skillset amongst nurses working at the sites; therefore, they were not necessarily 'interchangeable,' yet, this was not always considered when allocating nurses to appointment slots:

> *…somebody turned up for a diabetic check-up and the nurse who was on couldn't do it… (GP)*

A broader issue relating to substitutability (exchanging one type of worker for another) was highlighted by interviewees who described some individuals involved in the demonstrator as being more experienced, or more committed, than the average person in that role. This meant that the role could not be easily replicated. Many demonstrators flourished due to the contribution of individuals who are difficult to replace or replicate, due to their particular competences, ways of working and also the trusting relationships they had established with practices:

Simply adding six more nurses might not facilitate six times more to be achieved than what [postholder] has done, because she had an established relationship with practices, as well as being a good communicator, so she was trusted and accepted by the practices, so they were happy for her to have access to their systems. But this engagement will not happen automatically: GPs have to feel that they trust people that are doing the work for them. (GP site lead)

Thus, whilst many people worked hard to support the pilots, rolling out services more widely not only requires enough staff, but also requires understanding of issues of substitutability, working relationships and levels of interpersonal trust established over time.

Communications and engagement

The demonstrators involved complex networks of organisations; even the site with the smallest population coverage and narrowest focus involved seven different types of organisation. Establishing and maintaining engagement was mentioned by participants at all sites.

Some demonstrators built effectively upon existing relationships. Others, however, carried an over-optimistic expectation that people or organisations that had not worked together previously would immediately do so for the pilot, resulting in delays. Some GP site leads found practice managers and administrators somewhat self-protective when it came to operationalising the plans, reflecting limited trust between some practices:

The nursing appointments – we could fill them but ... [another practice] doesn't utilise their nurse appointments but won't let anybody else have them, and you get into this argy-bargy with practice managers then. 'Well can we use them?' 'No, we might use them.' 'But you're not using them'...what I call the general practice little bit of selfishness... they stick to their guns and say 'these are our appointments and we still want them.' (GP site lead)

Personal and direct communication with practices was felt to be vital, with letters to practices setting out plans highlighted as insufficient. Some practice managers reported being asked to carry out extra work at short notice, without having been involved in the planning stages of the project(s), nor their opinion sought. This manager, for example, ascribed 'teething troubles' at one site to an unanticipated request to arrange access to a computer system at short notice:

The first time I was aware (was when people arrived to set up IT access for a nurse practitioner) and (I thought) 'Oh right'...and that happened on at least three occasions. So three afternoons were completely trashed off...we were messing and mauling about trying to set things up, which irked me a bit, because... I'd not been privy to what this would mean, other than 'oh she's [the nurse] going to be able to access (the practice system)'. (Practice manager)

Sometimes, the demonstrators had acted to foster new relationships, or improve existing ones. For example, two practices providing additional appointments via a collaborative hub had historically tended to work independently. Here, the demonstrator process itself drove more collaborative working between them. Practice managers described how their initial engagement with each other had tended to be task-based, with division of responsibilities and limited discussion. However, their experience of working together led to closer working and managers described starting to telephone each other for advice on day-to-day practice issues not necessarily related to the demonstrator pilots. A strategic lead, who had worked with these practices, expressed a similar view, suggesting that the GPs seemed to have more genuine discussions:

Well, actually getting (several) practices in a room with two GPs and getting them to agree - that's not to be underestimated. And when I say agree, I mean agree in the room and agree outside the room. (Site lead)

Thus, engagement with the project and good communication went hand in hand. When it worked well, those involved felt both informed and consulted, with the ability to influence the pilot. While in some sites, a failure to take a dialogical approach, or to engage, resulted in resistance to changes, ongoing routine interaction through the demonstrators also generated collaborative relations and open, trusting relationships.

Supporting infrastructure

All demonstrators made use of current local infrastructure, using existing premises that were already equipped. As these were fixed-duration pilots, no demonstrator sought to acquire new premises, although the initiation of one demonstrator coincided with the establishment of a 'hub' location. The pilots operated within the wider health and social care infrastructure, with varying amounts of interaction with external organisations. Respondents across all demonstrators referenced local A&E departments, Out-of-Hours providers, the North West Ambulance Service and community pharmacies as important local services. Deciding which support services were needed was a pivotal decision for routine appointments provided during evenings and weekends. For

Table 2 interviewees by demonstrator and role[a]

Demonstrator	Role						
	Manager	Nurse	Doctor	Pharmacist	Support worker	Administrator/other[b]	total
A	7	1	2	1	1	1	13
B	13	0	5	1	1	0	20
C	7	0	3	0	0	1	11
D	9	1	4	0	1	1	16
E	6	1	6	0	0	2	15
F	18	1	1	1	5	0	26
Total	60	4	21	3	5	5	98[c]

[a]hybrid roles have been categorised by professional background of individual when they retain a clinical role (3) and by organisational role when they do not (3)
[b]occupational therapist (1) counsellor (1)
[c]8 individuals double-counted due to roles spanning sites D and E (7) and B, D and E (1)

financial and clinical reasons, there was recognition that such support would only entail 'sufficient' services and that it would be unfeasible to provide an entire health and social care system around the clock:

You don't need a full complement of staff in the evenings and weekends like you do during the day. What you do need is access to enough services to deliver a competent service...path lab stuff, transport and all that sorted out... a district nurse service in the evenings and weekends. (GP site lead)

Pathology collections during the evening were particularly important for the 'additional availability' demonstrators and one site reported positive experiences arranging this with a local hospital. Elsewhere, the lack of infrastructure support, in particular 'back office' support functions within the voluntary sector was highlighted. A manager employed by the local authority described some of the practical challenges she had faced when working with voluntary organisations; she seemed to lack confidence in the support available to make systems work together:

When they want to get onto the systems and get their emails, sometimes it works, sometimes it doesn't... and we all have a three way conversation to fix this problem in all the four organisations. That in itself is a ridiculously difficult thing to organise, and I'm struggling with it... (Local Authority Manager)

The time-limited nature of the demonstrators meant that they operated largely within the existing infrastructure, adapting to existing limitations. It was vital therefore that sites considered and planned both the level of necessary support and the level of resource available within external organisations.

Federations and alliances

Recently, groups of GP practices have started working together in more formal ways, often referred to as GP federations, defined as: groups 'of practices and primary care teams working together, sharing responsibility for developing and delivering high quality, patient-focussed services for their local communities' [26]. At two demonstrators, services were running through existing federations. Participants here identified several benefits from working as part of a federation: the ability to combine resources; increased population coverage; enhanced professional standards because of peer support and review; and the fostering of a common identity and purpose amongst practices. One pilot achieved full sharing of patient records, with read-write access between practices; this was singled out as resulting from the formal agreement between the practices in the federation:

[name] have full access to the patients' records. That's the unique bit. (Manager)

In both areas where demonstrators were run by federations, pre-existing relationships and historical joint working between practices were considered important in supporting the federation establishment. At the site with full shared records, previous joint working was seen as essential to this achievement; collaborators were familiar and trusted:

GPs are very protective of their patient data...but because the GPs are shareholders of this organisation...they've got a vested interest in this organisation, they work collaboratively and they know who they're sharing their data with...So in order to get that data sharing agreement you have to have some kind of collaboration going on in the background. (Manager)

As well as these immediate benefits, federations were seen by some as a way to protect primary care in the context of future policy demands, particularly around 'extended opening hours' and the associated likely demands on workload:

> *I think there's going to be a...coming together of practices. So going forward I can only see the federation will get bigger as individual practices struggle more to meet all the policy demands...if extended hours becomes the norm. It would be become really hard for an individual practice to do that. (Manager)*

Demonstrator pilots supported by local federations thus benefitted from existing joint working and trust between practices. Notably, these sites found it easier to overcome some of the challenges associated with IT, IG, workforce and communications than other sites, partly through better established relationships and trust and partly through having a formal mechanism to address such issues.

Discussion

Summary

This study explored the processes of implementing pilots focussed on access, integration and innovative use of technology in primary care through an evaluation of a programme initiated in Greater Manchester. Our analysis identified six factors which were influential in the implementation of the pilots: information technology; information governance; workforce and organisational development; communications and engagement; supporting infrastructure; and federations and alliances. Underpinning all of these factors was the issue of trust; there was consensus amongst our participants that trusting relationships were vital for collaboration.

Strengths and limitations

We accessed the experiences of people working at strategic and operational levels within a range of sectors, therefore gaining multiple perspectives on complex and poorly understood processes. Our interviews were mostly undertaken with people engaged with the pilots and therefore, overall, may represent a more 'interested' viewpoint. We did not capture patient experiences directly, which is a limitation of this study, although the quantitative component reported elsewhere included an analysis of items from the national GP Patient Survey [23].

Comparison with existing literature/implications for practice and areas for further research

There are commonalities between our findings and previous studies of implementation in healthcare, which have found factors such as information technology, relationships, communication and organisational culture to be important [7, 14, 16, 19]. Our study confirms these findings, but also extends them. Working relationships have been found to be vital, within and between various health and social care organisations; our data provide examples of the importance of these within general practice and show some of the ways in which these can be fostered. Whilst previous research [14] found relationships between people in senior leadership roles to be important, we found that relationships between practice managers in particular, as well as administrators, were also key. Research also emphasises the importance for change efforts of mobilising valued identities [19]. Disseminating the proposal brief direct to professionals (rather than cascading through commissioners in CCGs) helped to bypass some of the problems associated with resistance to change by professionals [27, 28]. Professionals then took ownership of 'their' projects and this helped create the positive and proactive dynamics and trust required to move beyond silos [14, 19]. Although there is a danger that this could also reproduce a narrow set of professional interests [29], the importance of trust to professional enrolment and professional-managerial boundary crossing was key. For example, whilst IT/IG issues were common, what determined whether or not they were surmountable was the extent to which trust existed, or could be developed, between the parties. Our study also provides further detailed evidence about the nature of IT/IG issues in joint working. Going beyond system interoperability (often the goal of integrated care programmes), we have shown that the issues of who can write to your records, who can read them and how decisions about the use of IT get made need careful consideration.

Whilst it is self-evident that communication is important in initiating and sustaining change programmes, our study aligns with existing research which highlights the need for a dialogical approach [30, 31]. By this we mean that it is not enough to simply passively disseminate information; participants need to feel that they are active contributors, understanding what is happening but also able to influence it and change the direction of a project should it be necessary. Some of our participants resented finding out about the projects only when they had to provide help at short notice, a finding which mirrors previous work on implementation in primary care, which found that staff did not feel involved in decision making and that a top-down approach was a negative factor [32, 33]. Furthermore, our data extends the existing research by providing evidence of how primary care implementation is experienced by practice managers. Moreover, our study suggests that, whilst federated working seemed helpful, this seemed to operate via the medium of shared history and the trust which arises out of practical experience of joint working in other spheres. This aligns with findings from research secondary care, which has emphasised the importance of both shared history and a shared purpose [34, 35]. The positive impact of existing federated working may simply reflect this shared history, and we would expect the question of shared purpose to be key to the success of future federations and other similar collaborative ventures.

Whilst we did not use a particular evaluation framework or tool in this study of implementation, there are parallels between our approach and findings and the constructs of the Consolidated Framework for Implementation Research (CFIR), an established framework used in evaluations of implementation [17]. In terms of approach, our focus on context and process fit with the inner and outer settings and process constructs in the CFIR. Our findings on the importance of relationships, communication and engagement in particular mirror the CFIR focus on engaging and involving individuals, networks and communication, culture and compatibility. It may be beneficial to consider the utility of frameworks such as CFIR in the design of future research on organisational change in primary care.

Conclusions

Taken together, our findings provide some very practical lessons for those seeking to initiate similar cross-boundary projects. Starting small, with trust building over time via the experience of shared working, is likely to be more effective than large scale projects imposed from above. Detailed consideration is also required not just of the mechanics of information technology ('the complicated easy stuff') and the legal aspects of information governance, but also issues of ownership, rights to log things to the record and facilitating the development of trust, particularly between general practices. It was crucial that GP practices trusted in the integrity of anyone external, particularly if they were to access data on the practice computer system. The schemes in question found ways to resolve their challenges, through provisional 'workarounds' or through more permanent negotiated solutions. This often relied upon the commitment and innovation of individuals within these pilots going beyond their established role both in scope (acting beyond the formal parameters of their role) and in scale (working longer hours). For future initiatives, it is important that all organisations and agencies involved in the design and delivery of innovative models of community-based primary care work to ensure that more suitable time periods for all aspects of project management are provided. Service providers and system leaders, in particular, should consider extended periods of operation, to further enable more sustained and more focused attempts at publicising the service. Having more appropriate time periods in which to plan and operate services would allow greater opportunity for engagement and communication, as well as managing inter/intra organisational expectation. With a clearer understanding of the complex and embedded practical challenges of collaboration developed through this evaluation, practitioners may be better positioned to anticipate and address these challenges. This is of increasing importance as the NHS rushes to implement a range of new models of care [9].

Abbreviations

A & E: Accident and emergency; CCG: Clinical commissioning group; CSU: Commissioning support unit; EMIS: Egton Medical Information Systems; GP: General Practitioner; IG: Information governance; IT: Information technology; MDG: Multi-disciplinary group; MDT: Multi-disciplinary team; NHS: National Health Service; UK: United Kingdom

Acknowledgements

We are very grateful to the participants who gave their time to be interviewed for the study. We also gratefully acknowledge the support of the wider research team who worked on other aspects of this project; Dr. Will Whittaker, Dr. Laura Anselmi, Dr. Jonathan Stokes, Dr. Soren Rud Kristensen, and Prof. Peter Bower and Prof. Ruth Boaden for broader research advice.

Funding

This project is funded by NHS England (Greater Manchester) and the National Institute for Health Research Collaboration for Leadership in Applied Health Research and Care (NIHR CLAHRC) Greater Manchester. The views expressed in this article are those of the author and not necessarily those of the NHS, NIHR or the Department of Health.

Authors' contributions

DH, SB, KC, AM and KR designed the study. RE, SB and DH collected the data, RE, SB, KC, AM, SP, KR and DH analysed the data and contributed to writing this paper. All authors read and approved the final manuscript.

Competing interests

The authors declare that they have no competing interests.

Author details

[1]The University of Manchester, Oxford Road, Manchester M13 9PL, UK. [2]Radcliffe Observatory Quarter, University of Oxford, Woodstock Road, Oxford OX2 6GG, UK. [3]NIHR Collaboration for Leadership in Applied Health Research and Care (CLAHRC), Salford Royal Foundation Trust, Stott Lane, Salford M6 8HD, UK.

References

1. Department of Health. The NHS Plan, a plan for investment, a plan for reform 2000. Available from: http://webarchive.nationalarchives.gov.uk/+/www.dh.gov.uk/en/publicationsandstatistics/publications/publicationspolicyandguidance/dh_4002960. Accessed 3 Mar 2018.
2. Glendinning C. Breaking down barriers: integrating health and care services. Health Policy. 2003;65(2):139–51.
3. Department of Health. Our health our care our say: a new direction for community services 2006. Available from: https://www.gov.uk/government/publications/our-health-our-care-our-say-a-new-direction-for-community-services. Accessed 3 Mar 2018.
4. Department of Health. Transforming primary care 2014. Available from: https://www.gov.uk/government/publications/plans-to-improve-primary-care. Accessed 3 Mar 2018.
5. NHS England. Better care fund 2015. Available from: https://www.england.nhs.uk/ourwork/part-rel/transformation-fund/bcf-plan/. Accessed 3 Mar 2018.
6. Newman S,Bardsley M, Barlow J, Beecham J, Beynon M, Billings J et al. The whole system demonstrator programme. Available from: https://www.city.ac.uk/__data/assets/pdf_file/0004/243067/WSD_report_Final_27th_20Aug.PDF. Accessed 3 Mar 2018.

7. Hendy J, Chrysanthaki T, Barlow J, Knapp M, Rogers A, Sanders C, et al. An organisational analysis of the implementation of telecare and telehealth: the whole systems demonstrator. BMC Health Serv Res. 2012; https://doi.org/10.1186/1472-6963-12-403.
8. Department of Health. Five Year Forward View 2014. Available from: https://www.england.nhs.uk/ourwork/futurenhs/. Accessed 8 Mar 2018.
9. NHS England. New care models – vanguard sites. Available from: https://www.england.nhs.uk/ourwork/futurenhs/new-care-models/. Accessed 8 Mar 2018.
10. NHS England. Prime Minister's GP Access Fund. Available from: https://www.england.nhs.uk/ourwork/futurenhs/pm-ext-access/. Accessed 8 Mar 2018.
11. NHS England. Our 5 year strategy for improving primary care within greater Manchester, supporting the development of community based care 2014–2018; 2014 Available from http://www.gmhsc.org.uk/assets/GMHSC-Partnership-Primary-Care-Strategy.pdf. Accessed 8 Mar 2018.
12. Healthier Together. A review of health and care in Greater Manchester. Available from: https://healthiertogethergm.nhs.uk/. Accessed 10 July 2016.
13. NHS England. Greater Manchester primary care demonstrators briefing note. Available from: https://healthiertogethergm.nhs.uk/files/8113/9704/3908/Briefing_Note_-_1_October.pdf. Accessed 8 Mar 2018.
14. Ling T, Brereton L, Conklin A, Newbould J, Roland M. Barriers and facilitators to integrating care: experiences from the English integrated care pilots. Int J Integr Care. 2012;12(5) https://doi.org/10.5334/ijic.982.
15. MacNeill V, Sanders C, Fitzpatrick R, Hendy J, Barlow J, Knapp M, et al. Experiences of front-line health professionals in the delivery of telehealth: a qualitative study. Br J Gen Pract. 2014; https://doi.org/10.3399/bjgp14X680485.
16. Mott MacDonald. Prime Minister's Challenge Fund: Improving Access to General Practice, First Evaluation Report: 2015. Available from:https://www.england.nhs.uk/wp-content/uploads/2015/10/pmcf-wv-one-eval-report.pdf. Accessed 8 Mar 2018.
17. CFIR Research Team. CFIR constructs. Consolidated framework for implementation research. Available at http://www.cfirguide.org/constructs.html. Accessed 8 Mar 2018.
18. Lau R, Stevenson F, Ong BN, Dziedzic K, Treweek S, Eldridge S, et al. Achieving change in primary care—effectiveness of strategies for improving implementation of complex interventions: systematic review of reviews. BMJ Open. 2015;5:e009993. https://doi.org/10.1136/bmjopen-2015-009993.
19. Kreindler SA, Dowd DA, Dana Star N, Gottschalk T. Silos and social identity: the social identity approach as a framework for understanding and overcoming divisions in health care. Milbank Q. 2012;90(2):347–74. https://doi.org/10.1111/j.1468-0009.2012.00666.x.
20. Greenhalgh T, Robert G, MacFarlane F, Bate P, Kyriakidou O. Diffusion of innovations in service Organisations: systematic review and recommendations. Milbank Q. 2004;82(4):581–629.
21. Huntley A, Lasserson D, Wye L, Morris R, Checkland K, England H, et al. Which features of primary care affect unscheduled secondary care use? A systematic review. BMJ Open. 2014;4(5):e004746. https://doi.org/10.1136/bmjopen-2013-004746.
22. Checkland K, Harrison S, Marshall M. Is the metaphor of 'barriers to change' useful in understanding implementation? Evidence from general medical practice. J Health Serv Res Policy. 2007;12(2):95–100.
23. National Institute for Health Research Collaboration for Leadership in Applied Health Research and Care (NIHR CLAHRC) for Greater Manchester. NHS Greater Manchester Primary Care Demonstrators Evaluation Final Report 2015. Available from: http://clahrc-gm.nihr.ac.uk/wp-content/uploads/PCDE-final-report-full-final.pdf. Accessed 8 Mar 2018.
24. Whittaker W, Anselmi L, Kristensen KR, Lau Y-S, Bailey S, Bower P, et al. Associations between extending access to primary care and emergency department visits: a difference-in-differences analysis. PLoS Med. 2016;13(9):e1002113. https://doi.org/10.1371/journal.pmed.1002113.
25. Silverman S. Interpreting qualitative data: methods for Analysing talk, text and interaction. London: Thousand Oaks; 2001.
26. Imison C, Williams S, Smith J, Dingwall C. Toolkit to support the development of Primary Care federations. Royal College of General Practitioners. Available from: http://www.rcgp.org.uk/clinical-and-research/a-to-z-clinical-resources/primary-care-federations-toolkit.aspx. Accessed 8 Mar 2018.
27. Currie G, Finn R, Martin G. Role transition and the interaction of relational and social identity: new nursing roles in the English NHS. Organ Stud. 2010;31(7):941–61.
28. Finn R, Currie G, Martin G. Team work in context: institutional mediation in the public-service professional bureaucracy. Organ Stud. 2010;31(8):1069–97.
29. McDonald R, Harrison S, Checkland K. Identity, contract and Enterprise in a Primary Care Setting: an English general practice case study. Organization. 2008;15(3):355–70.
30. Greener I, Harrington B, Hunter D, Mannion R, Powell M. A realistic review of clinico-managerial relationships in the NHS: 1991–2010: National Institute for Health Research, Service Delivery & Organisation programme; 2011, 2011.
31. Iles V, Sutherland K. Managing change in the NHS. Organisational change. A review for health care managers, professionals and researchers. London: National co-ordinating centre for NHS Service Delivery and Organisation R & D; 2001.
32. McDonald R. Individual identity and organisational control: empowerment and modernisation in a primary care trust. Sociology of Health & Illness. 2004;26(7):925–50.
33. Carlfjord S, Lindberg M, Bendtsen P, Nilsen P, Andersson A. Key factors influencing adoption of an innovation in primary health care: a qualitative study based on implementation theory. BMC Fam Pract. 2010;11(60) https://doi.org/10.1186/1471-2296-11-60.
34. Kirkpatrick, I., B. Malby, I. Neogy, with M. Dent and the Inquiry Panel. 2007. National Inquiry into Management and Medicine. Leeds: Centre for Innovation in Health Management.
35. Graham A, Steele J. Optimising Value: The Motivation of Doctors and Managers in the NHS. London: Public Management Foundation; 2001.

11

Changes of the perceived quality of care for older patients with hypertension by community health centers in Shanghai

Haitao Li[1], Xiaolin Wei[2*] and Martin C. S. Wong[3]

Abstract

Background: Monitoring and evaluating changes of quality of primary care for older adult hypertensive patients is part of effective delivery of primary care. This study aimed to investigate changes of older adult hypertensive patients' perceived quality of primary care over time in Shanghai.

Methods: Two rounds of cross-sectional questionnaire surveys were conducted in Shanghai in November 2011 and June 2013. A total of 437 patients participated in the first Round survey and 443 in the second. Primary care attributes were collected from Community Health Center users through on-site face-to-face interview surveys using the validated Primary Care Assessment Tool. Multiple linear regressions were used to determine whether there was any difference in primary quality of care scores between 2011 and 2013 surveys.

Results: Compared with those in the first Round, participants in the second Round reported higher scores in total primary care quality (28.73 vs. 27.75, $P < 0.001$), as well as primary care attributes including first-contact utilization (2.81 vs. 2.60, $P < 0.001$) and accessibility (2.48 vs. 2.44, $P < 0.05$), continuity of care (3.38 vs. 3.27, $P < 0.001$), coordination of information (3.82 vs. 3.67, $P < 0.001$), comprehensiveness of service availability (3.51 vs. 3.39, $P < 0.001$) and provision (2.69 vs. 2.43, $P < 0.001$), and cultural competence (2.67 vs. 2.49, $P < 0.05$), but a lower score in coordination of services (2.45 vs. 2.55, $P < 0.05$).

Conclusion: Older adult hypertensive patients perceived better primary care quality from 2011 to 2013 in Shanghai. This may be associated with the general practitioner team service in Shanghai where hypertensive patients were targeted.

Keywords: Primary care, Quality of care, Hypertension, High blood pressure

Background

China is a rapidly aging society, where older population aged 60 years and above accounted for over 200 million in 2013 [1]. Hypertension is found to be the commonest chronic disease among this age group [2]. An estimated hypertension prevalence among Chinese aged from 60 to 69 years onwards was more than 50% [3]. Hypertension prevalence keeps rising in old age [3, 4]. However, hypertension control remains sub-optimal worldwide [5, 6], including China [3, 7, 8]. Therefore, understanding quality of care for older adult hypertensive patients has important implications for policy makers.

Key features of primary care quality include accessibility, continuity, coordination and comprehensiveness and patient centered care [9]. Accessibility has been found positively correlated with population health. Higher accessibility has also been shown leading to reduced socioeconomic and racial disparities in health. Coordination of care has been found have mixed results with respect to health. Patient satisfaction is correlated to certain features of the coordination of care. A strong association between continuity of care and improved patient satisfaction has been established. It was also found that continuity of care is cost-effective in primary care, and ensures greater efficiency of services.

* Correspondence: Xiaolin.wei@utoronto.ca
[2]Division of Clinical Public Health and Institute of Health Policy, Management and Evaluation, Dalla Lana School of Public Health, University of Toronto, 155 College St, Toronto, ON M5T 3M7, Canada

There is also a strong relevance of continuity of care to decreased hospitalization and improved early diagnosis. The delivery of a wide range of primary care services is associated with improved health outcomes [10]. Researchers have demonstrated the relevance of accessibility, continuity, coordination and comprehensiveness to the quality of management of hypertension [11].

In urban China, Community Health Centers (CHCs) are the major primary care providers to residents. Shanghai is a pioneer in exploring and developing CHCs in China. Early-built CHCs in Shanghai are transformed from first-level hospitals, while newly-built ones are established directly by the government [12]. By the end of 2010, there were 227 CHCs in Shanghai. These CHCs act as independent entities, funded fully and managed directly by the district government, rendering them not-for-profit [13].

Chronic disease management, including hypertension and diabetes, is one of the six integrated health services provided by CHCs since the launch of the primary care program in 1997. The Health Care Reform Plan Policy launched by the State Council of China in 2009 re-emphasized the relevance of the primary care approach in managing chronic diseases including hypertension [14]. Hypertensive patients can be detected through screening of health records or free health examination. An alternative for detection of hypertension is through mandatory BP tests of all patients over 35 years old in CHCs. All diagnosed hypertensive patients are registered and managed in their CHCs. CHCs are responsible for establishing a separate health record for standard management of hypertension, including regular monitoring of BP and complications, lifestyle modification advises, medication refill etc. The work is provided by a team led by the general practitioners, with doctors trained in Traditional Chinese Medicine, nurses and public health doctors. These strategies may impact the utilization of primary care by older hypertensive patients.

From 2011, residents are promoted to enroll in the general practitioner team to manage their health [15]. The team provides a free package of clinical and preventive care, including hypertension management. They, together with community organizations, also provide health education such as healthy diet and smoking cessation, which may improve comprehensiveness of service in CHCs. Capitation payment and pay-for-performance have been introduced [16]. Performance is determined by volume of services provided, their quality and patient satisfaction. The older adult hypertensive patients are thus easier to obtain needed care for better hypertension management (i.e., improved accessibility and continuity of care) [16].

Monitoring and evaluating changes of quality of primary care for older patients with hypertension is part of assurance of effective primary care delivery, and in maximizing its full potential. This study aimed to investigate changes in primary care quality perceived by older adult hypertensive patients from 2011 to 2013 in Shanghai. It also examined whether household income and multi-morbidity had any effect on perceived primary care quality in 2011 and 2013.

Methods

Ethics approval

Ethical approval was obtained from the Joint Chinese University of Hong Kong and New Territories East Cluster Clinical Research Ethnics Committee (Ref. No. CRE-2010.441). Shanghai Association of Community Health Care (SACH) reviewed the ethical point and approved it in 2011 until 2014 (SACH201103) (the whole study period).

Participants and procedures

Two rounds of cross-sectional surveys were conducted in Shanghai in November 2011 and June 2013, respectively. Multistage stratified random sampling method was used to select CHCs as study settings. Firstly, four districts, namely Jing'an, Changning, Xuhui and Pudong, were selected randomly from four geographic areas. Secondly, one CHC was selected at random from each district, arriving at a total of 4 CHCs. Both rounds of surveys were performed in the same CHCs.

The sampling frame was the users' population in the CHCs, with a planned sample size of 614. The sample size was estimated for additional planned analyses which is not the focus of this paper, but further information can be found in our previous publication [16]. Eight hundred subjects were intended to be interviewed when considering a 90% response rate and an 85% of usual CHC users. The inclusion criteria of the participants consisted of subjects who were: 1) age ≥ 18 years; 2) able to communicate and give informed consent; and 3) paid ≥1 CHC visit before the survey. Employing systematic sampling methods, at least 200 participants were recruited from each CHC in each round of the survey. The samples between the two rounds of surveys were different. Extensively trained interviewers performed on-site face-to-face interview surveys. Written informed consent from CHCs and participants was obtained before the surveys were commenced. In total, 811 and 795 participants completed the survey in Rounds 1 and 2 respectively, with response rates of 94% and 92%. We selected the subset for older hypertensive patients as this is the core group of patients managed in CHCs. There was a total of 437 and 443 participants were aged ≥60 years and had physician-diagnosed hypertension. This study was a pre-specified sub-analysis where the full dataset was reported elsewhere [16].

Key measures

Primary Care Assessment Tool (PCAT) [17], which was translated, adapted and validated at Chinese primary care settings [18, 19], was used to measure quality of primary care for older patients with hypertension. The questionnaire asked about primary care attributes which were recognized as the structural bases of primary care process. These attributes included first contact utilization, first contact accessibility, continuity of care, coordination of services, coordination of information, comprehensiveness of service availability, comprehensiveness of service provision, patient focused care, community oriented and cultural competence. The answers to each question were based on a four-point Likert-type scale (definitely, probably, probably not, definitely not). Scores were calculated for each question, with a higher score indicating a better quality. Attributes scores were calculated as a mean score for all questions under the subject heading (range, 1–4). A total score was calculated by adding the scores for each attribute (range, 10–40). PCAT has been used as a tool for measuring changes in primary care quality over time [20, 21].

Socioeconomic and demographic characteristics of study subjects were collected in the survey including gender, age, self-reported health status, hypertension related co-morbidities, registration status, education level, occupation, monthly household income and health insurance. Health care utilization measures were also collected by asking two questions: 1) number of CHC visits during the past one year; and 2) length of time with the visited CHC since their first visit.

Statistical analysis

The differences in individual and total primary care attributes scores between the two rounds of surveys were examined first by using independent two samples *t*-tests and then by multiple linear regression models after controlling possible confounders. We compared individual and total primary care attributes scores among the participants with different household income levels, and between the participants with and without multi-morbidities in each round of survey. Interaction between variables was also tested by including an appropriate term in the model. Potential confounders in the multiple linear regression models included socio-demographic characteristics (i.e., gender, self-reported health status, presence of multi-morbidities, registration status, education level, occupation, household income, health insurance) and health care utilization measures (number of CHC visits and length of time with the CHC). The assumptions of multiple linear regression models such as linearity, independence of errors, equal variance of errors, as well as normality of errors were tested. Model fittings were conducted by using backward elimination with a threshold of 0.10 for variable inclusion in the model. For all tests conducted in the study, a P value of <0.05 was regarded as statistically significant. All analyses were performed using SPSS20.0.

Results

No significant differences were identified in terms of gender, self-reported health status, registration status, education level, occupation, health insurance, as well as number of CHC visits between study participants in the two rounds. However, compared with the participants in the Round 1, the subjects in the Round 2 were less likely to have multi-morbidities (63.8% vs. 50.3%, $P < 0.001$). The participants in the Round 2 tended to have a higher income than those in the Round 1 ($P < 0.001$). The participants in the Round 2 had been utilizing services provided by the CHCs for a longer period when compared with those in the Round 1 ($P = 0.002$) (Table 1).

Participants in the Round 2 reported a higher score in first contact utilization (2.81 vs. 2.60, $P < 0.001$), continuity of care (3.38 vs. 3.27, $P < 0.001$), coordination of information (3.82 vs. 3.67, $P < 0.001$), comprehensiveness of service availability (3.51 vs. 3.39, $P < 0.001$) and provision (2.69 vs. 2.43, $P < 0.001$), as well as cultural competence (2.67 vs. 2.49, $P < 0.05$), while a lower score in coordination of services (2.45 vs. 2.55, $P < 0.05$) when compared with those in the Round 1. The total score reported by participants in the Round 2 was also higher than that in the Round 1, 28.73 and 27.75 respectively ($P < 0.001$). These significant differences still remained after controlling for confounding variables. Additionally, multiple regression analysis identified a significantly higher score among participants in Round 2 when compared with those in Round 1 with respect to first contact accessibility (2.48 vs. 2.44; $\beta = 0.045$, 95% CI: 0.002–0.088) (Table 2).

In the Round 1, compared with the participants having a higher household income level, those in the low income group reported a higher score in first contact utilization ($P < 0.05$), while lower scores in continuity of care ($P < 0.05$) and comprehensiveness of service availability ($P < 0.05$). In the Round 2, the participants in the higher income group than in the lower income group were found to have a higher score regarding comprehensiveness of service availability ($P < 0.05$) and family centeredness ($P < 0.05$), but a lower score in coordination of information ($P < 0.05$). However, no significant difference was identified in total primary care quality score among the participants with different household income levels in both rounds of surveys (Table 3).

In the first round of survey, there were no significant differences in all individual and total primary care attributes scores between the participants with and without multi-morbidities. However, in the second round of survey, the participants with multi-morbidities reported a higher score in coordination of services (2.47 vs. 2.44, $P < 0.001$) and coordination of information (3.84 vs. 3.80, $P < 0.001$) when compared with those without multi-morbidities (Table 4).

Table 1 Socioeconomic and demographic characteristics, and health care utilization measures of the older patients with hypertension in Round 1 and Round 2 surveys

Characteristics	Round 1 ($N=437$) n(%)	Round 2 ($N=443$) n(%)	*P* value
Demographics			
Gender			0.618
Female	293(67.0)	289(65.2)	
Male	144(33.0)	154(34.8)	
Self reported health status			0.450
Good and above	75(17.2)	84(19.0)	
Fair	283(65.8)	292(65.9)	
Poor	79(18.1)	67(15.1)	
Presence of multi-morbidities[a]			*<0.001*
Yes	279(63.8)	223(50.3)	
No	158(36.2)	220(49.7)	
Socioeconomics			
Registration[b]			1.000
Locals	421(96.3)	426(96.2)	
Migrants	16(3.7)	17(3.8)	
Education			0.120
5-year university and above	46(10.5)	65(14.7)	
3-year college	45(10.3)	55(12.4)	
High school and equivalent	126(28.8)	134(30.2)	
Middle school	154(35.2)	126(28.4)	
Primary school and below	66(15.1)	63(14.2)	
Occupation[c]			0.298
Have a job	5(1.1)	10(2.3)	
Do not have a job	432(98.9)	433(97.7)	
Household income[d]			*<0.001*
Below poverty line	75(17.2)	48(10.8)	
Between poverty line and median	328(75.1)	323(72.9)	
Above median	34(7.8)	72(16.3)	
Health insurance[e]			0.093
Yes	432(98.9)	430(97.1)	
No	5(1.1)	13(2.9)	
Visits to the primary care provider			
Number of visits in the last year, n(%)			0.167
≤ 12 visits	94(21.5)	110(24.8)	
13–24 visits	88(20.1)	101(22.8)	
25–36 visits	68(15.6)	75(16.9)	
≥ 37 visits	187(42.8)	157(35.4)	
Length of time with the health facility			*0.002*
≤ 1 year	25(5.7)	16(3.6)	
1~2 years	49(11.2)	23(5.2)	
3~4 years	55(12.6)	49(11.1)	
≥ 5 years	308(70.5)	355(80.1)	

Table 1 Socioeconomic and demographic characteristics, and health care utilization measures of the older patients with hypertension in Round 1 and Round 2 surveys *(Continued)*

[a]Hypertension related co-morbidities included cerebrovascular disease, diabetes, heart disease, kidney disease and high cholesterol

[b]Registration status dividedthe participants into two groups – migrants and locals – based on their *hukou* status, which was usually used to identify a person's official place of residence [28]

[c]The participants were classified into two groups, those who had a job (including employed and self-employed) and those who did not have a job (including the retired, students, unemployed and housewives)

[d]The participants were allocatedinto three economic groups according to monthly household poverty line (RMB3,000/US$484) and mean household income level (RMB10,000/US$1282) in 2011 [30]

[e]The participants with health insurance referred to those covered by local health insurance schemes including Basic Medical Insurance Scheme for Urban Employees and Basic Medical Insurance Scheme for Urban Residents

Discussion

This study in Shanghai found that total primary care quality perceived by older patients with hypertension improved significantly from 2011 to 2013, as reflected in improved total scores of care quality and its key attributes such as first contact utilization and accessibility, continuity of care, coordination of information, comprehensiveness of service availability and provision, and cultural competence. However, coordination of services score was lower in 2013compared to that in 2011. Although no significant difference was identified in total primary care quality score among the participants with different household income levels in each round of survey, there was some association between lower household income and lower scores in specific PCAT domains.

Increased scores in first contact suggests an improved gate-keeping role played by CHC provided primary care. This may be linked to improved patient confidence of CHC doctors due to its better capacity through training [22]. Improved scores in first contact accessibility and continuity of care echoed a previous study of all primary care users in Shanghai [16]. From 2011, older adult hypertensive patients are promoted to enroll in the general practitioner team service in CHCs [15]. The enrollees can receive hypertension management and elderly care free of charge. A free annual risk assessment and a longer duration per prescription, from two weeks to up to eight weeks, are also the benefits to enrollees. Capitation payment and pay-for-performance have been introduced [16]. Performance is determined by volume of services provided, their quality and patient satisfaction. The older adult hypertensive patients are thus easier to obtain needed care for better hypertension management (i.e., improved accessibility) [16]. The strategy encourages CHC doctors to improve continuity of care for

Table 2 Individual and total primary care attributes scores reported by the older patients with hypertension in Round 1 and Round 2 surveys

Attributes	Round 1(SE) ($N = 437$)	Round 2(SE)[a] ($N = 443$)	Adjusted β(95% CI)[b]
First contact-utilization	2.60(0.028)	2.81(0.026)***	0.206(0.132,0.280)***
First contact-accessibility	2.44(0.014)	2.48(0.016)	0.045(0.002,0.088)*
Continuity of care	3.27(0.020)	3.38(0.021)***	0.132(0.076,0.188)***
Coordination of services	2.55(0.026)	2.45(0.030)*	−0.105(−0.184,-0.025)*
Coordination of information	3.67(0.021)	3.82(0.018)***	0.147(0.090,0.204)***
Comprehensiveness- service availability	3.39(0.019)	3.51(0.015)***	0.092(0.044,0.139)***
Comprehensiveness- service provided	2.43(0.028)	2.69(0.027)***	0.260(0.182,0.339)***
Family centeredness	2.79(0.040)	2.73(0.040)	−0.059(−0.172,0.053)
Community orientation	2.11(0.033)	2.18(0.037)	0.070(−0.029,0.170)
Cultural competence	2.49(0.051)	2.67(0.052)*	0.181(0.035,0.328))*
Total score	27.75(0.172)	28.73(0.166)***	0.969(0.501,1.438)***

SE Standard error, *CI* Confidence level;
[a]Independent two-sample *t*-test,
[b]Multiple linear regression analysis where dependent variables were individual and total primary care attributes scores, while covariates were gender, self-reported health status, presence of multi-morbidities, registration, education, occupation, household income, health insurance, number of CHC visits and length of time with the CHC;
β: Calculated with Round 1 as the reference;
*$P < 0.05$;
***$P < 0.001$

improved performance. Studies showed improved overall care scores in Shanghai as compared with Shenzhen [16] and Kunming [23] where the general practitioner team policy was not or partially implemented.

We found improved score in coordination of information, but decreased score in coordination of services. The former may be linked with the establishment of a single medical insurance card that contains all medical consultations in Shanghai, which may help CHC doctors to recognize older adult hypertensive patients' multi-morbidities and their past medical history [16, 24]. The latter may be related to the relatively slow progress regarding the referral system between public hospitals and CHCs. This may be due to the competition among medical institutions for patients and profits and the lack of incentives from public hospitals to collaborate with CHCs [25].

Table 3 Individual and total primary care attributes scores reported by the older patients with hypertension with different household income levels in the two rounds of surveys

Attributes	Round 1, mean(SE)[a]			Round 2, mean(SE)[a]		
	Low($N = 75$)	Middle($N = 328$)	High($N = 34$)	Low($N = 48$)	Middle($N = 323$)	High($N = 72$)
First contact-utilization	2.74(0.064)	2.58(0.032)*	2.51(0.104)*	2.83(0.081)	2.80(0.031)	2.84(0.062)
First contact-accessibility	2.46(0.033)	2.43(0.016)	2.48(0.057)	2.47(0.049)	2.50(0.019)	2.44(0.039)
Continuity of care	3.23(0.049)	3.27(0.023)	3.37(0.067)*	3.33(0.078)	3.40(0.023)	3.28(0.061)
Coordination of services	2.56(0.055)	2.56(0.030)	2.47(0.092)	2.55(0.090)	2.43(0.037)	2.51(0.066)
Coordination of information	3.62(0.059)	3.68(0.024)	3.74(0.066)	3.89(0.038)	3.83(0.020)	3.73(0.064)*
Comprehensiveness- service availability	3.29(0.052)	3.41(0.021)*	3.41(0.076)*	3.43(0.038)	3.52(0.018)*	3.52(0.034)*
Comprehensiveness-service provided	2.47(0.067)	2.43(0.032)	2.36(0.105)	2.64(0.085)	2.68(0.032)	2.77(0.072)
Family centeredness	2.64(0.086)	2.82(0.047)	2.84(0.134)	2.58(0.116)	2.71(0.047)	2.92(0.099)*
Community orientation	2.25(0.077)	2.07(0.038)	2.14(0.117)	2.09(0.116)	2.17(0.042)	2.30(0.106)
Cultural competence	2.48(0.108)	2.47(0.061)	2.61(0.173)	2.79(0.151)	2.63(0.061)	2.76(0.135)
Total score	27.75(0.391)	27.73(0.204)	27.94(0.562)	28.59(0.525)	28.67(0.186)	29.09(0.472)

SE Standard error;
[a]Multiple linear regression analysis where dependent variables were individual and total primary care attributes scores, while independent variables were gender, self-reported health status, presence of multi-morbidities, registration, education, occupation, household income, health insurance, number of CHC visits and length of time with the CHC;
Respondents with low income were used as reference group;
*$P < 0.05$

Table 4 Individual and total primary care attributes scores reported by the older patients with hypertension with and without multi-morbidities in the two rounds of surveys

Attributes	Round 1, mean(SE)[a]		Round 2, mean(SE)[a]	
	Without($N = 158$)	With($N = 279$)	Without($N = 220$)	With($N = 223$)
First contact-utilization	2.59(0.047)	2.60(0.034)	2.84(0.036)	2.78(0.038)
First contact-accessibility	2.44(0.024)	2.44(0.018)	2.47(0.023)	2.49(0.023)
Continuity of care	3.23(0.034)	3.29(0.024)	3.41(0.030)	3.35(0.030)
Coordination of services	2.59(0.041)	2.54(0.033)	2.44(0.044)	2.47(0.042)*
Coordination of information	3.71(0.033)	3.65(0.027)	3.80(0.028)	3.84(0.024)*
Comprehensiveness- service availability	3.40(0.034)	3.39(0.023)	3.50(0.019)	3.51(0.023)
Comprehensiveness-service provided	2.39(0.049)	2.46(0.034)	2.70(0.039)	2.67(0.039)
Family centeredness	2.84(0.067)	2.76(0.050)	2.78(0.058)	2.69(0.055)
Community orientation	2.11(0.058)	2.11(0.040)	2.21(0.053)	2.16(0.053)
Cultural competence	2.57(0.088)	2.44(0.063)	2.66(0.075)	2.69(0.072)
Total score	27.86(0.297)	27.69(0.212)	28.81(0.238)	28.65(0.230)

SE: Standard error;
[a]Multiple linear regression analysis where dependent variables were individual and total primary care attributes scores, while independent variables were gender, self-reported health status, presence of multi-morbidities, registration, education, occupation, household income, health insurance, number of CHC visits and length of time with the CHC;
Respondents without multi-morbidities were used as reference group;
*$P < 0.05$

We reported improved scores in comprehensiveness of service availability and provision, suggesting that it is more likely for older adult hypertensive patients to receive non-pharmacological and pharmacological treatments to control the disease. Primary care provider team in CHCs provides a free package of clinical and preventive care for the enrolled older adult hypertensive patients. They, together with community organizations, also provide health education such as healthy diet and smoking cessation, which may improve comprehensiveness of service availability and provision. A previous study showed that hypertensive patients in Shanghai received more pharmaceutical care compared with those in Shenzhen [12]. Life-style modification initiatives are complementary to pharmaceutical treatment, and needs to be incorporated at the point of care delivery [26].

Our study did not find significant differences in total perceived primary care quality among the older adult hypertensive patients with different household income levels in both Round 1 and Round 2, which are consistent with the findings of previous studies [16, 27]. However, we did found that patients with lower household income reported lower scores for first contact utilization, continuity of care, comprehensiveness availability and family centeredness. This may reflect the inequalities of primary care quality in Shanghai primary care settings. From the health system point of view, Shanghai's primary care is fully publicly owned and operated, and showed less inequality among different income groups compared with Shenzhen, where CHCs are hospital-owned and privately operated [16]. Other studies showed that Shanghai's primary care is more equitable compared with that of Hong Kong, where public service only account for 20%, [22, 25] and Shenzhen, where a large proportion of its users, such as migrants, were not entitled to health insurance schemes [28]. Perceived quality of primary care tends to be equitable in public and no-profit primary care oriented systems such as UK, but not in countries with a large for-profit private sector in primary care [29].

The limitations of the study should be mentioned. Firstly, the generalizability of findings is limited since only 4 out of more than 200 CHCs were selected as study settings which may introduce sampling bias. Secondly, the participants were CHC users and were selected based on random cluster sampling methods, which prevents the findings from extending to the general older hypertensive patients who did not utilize services in CHCs. Thirdly, the patient-reported PCAT scores may be subject to recall bias. Finally, since this study compared findings between two cross-sectional surveys but not followed the subjects longitudinally, cause-and-effect relationship might not be directly ascertained.

Conclusions

We found that older adult hypertensive patients in Shanghai had better experiences of primary care over time, especially with respect to first contact utilization and accessibility, continuity of care, coordination of information, comprehensiveness of service availability and provision, as well as cultural competence. Our findings on better perceived quality of primary care from 2011 to 2013 may be associated with the introduction of the general practitioner team service in Shanghai since 2011.

Abbreviations
B: Blood pressure; CHCs: Community Health Centers; PCAT: Primary Care Assessment Tool

Acknowledgements
We would express thanks to all co-investigators of the project who have participated in the design of the overall study. We are also grateful to the Shanghai Association of Community Health Care for their co-ordination in data collection. There is no prior presentation in any conferences regarding this paper.

Funding
The authors would like to acknowledge the Strategic Public Policy Research of the Research Grants Council (RGC), Hong Kong [grant number 4002 SPPR 10] in providing financial support to collect the data. However, the data-analysis and writing were supported from routine University funds and Shenzhen Basic Research Program (Grant number JCYJ20160427183317387).

Authors' contributions
XW conceived of the study. XW and HL took part in the study's design. XW and HL participated in the data collection and analysis. HL, XW and MW drafted the manuscript and were responsible for data interpretation. MW provided significant comments. All authors read and approved the final manuscript.

Consent for publication
Not applicable

Competing interests
The authors declare that they have no competing interests.

Author details
[1]School of Medicine, Shenzhen University, Shenzhen, China. [2]Division of Clinical Public Health and Institute of Health Policy, Management and Evaluation, Dalla Lana School of Public Health, University of Toronto, 155 College St, Toronto, ON M5T 3M7, Canada. [3]The Jockey Club School of Public Health and Primary Care, Faculty of Medicine, The Chinese University of Hong Kong, Hong Kong, SAR, China.

References

1. Chen S, Conwell Y, Chiu HF. Loneliness and aging in China–a public health problem in need of solutions. Int Psychogeriatr. 2014;26(11):1771–2.
2. Bisognano JD, Townsend KA, Skyles AJ, Samuels KM. Prevalence of comorbidities and their influence on blood pressure goal attainment in geriatric patients. Am J Geriatr Cardiol. 2007;16(1):24–9.
3. Li D, Lv J, Liu F, Liu P, Yang X, Feng Y, Chen G, Hao M. Hypertension burden and control in mainland China: analysis of nationwide data 2003-2012. Int J Cardiol. 2015;184:637–44.
4. Wu X, Duan X, Gu D, Hao J, Tao S, Fan D. Prevalence of hypertension and its trends in Chinese populations. Int J Cardiol. 1995;52(1):39–44.
5. Hajjar I, Kotchen TA. Trends in prevalence, awareness, treatment, and control of hypertension in the United States, 1988-2000. JAMA. 2003;290(2):199–206.
6. Kearney PM, Whelton M, Reynolds K, Muntner P, Whelton PK, He J. Global burden of hypertension: analysis of worldwide data. Lancet. 2005;365(9455):217–23.
7. Li H, Wei X, Wong MC, Yang N, Wong SY, Lao X, Griffiths SM. A comparison of the quality of hypertension management in primary care between shanghai and Shenzhen: a cohort study of 3196 patients. Medicine. 2015;94(5):e455.
8. Feng XL, Pang M, Beard J. Health system strengthening and hypertension awareness, treatment and control: data from the China health and retirement longitudinal study. Bull World Health Organ. 2014;92(1):1–76.
9. Starfield B. Primary care: balancing health needs, services, and technology. New York: Oxford University Press; 1998.
10. Starfield B, Shi L, Macinko J. Contribution of primary care to health systems and health. Milbank Q. 2005;83(3):457–502.
11. D'Avila OP, Pinto LF, Hauser L, Goncalves MR, Harzheim E. The use of the primary care assessment tool (PCAT): an integrative review and proposed update. Cien Saude Colet. 2017;22(3):855–65.
12. Wei X, Zakus D, Liang H, Sun X. The shanghai case: a qualitative evaluation of community health reform in response to the challenge of population ageing. Int J Health Plann Manag. 2005;20(3):269–86.
13. Wei X, Yang N, Gao Y, Wong SY, Wong MC, Wang J, Wang HH, Li DK, Tang J, Griffiths SM. Comparison of three models of ownership of community health centres in China: a qualitative study. J Health Serv Res Policy. 2015;20(3):162–9.
14. Liu Q, Wang B, Kong Y, Cheng KK. China's primary health-care reform. Lancet. 2011;377(9783):2064–6.
15. Guiding principles on establishing the general practitioner service model. In. Edited by Council S. Beijing; 2011.
16. Wei X, Li H, Yang N, Wong SY, Chong MK, Shi L, Wong MC, Xu J, Zhang D, Tang J, et al. Changes in the perceived quality of primary care in shanghai and Shenzhen, China: a difference-in-difference analysis. Bull World Health Organ. 2015;93:407–16.
17. Shi L, Starfield B, Xu J, Politzer R, Regan J. Primary care quality: community health center and health maintenance organization. South Med J. 2003;96(8):787–95.
18. Wang HH, Wong SY, Wong MC, Wei XL, Wang JJ, Li DK, Tang JL, Gao GY, Griffiths SM. Patients' experiences in different models of community health centers in southern China. Ann Fam Med. 2013;11(6):517–26.
19. Yang H, Shi L, Lebrun LA, Zhou X, Liu J, Wang H. Development of the Chinese primary care assessment tool: data quality and measurement properties. Int J Qual Health Care. 2013;25(1):92–105.
20. Tourigny A, Aubin M, Haggerty J, Bonin L, Morin D, Reinharz D, Leduc Y, St-Pierre M, Houle N, Giguere A, et al. Patients' perceptions of the quality of care after primary care reform: family medicine groups in Quebec. Can Fam Physician. 2010;56(7):e273–82.
21. Yin J, Wei X, Li H, Jiang Y, Mao C. Assessing the impact of general practitioner team service on perceived quality of care among patients with non-communicable diseases in China: a natural experimental study. Int J Qual Health Care. 2016;28(5):554–60.
22 Wei X, Li H, Yang N, Wong SY, Owolabi O, Xu J, Shi L, Tang J, Li D, Griffiths SM. Comparing quality of public primary care between Hong Kong and shanghai using validated patient assessment tools. PLoS One. 2015;10(3):e0121269.
23 Yin J, Wei X, Li H, Jiang Y, Mao C. Assessing the impact of general practitioner team service on perceived quality of care among patients with non-communicable diseases in China: a natural experimental study. Int J Qual Health Care. 2016:1–7.
24 Yip WC, Hsiao WC, Chen W, Hu S, Ma J, Maynard A. Early appraisal of China's huge and complex health-care reforms. Lancet. 2012;379(9818):833–42.
25 Wei X, Yin J, Wong SY, Griffiths SM, Zou G, Shi L. Private ownership of primary care providers associated with patient perceived quality of care: a comparative cross-sectional survey in three big Chinese cities. Medicine. 2017;96(1):e5755.
26 Zou G, Zhang Z, Walley J, Gong W, Yu Y, Hu R, Yin J, Yu M, Wei X. Use of medications and lifestyles of hypertensive patients with high risk of cardiovascular disease in rural china. PLoS One. 2015;10(5):e0124484.
27 Li H, Wei X, Wong MC, Wong SY, Yang N, Griffiths SM, Cross-Sectional Comparison A. Of perceived quality of primary care by hypertensive patients in shanghai and Shenzhen, China. Medicine. 2015;94(34):e1388.
28 Li H, Chung RY, Wei X, Mou J, Wong SY, Wong MC, Zhang D, Zhang Y, Griffiths S. Comparison of perceived quality amongst migrant and local patients using primary health care delivered by community health centres in Shenzhen, China. BMC Fam Pract. 2014;15:76.
29 Mills A, Brugha R, Hanson K, McPake B. What can be done about the private health sector in low-income countries? Bull World Health Organ. 2002;80(4): 325–30.
30 Shanghai Statistical Bureau: Report of income growth in shanghai. In.; 2011.

12

Clinical effectiveness of care managers in collaborative care for patients with depression in Swedish primary health care

Cecilia Björkelund[1,9*], Irene Svenningsson[1], Dominique Hange[1], Camilla Udo[2], Eva-Lisa Petersson[1,3], Nashmil Ariai[1], Shabnam Nejati[1], Catrin Wessman[4], Carl Wikberg[1], Malin André[5], Lars Wallin[2,6,7] and Jeanette Westman[8]

Abstract

Background: Depression is one of the leading causes of disability and affects 10-15% of the population. The majority of people with depressive symptoms seek care and are treated in primary care. Evidence internationally for high quality care supports collaborative care with a care manager. Our aim was to study clinical effectiveness of a care manager intervention in management of primary care patients with depression in Sweden.

Methods: In a pragmatic cluster randomized controlled trial 23 primary care centers (PCCs), urban and rural, included patients aged ≥ 18 years with a new (< 1 month) depression diagnosis. Intervention consisted of Care management including continuous contact between care manager and patient, a structured management plan, and behavioral activation, altogether around 6-7 contacts over 12 weeks. Control condition was care as usual (CAU). Outcome measures: Depression symptoms (measured by Mongomery-Asberg depression score-self (MADRS-S) and BDI-II), quality of life (QoL) (EQ-5D), return to work and sick leave, service satisfaction, and antidepressant medication. Data were analyzed with the intention-to-treat principle.

Results: One hundred ninety two patients with depression at PCCs with care managers were allocated to the intervention group, and 184 patients at control PCCs were allocated to the control group. Mean depression score measured by MADRS-S was 2.17 lower in the intervention vs. the control group (95% CI [0.56; 3.79], $p = 0.009$) at 3 months and 2.27 lower (95% CI [0.59; 3.95], $p = 0.008$) at 6 months; corresponding BDI-II scores were 1.96 lower (95% CI [− 0.19; 4.11], $p = 0.07$) in the intervention vs. control group at 6 months. Remission was significantly higher in the intervention group at 6 months (61% vs. 47%, $p = 0.006$). QoL showed a steeper increase in the intervention group at 3 months ($p = 0.01$). During the first 3 months, return to work was significantly higher in the intervention vs. the control group. Patients in the intervention group were more consistently on antidepressant medication than patients in the control group.

(Continued on next page)

* Correspondence: Cecilia.bjorkelund@allmed.gu.se
[1]Department of Primary Health Care, Institute of Medicine, The Sahlgrenska Academy, University of Gothenburg, Gothenburg, Sweden
[9]Department of Primary Health Care, Institute of Medicine, The Sahlgrenska Academy, University of Gothenburg, Box 454, 40530 Göteborg, Sweden
Full list of author information is available at the end of the article

(Continued from previous page)

Conclusions: Care managers for depression treatment have positive effects on depression course, return to work, remission frequency, antidepressant frequency, and quality of life compared to usual care and is valued by the patients.

Keywords: Depression, Primary care, Care manager, Collaborative care, Sick-leave, Quality-of- life

Background

Depression is one of the leading causes of disability and affects 10-15% of the population [1, 2]. According to WHO, unipolar depressive disorders are the leading cause of years of healthy life lost due to disability in both men and women [2]. The majority of people with depressive symptoms seek care and are treated in primary care [1–5]. Most patients with depression have mild, moderate, or greater functional impairment that is not always congruent with the severity of the depression [6, 7]. In working life today, which is characterized by increasing high demands on cognitive performance [8], depression is one of the most common reasons for sick leave and is costly not only for the individual but also for society [9].

Depression is a common problem among patients visiting primary care. At present, best evidence internationally for high quality care and effectiveness in care of patients with depression supports collaborative care with a care manager [9].

Collaborative care interventions with care managers are organizational interventions to improve patient care by leadership support, decision support developed within the PCC, linkage to psychiatry specialist resources and community resources, and, most importantly, by engagement of the patients in their care through self-management support [10, 11]. Research shows that isolated, separate interventions are not effective for improving the treatment and management of depression in primary care [12, 13]. This means that increased waiting room screening, development of clinical guidelines, and training in refined diagnostics as separate interventions do not generate better efficiency or quality in the management and treatment of patients with depression compared to usual primary care [12, 13]. Literature reviews have shown that only those organizational measures known as collaborative care that include complex interventions can reduce depression and improve patient satisfaction and quality of life more than usual care [13–16]. Such complex interventions include measures such as education for all personnel at the primary care center (PCC) about guidelines on depression treatment and prevention; strengthening the role of nurses (care managers) who carry out telephone counseling, give treatment advice, and develop call systems; and increasing the integration between primary care and specialized care [13].

The care manager puts collaborative care into practice. Care management combines increased accessibility to the PCC via patient contacts with continuity of care for the patient and organizational and educational development at the PCC. Care management thus facilitates the care of patients with depression, improves team communication, and improves communication with secondary care (and thus continuity of care) [16]. Care managers are responsible for providing support to and maintaining continuous contact with patients with depression, training the care team, and providing feedback on the course of the patient's depression to the physician. Studies have shown that care management is an effective strategy for successfully organizing depression treatment in primary care [13–16]. Care management increased the adequacy of antidepressant prescription, reduced patients' symptom burden, and was cost effective [13]. However, after noting that there is a knowledge gap about care management and care managers in depression primary care treatment in Sweden, the national health care authorities called for clinical studies in Swedish primary care to evaluate the effectiveness of care management [14].

Complex interventions including organizational changes are context bound. Swedish primary care is publicly financed with salary paid GPs, organized in rather large group practices also with specialized nurses, and often including psychotherapists. Patients' visits are fewer and longer compared to other Western countries [17].Thus, it was important to test care management in Swedish primary care to study whether it could provide more effective treatment for patients with depression than care as usual (CAU). We set out to investigate whether specially trained district nurses could facilitate effective, person-centered treatment that is concordant with evidence-based guidelines for treatment of depression in primary care.

The aim of the present study was to compare the short- and long-term effects of care management and care as usual upon remission of depressive symptoms, return to work, treatment adherence, quality of life, and patients' satisfaction with care.

Methods

The study was designed as a pragmatic cluster randomized controlled trial of two groups (intervention and control), named the PRIM-CARE RCT (PRImary care CARE manager). The randomization was at the level of the primary care centers (PCCs). All PCCs without an onsite function at the PCC equal or comparable to a care manager in the Region Västra Götaland (VG Region) were invited to participate in the implementation of a care manager at the PCC. The implementation was designed in cooperation between the Region's care manager implementation team and the research team, based on available evidence [7–11, 13–15], and the first wave of the implementation was carried out as the PRIM-CARE RCT. The implementation was planned to be extended to all other interested PCCs after the completion of the PRIM-CARE study. In VG Region, 160 PCCs declared an interest in participating in the implementation, and 23 of these PCCs were also interested in taking part in the research trial. Four PCCs in Region Dalarna also declared interest and were included in the study. For organizational reasons, 4 PCCs in VG Region declined participation. Consequently, the PCCs in this final group of 23 PCCs who were randomized to intervention PCCs were the first PCCs to implement a care manager function. The intervention consisted of care manager contact during 12 weeks at 11 PCCs. Control was care as usual (CAU) at 12 PCCs. Data on the PCCs are presented in Fig. 1 [18].

Population

Patients attending 23 different urban and rural PCCs, aged ≥ 18 years, diagnosed with a new (< 1 month) mild or moderate (according to Montgomery-Åsberg Depression Rating Scale- Self assessment (MADRS-S) < 35) depression (ICD-10 diagnosis F32, F33) [19] and not diagnosed with bipolar disorder, psychosis, addiction, or cognitive impairment were included. Those not speaking/understanding Swedish were excluded. Start of inclusion was December 2014.

Outcome

Primary outcome was patient's depressive symptoms (measured by MADRS-S [19, 20] and BDI-II [21]) at 6 months.

Secondary outcomes were patient's quality of life (EuroQoL-5D 3 L scale, English tariff [22]), sick leave

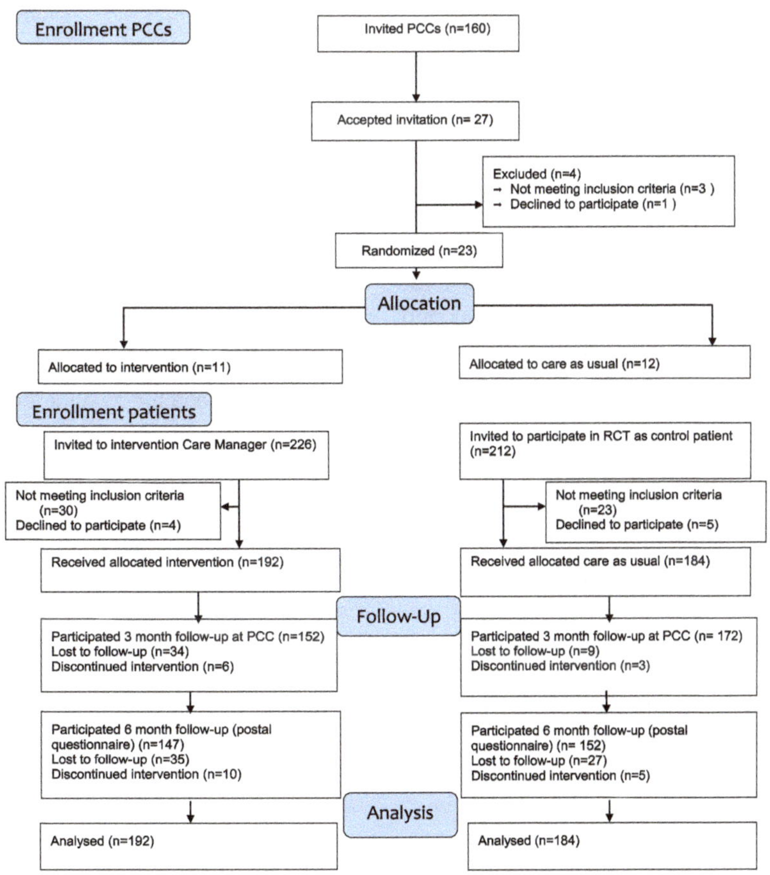

Fig. 1 Consort flow chart of the PRIM-CARE RCT. PCCs engaged in the study and patients recruited in the study at the intervention and control PCCs from baseline and 3 and 6 months follow-up (15)

(days), percentage return to work (RTW), antidepressant medication, and patient satisfaction (from Psychiatric Outpatient Satisfaction Scale [23]) at 3 and 6 months.

Initial data collection included age, gender, socio-demographic and economic variables, alcohol consumption, physical activity, and ethnicity. In the 3 and 6 month follow-ups, sick leave status, RTW, data on medication, comorbidity and other treatment (psychological, counseling, or other) were collected. For somatic health reasons, blood pressure and p-glucose were monitored.

Randomization

The 23 health care centers were stratified into two strata; rural (12 health care centers) and urban (11 health care centers). Each stratum was allocated into six blocks consisting of two health care centers, in which one was randomly assigned to implement the care manager function.

Intervention

At the intervention PCCs, a nurse devoted around 20-25% of working time as care manager for management of care for the patients with depression. Before patient recruitment began, GPs and the nurse/district nurse (care manager) participated in sessions (for GPs 2 one-day sessions and for care managers 1 three-days session before start of intervention + 2 one-day sessions during initial part of intervention) for training in providing clinical services. During the study every PCC, both intervention and control PCCs, was regularly, at least once a week, visited by the research assistants (all specialized nurses) and in addition, solely for intervention PCCs, regular follow-up meetings were held every second month where all care managers participated and where difficulties, obstacles, and successes were discussed and dealt with together with the research team and the Region's implementation team.

Clinical services for the care manager consisted of creating an individual care plan (1 h session with patient) and further telephone contacts between nurse and patient at least 6-8 times (around 15-30 min each) during 12 weeks, with person-centered communication around depressive symptoms based on the patient's current depression symptom assessment with a self-assessment instrument in connection with the regular telephone call, as well as behavioral activation [19, 24]. Thus, the intervention group received care as usual plus the intervention. All patients could directly contact the care manager between the scheduled telephone contacts if they needed. The care manager had direct and regular contact with the General Practitioner (GP), therapist, or other PCC personnel who were involved in the care of the patient. The care manager did not include any type of psycho-therapy in her/his care of the patient, but supported the patient and increased the accessibility and continuity of the PCC's care for the patient, coupled with organizational changes that would facilitate care for the patient with depression (see Table 1).

Control

Participants at the control PCCs received care as usual (CAU) according to standard protocol and procedures. The Swedish National Guidelines for Depression and Anxiety Disorders recommend high accessibility and continuity, early next appointment, guided self-help, cognitive behavior therapy (CBT) (face-to-face or internet delivered), interpersonal therapy, and/or antidepressants as first and second steps in a stepped care model [3].

Table 1 The care manager function in the PRIM-CARE trial: Function for the patient and function for the PCC's organization of depression care

Care manager function for the patient	Care manger function for the PCC's organization of depression care
Is the contact nurse for patients with depression at the PCC and facilitates the continuity and accessibility of care	Supports development of an organization for collaborative care cooperation (physician, psychologist, psychotherapist, counselor, rehabilitation personnel etc.)
Makes a structured management plan together with the patient	Facilitates cooperation with psychiatry, secondary care, community services, etc.
Keeps close cooperation with the patient's GP and inter-professional communication	Facilitates continuity and accessibility
Follows patient symptoms by scheduled follow-ups	
Follows antidepressant treatment and possible side effects	
Pays attention to the needs of changed antidepressants or other treatment if the patient does not improve - and notifies the physician	
Provides advice on self-care and encourages behavioral activation such as planning for physical activity and pleasant events	
Informs about psychotherapy and other treatment	
Educates patients (and their families) about depression	

Enrollment of patients and diagnostic procedure
All patients ≥ 18 years seeking care at the PCCs and who were judged to have a probable diagnosis of new (< 1 month) depression in connection with a visit to a doctor, nurse, or therapist and not judged to have any of the exclusion criteria were asked and informed about participation. The patients who accepted to participate immediately received a visit to the PCC's care manager (intervention PCC), alternatively to a research nurse (control PCC), for diagnosis confirmation and research baseline data purposes. The depression diagnosis was confirmed by use of PRIME-MD (depression module) in accordance with DSM-IV criteria for mild/moderate depressive disorder [25].

Statistical analysis
Standard statistical methods were used for descriptive statistics. Continuous variables were analyzed by independent sample t-test or Mann-Whitney U test and categorical variables or frequencies by Pearson chi-square test. Means of intra-individual change of depressive symptoms, and quality of life (QoL) scores were compared between the intervention group and the TAU group by using mixed model analysis with repeated measures. These analyses were adjusted for the type of PCC, age, sex, education, antidepressants at inclusion, and response variable at baseline.

The statistical analyses were made using statistical software SPSS, version 23 and SAS, version 9.4. Statistical significance was set at $p < 0.05$. No multiple adjustments were considered. We did not adjust for the cluster randomization due to sparse data in some of the health centers.

Power calculation
The primary variable was the level of depression (as measured by MADRS-S and BDI-II) and analyzed in an ANCOVA model with repeated measures. In order to detect an effect of 3 units in the difference between the two groups, with a power of 80% and a significance level of 10% (two-sided), around 200 patients were needed in each group. The underlying assumption was a standard deviation in the group of 10 units, a within-subject correlation of 0.4, and a within-cluster correlation of 0.1, i.e. a design effect of 1.9 to correct for having a cluster analysis.

Results

The inclusion of patients started in December 2014 and continued until January 2016, and 6 months follow-up was completed by August 2016. In all, 192 patients with mild-moderate depression (according to MADRS-S < 35) were included at the intervention PCCs with care manager and 184 patients at the control PCCs with CAU. Participation of PCCs and patients from baseline and at 3 and 6 months are shown in Fig. 1. At the 3 month follow-up, 86% participated: 79% at the intervention PCCs and 93% at control PCCs, and at 6 months 76% and 83%, respectively (postal questionnaire) (Fig. 1). Table 2 shows baseline data for intervention and control patients. There were no statistically significant differences between participants in the intervention and control patient groups at baseline concerning age, gender, lifestyle, education, occupation, sick leave, depression symptom scores (MADRS-S and BDI), or QoL.

Non-participants
A total of 34 patients did not participate in the 3 and 6 months follow-up, 29 in the intervention group and 5 in the control group. Patients lost to follow-up were not reached despite several contacts by mail and telephone. There were statistically significant differences ($p < 0.05$) at baseline concerning age (non- participants: mean age around 10 years younger), MADRS-S (non- participants: mean value around 4 units higher) and BDI-II (non- participants: mean value around 4 units higher), and in the intervention group, a greater proportion of the non-participants were students. There were no other significant differences between participants and non-participants concerning demographic data described in Table 2.

The course of depression and QoL is shown in Fig. 2a, b, and c. There was a substantial reduction of depression scores both in intervention and control groups, but the reduction was significantly greater in the intervention group compared to control group when measured with MADRS-S, and the difference still progressed during the period 4-6 months, although the care manager intervention was terminated at 3 months. Mean depression score measured by MADRS-S was 2.17 lower (95% CI [0.56; 3.79], $p = 0.009$) at 3 months and 2.27 lower (95% CI [0.59; 3.95], $p = 0.008$) at 6 months. The QoL also showed a steeper increase in the intervention group from baseline to 3 months (statistically significant difference between intervention and control at 3 months, $p = 0.01$), but this leveled off at the 6 months follow-up. Depression score reduction measured by BDI-II did not reach significance. Mean depression score measured by BDI-II was 0.44 lower (95% CI [– 1.62; 2.50], $p = 0.67$) at 3 months, and 1.96 lower (95% CI [– 0.19; 4.11], $p = 0.07$) at 6 months.

Table 3 shows remission frequency, defined as MADRS-S ≤ 12, in intervention and control group at 3 and 6 months follow-up. There was a statistically significant higher remission frequency in the intervention group at 6 months follow-up, 67% compared to 47% in the control CAU group, also illustrating the progress of

Table 2 Demographics at baseline for primary care patients in the intervention group (care manager during depression) and the control group (care as usual during depression). Figures indicate numbers and percentage (%) of patients

	Intervention $n = 192$	Control $n = 184$	Total $n = 376$	p
Age				
Mean (SD)	40.8 (15.0)	41.6 (15,4)	41.2 (15.2)	0.61
Gender, n(%)				
Women	131 (68.2)	137 (74.5)	268 (71.3)	0.18
Men	61 (56.0)	47 (44.0)	108 (28.7)	
BMI				
Mean (SD)	25.6 (5.57)	25.8 (5.2)	25.6 (5.6)	0.73
Occupation n (%)				
Working	137 (72.9)	122 (66.3)	259 (69.6)	
Studying	18 (9.6)	19 (10.3)	37 (9.9)	
In search of work/other	23 (17.6)	43 (23.4)	76 (20.5)	0.52
Working, n (%)				
Full-time	157 (87.7)	149 (87.6)	306 (87.7)	0.98
Other (25-75%)	22 (12.3)	21 (12.4)	43 (12.3)	
Marital status, n (%)				
Cohabiting	122 (67)	122 (68)	244 (67)	0.82
Single	61 (33)	58 (32)	119 (33)	
Born				
Outside Nordic Country n (%)	18 (9.4)	21 (11.5)	39 (10.4)	0.63
Educational level n (%)				
Primary education	17 (8.9)	27 (14.8)	44 (11.8)	
Secondary education	103 (53.9)	90 (49.2)	193 (51.9)	
University or college	71 (37.2)	66 (36.1)	137 (36.6)	0.21
Physical activity leisure time n (%)				
Sedentary	25 (13.1)	33 (17.9)	58 (15.5)	0.44
Smoking n (%)				0.26
Yes+ sometimes	45 (23.5)	56 (30.5)	101 (26.9)	
Alcohol n (%)				
once a week	14 (7.4)	14 (7.7)	28 (7.5)	0.92
Sick leave n (%)				
Sick leave last year (Yes)	83 (45.6)	66 (37.9)	149 (41.9)	0.14
On sick leave baseline	93 (50.5)	94 (55.0)	187 (52.7)	0.40
MADRS-S m (SD)	20.8 (7.2)	21.9 (7.1)	21.4 (7.1)	0.12
BDI-II m (SD)	23.9 (8.7)	25.1 (8.5)	24.5 (8.7)	0.16
EQ-5D m (SD)	0.58 (0.24)	0.56 (0.25)	0.57 (0.24)	0.41

depression symptom score reduction during the 4-6 months period in the intervention group.

Use of antidepressants was present at inclusion in 53% and 63% of the intervention and control group patients, respectively, and continued at the same level in the intervention group (51%), but significantly increased to 67% in the control group at 3 months follow-up (see Table 3). However, at 6 months follow-up, the antidepressant medication frequency in the control group was somewhat reduced to 61%, while the antidepressant medication frequency in the intervention group still remained stable at 51%.

At inclusion, 53% of the patients were on sick leave, with no significant difference between intervention and control patients (50.5% and 55%, respectively) (Fig. 3). During the period between baseline and 3 months

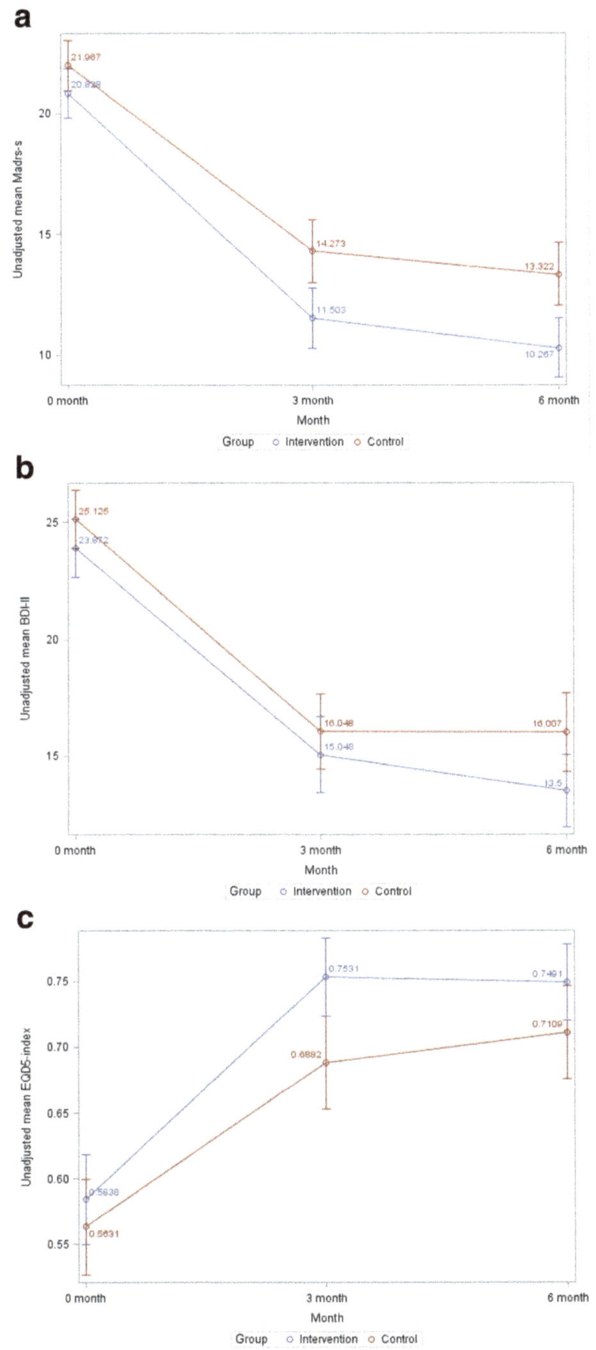

Fig. 2 a Unadjusted mean of patient depression scores measured with MADRS-S at baseline, 3 and 6 months follow-up, with unadjusted confidence bars at each occasion. Statistically significant adjusted differences between intervention and control at 3 months ($p = 0.009$) and 6 months ($p = 0.008$) follow-up. **b** Unadjusted mean of patient depression scores measured with BDI-II at baseline, at 3 months ($p = 0.67$) and 6 months follow-up ($p = 0.07$) with unadjusted confidence bars at each occasion. **c** Unadjusted mean of patient quality of life scores measured with EQ-5D at baseline, at 3 months ($p = 0.01$) and 6 months follow-up (NS) with unadjusted confidence bars at each occasion

follow-up, 55% of patients in the intervention group (83/152) and 51% (88/172) in the control group were on sick leave (ranging between 25 and 100% sick leave); mean number of sick leave days was 69.2 (intervention) and 66.2 (control). During the 4-6 months, 40% (59/147) of the intervention and 42% (64/152) of the control group patients were on sick leave for 60 and 62 mean days, respectively (Fig 3). However, significantly more patients in the intervention group returned to work during baseline to 3 months follow-up (62% vs 43%, $p = 0.028$), as significantly more patients in the intervention group returned via part-time sick leave (in Sweden 25, 50, and 75%) (Table 3, and Fig. 3).

Patients were asked by a questionnaire distributed by the research personnel (postal questionnaire at the 6 months follow-up) about the helpfulness, perception of waiting time, information given, and whether they would recommend the treatment to family members and/or close friends [23]. There were statistically significant differences between intervention and control patients concerning recommending the treatment to close friends and relatives (Table 4), but on the whole most patients were satisfied with the care given at the PCCs.

Discussion

This study showed that PCCs that establish organizational changes concerning depression care through the implementation of a care manager improve the quality of care within a 6 month perspective, as indicated by significant reduction of depression (based on MADRS-S score), significant increase of remission frequency, QoL, and RTW compared to PCCs with care as usual for the depressed patient. Further, the patients' antidepressant medication continued in accordance with guideline recommendations, and antidepressant medication frequency was more continuously stable when a care manager had been engaged. Patient reported satisfaction was also more favorable in PCCs with a care manager.

Strengths and limitations

The majority of all PCCs in a region with 1.6 million inhabitants were invited to this trial. The participating PCCs, constituting around 10% of all PCCs, were representative of the region as a whole, with both urban and rural PCCs scattered over the region. Thus, the participating PCCs can be regarded as representative for Swedish primary care (total number 1200 PCCs). The number of patients recruited by the PCCs was satisfactory for attaining the pre-determined level of statistical power. The results of this trial could consequently be generalizable and representative for Swedish primary care. The attrition rate was low, and through access to the electronic patient records, complementary data

Table 3 Remission frequency and use of antidepressant frequency at 3 and 6 months follow-up in the PRIM-CARE RCT. Remission defined as MADRS-S ≤ 12

	3 months Intervention N = 149	3 months Control N = 152	p	6 months Intervention N = 146	6 months Control N = 152	p
	n (%)	n (%)		n (%)	n (%)	
Remission according to MADRS-S (≤ 12)	74 (49.7)	73 (42.4)	0.20	98 (67)	72 (47)	*0.001*
Use of antidepressants	77 (50.7)	116(67.4)	*0.02*	75 (51.0)	92(60.5)	0.10
Individuals (n; %) on sick leave	83 (54.6)	88 (51.2)	0.54	59 (40.1)	64 (42.1)	0.73
Individuals (n;%) with return to work (full or part-time)	40(62.5)	33(42.9)	*0.02*	7 (33)	10 (33)	1.0

Italic figures; statistically significant difference between intervention and control group

especially concerning medication and sick certification were also collected.

However, there were also limitations. Due to the comprehensive organizational changes that the establishment of a care manager entailed for a PCC, concealment of the intervention status of the PCC was not possible, and all personnel at the intervention PCCs were thoroughly informed about the aim of the study and the care manager organization. The 3 months assessment at the intervention PCCs was carried out by research personnel unknown to the patient, as it could have been a possible source of bias if the assessment was made by the local care manager. At the control PCCs, the 3 months assessment was administered by a specially trained research nurse. Further, we used both MADRS-S and BDI-II as measures of depression symptom outcomes, but only MADRS-S outcomes showed statistically significant differences between the intervention and control group, although BDI-II outcomes showed similar tendencies. However, MADRS-S is an instrument specially constructed to measure change in depression course, while BDI-II is an instrument developed primarily for measuring level of depression. The instruments are complementary and show good correspondence in primary care [26], but MADRS-S is more clinically applicable for primary care and more clinically relevant concerning measurement of depression level severity [26]. Another limitation is the follow-up duration, which only covered 6 months. Important health economic consequences concerning especially care consumption, sick leave duration, and RTW for mild/medium depressed individuals should preferably be evaluated within a longer time perspective. However, in a 6 month perspective, this PRIM-CARE RCT already has shown important significant effects concerning full recovery from depression and earlier RTW, despite lower antidepressant medication frequency.

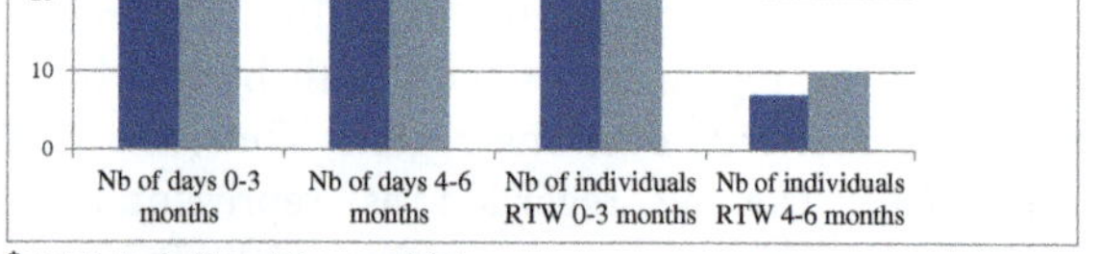

* statistically significant difference, p=0.028

Fig. 3 Mean number of days on sick leave from baseline to 3 months and 4 to 6 months for intervention and control group in the PRIM-CARE trial, as well as number of individuals who returned to work from baseline to 3 months, and 4 to 6 months for intervention and control group. Statistically significantly more patients in the intervention group returned via part-time sick leave to work during baseline to 3 months follow-up (62% vs 43%, $p = 0.028$)

The care manager's function at the PCC is to combine patient contacts for increased accessibility and continuity for the patient as well as facilitate support for the depressed patient through organizational changes [11]. Swedish primary care has high quality concerning medical and psycho-therapeutic competence, which is shown by the relatively modest differences between the results in the intervention and control groups. However, cornerstones of primary care such as accessibility and continuity are not sufficiently met in Swedish primary care [27], and in that respect a care manager can make a difference, especially for the group of patients with depression and anxiety, who often have low access to care due to the symptoms of the disorder. Quality improvements in Swedish primary care should also strongly enhance non-psycho-therapeutic care components to support the patient's recovery by facilitating the patient's own course to remission [3, 14, 15]. Further, those individuals who do not improve or deteriorate in their depression course are earlier identified by the continuous care manager contact [14].

Recently, several trials and literature reviews have been published on collaborative care with care managers in primary care [16, 28, 29]. Studies show that mental illness often negatively affects other somatic conditions, and a care manager who coordinates the care by

Table 4 Patient reported outcomes (Psychiatric Outpatient Satisfaction Scale) concerning perceived helpfulness, waiting time, information, respect of patient's opinion, and whether the patient would recommend the treatment to family members and/or close friends

	Intervention		Control		
Opinion on	Good/excellent n (%)	Insufficient n (%)	Good/excellent n (%)	Insufficient n (%)	*p*
Helpfulness of PCC (baseline)	169 (100)	0(0)	179 (98.9)	2 (1.1)	0.17
Waiting time to visit (baseline)	165 (98.2)	3 (1.8)	165 (95.4)	8 (4.6)	0.14
Information given to you about your problem (baseline)	161 (98.2)	3 (1.8)	167 (96)	7 (4)	0.23
Information given to you about your problem (3 months)	138 (96.5)	5 (3.5)	138 91.4	13 (8.6)	0.07
Respect shown for your opinions about treatment (baseline)	163 (99.4)	1 (0.6)	163 (98.8)	2 (1.2)	0.56
Respect shown for your opinions about treatment (3 months)	130 (95.6)	6 (4.4)	140 (95.9)	6 (4.1)	0.9
Would you recommend this treatment to a friend or family member (baseline)	170 (98.8)	2 (1.2)	168 (96.0)	7 (4.0)	0.10
Would you recommend this treatment to a friend or family member (3 months)	137 (95.8)	6 (4.2)	137 (89.0)	17 (11.0)	0.03
Would you recommend this treatment to a friend or family member (6 months)	131 (97.8)	3 (2.2)	126 (86.9)	19 (13.1)	0.001

maintaining a close and regular contact with patients and aligns efforts for their individual needs is shown not only to generate improvement of the depression but also improvement of the physical health [16]. A recent systematic review of measures in primary care leading to improved RTW also showed, similar to our study, that adding a care manager to the PCC organization is one of few factors that increase RTW for the individual [9].

The distinguishing features of a collaborative care organization with a care manager in contrast to most other types of measures already undertaken in primary care are the provision of high accessibility and continuity for the individual but also the opportunity afforded for individuals to gain knowledge about their disease, as well as the increased ability to customize care interventions to the individual's specific needs [1, 14]. This type of care organization also allows for a better engagement of the entire PCC in terms of resources and contacts with other health care levels and society in general and provides opportunities for the continuity of these contacts. Such an organization facilitates health care that is adapted to the patient's specific needs over time in close collaboration with the patient [14, 28, 29] and thus allows for complexity, person-centered care, and interaction on multiple levels.

Conclusions

Our evaluation of the implementation of a care manager organization at the Swedish PCC within a 6 month perspective has shown important significant effects concerning full recovery from depression and earlier RTW for the patient, despite lower antidepressant medication frequency. The care manager organization represents a cost for the PCC in order to attain increased quality of care, especially concerning increased accessibility and continuity for the patient, and this cost should in some way be reimbursed. Further information on outcomes concerning depression, RTW, function and sick leave will be obtained in the upcoming 12 month follow-up, as well as in a health economic evaluation. The feasibility and the effectiveness of a care manager function for depressed patients also in ordinary Swedish primary care could be regarded as proven in this pragmatic RCT.

Abbreviations

BDI-II: Beck Depression Inventory II; CAU: Care as usual; CI: Confidence interval; EQ-5D: EuroQol 5 Dimensions; GP: General Practitioner; ICD-10: International Classification of Diagnoses; MADRS-S: Montgomery-Asberg Depression Rating Scale-Self (Self-administered); NS: Not statistically significant; PCC: Primary care centers; PRIM-CARE: PRIMary care CARE manager; QoL: Quality of Life; RCT: Randomized Controlled Trial; RTW: Return to work; TMG: Trial management group; VG Region: Region Västra Götaland

Acknowledgements

The authors are grateful to the participating PCCs, all patients and all personnel. We are also grateful for support and cooperation with Region Västra Götaland, the Region's implementation team, and Närhälsan Research and Development Primary Health Care.

Funding

The study was financed by grants from the Västra Götaland Region of Sweden. The study sponsors had no role in the collection, analysis, interpretation of data, or the writing of the report or the decision to submit the article for publication. All authors were independent from funders.

Authors' contributions

CB was chief investigator and initiated the project, designed the RCT, chaired the Trial Management Group (TMG), drafted and revised the paper and is guarantor. JW, IS, DH, E-LP, participated in the design of the RCT, was member of the TMG, assisted during the whole conduct of the RCT at the PCCs sites, monitored data, drafted and revised the paper. CWi, CU and SN assisted during the whole conduct of the RCT at the PCCs sites, monitored data, drafted and revised the paper and were members of the TMG. NA, CWe, MA and LW were members of the TMG, contributed to the trial design, drafted and revised the paper. All authors had full access to all of the study data and take responsibility for the integrity and accuracy of the data. All authors have read and approved the final version of the paper.

Consent for publication

Not applicable.

Competing interests

All authors declare that they have no competing interest.

Author details

[1]Department of Primary Health Care, Institute of Medicine, The Sahlgrenska Academy, University of Gothenburg, Gothenburg, Sweden. [2]School of Education, Health and Social Studies, Dalarna University, Falun, Sweden. [3]Region Västra Götaland, Närhälsan Research and Development Primary Health Care, Gothenburg, Sweden. [4]Health Metrics Unit, Sahlgrenska Academy, University of Gothenburg, Gothenburg, Sweden. [5]Department of Public Health and Caring Sciences - Family Medicine and Preventive Medicine, Uppsala University, Uppsala, Sweden. [6]Department of Health and Care Sciences, The Sahlgrenska Academy, University of Gothenburg, Gothenburg, Sweden. [7]Division of Nursing, Department of Neurobiology, Care Sciences and Society, Karolinska Institute, Stockholm, Sweden. [8]Division of Family Medicine, Department of Neurobiology, Care Sciences and Society, Karolinska Institute, Stockholm, Sweden. [9]Department of Primary Health Care, Institute of Medicine, The Sahlgrenska Academy, University of Gothenburg, Box 454, 40530 Göteborg, Sweden.

References

1. Swedish Council on Health Technology Assessment. Treatment of depressive disorders – a literature review. Report 166. Stockholm: 2004. p. 1.
2. WHO. Methods and data sources for global burden of disease estimates 2000-2011. Geneva: WHO; 2013. http://www.who.int/healthinfo/statistics/GlobalDALYmethods_2000_2011.pdf. Accessed 25 May 2017.
3. National Guidelines for depression and anxiety syndromes. The Swedish National Board of Health and Welfare. Stockholm; 2010. http://www.angest-stockholm.se/wp-content/uploads/2009/08/Socialstyrelsens-riktlinjer-depression-och-angestsyndrom.pdf. Accessed 27 Jan 2018.
4. Månsson J, Nilsson G, Strender LE, Björkelund C. Reasons for encounters, investigations, referrals, diagnoses and treatments in general practice in Sweden–a multicentre pilot study using electronic patient records. Euro J Gen Pract. 2011;17(2):87–94.
5. Roca M, Gill M, Garcia-Garcia M, Salva J, Ylves M, Garcia Campayo J, et al. Prevalence and comorbidity of common mental disorders in primary care. J Affect Disord. 2009;119(1):52–8.
6. Rost K, Nutting P, Smith J, Werner J, Duan N. Improving depression outcomes in community primary care practice: a randomized trial of the quEST intervention. Quality enhancement by strategic teaming. J Gen Intern Med. 2001;16:143–9.
7. Adler DA, TJ ML, Rogers WH, Chang H, Lapitsky L, Lerner D. Job performance deficits due to depression. Am J Psychiatry. 2006;163(9):1569–76.
8. Willis RJ. The cognitive demands of work and the length of working life: the case of computerization. Stanford: Stanford Inst. for Economic Policy Research; 2013. http://siepr.stanford.edu/sites/default/files/publications/Cognitive_Demands_v10_7_13_0.pdf. Accessed 25 May 2017.
9. Nieuwenhuijsen K, Faber B, Verbeek JH, Neumeyer-Gromen A, Hees HL, Verhoeven AC, et al. Interventions to improve return to work in depressed people. Cochrane Database Syst. Rev. 2014;12:CD006237.
10. Archer J, Bower P, Gilbody S, Lovell K, Richards D, Gask L, et al. Collaborative care for depression and anxiety problems. Cochrane Database Syst. Rev. 2012;10:Cd006525.
11. Goodrich DE, Kilbourne AM, Nord KM, Bauer MS. Mental health collaborative care and its role in primary care settings. Curr Psychiat Rep. 2013;15(8):383.
12. Gilbody S, Sheldon T, House A. Screening and case-finding instruments for depression: a meta-analysis. CMAJ. 2008;178(8):997.
13. Gilbody S, Whitty P, Grimshaw J, Thomas R. Educational and organizational interventions to improve the management of depression in primary care. A systematic review. JAMA. 2003;289:3145–51.
14. The Swedish Council on Health Technology Assessment. Implementation support for psychiatric evidence in primary care. Report 211. Stockholm 2012.
15. Sighinolfi C, Nespeca C, Menchetti M, Levantesi P, Belvederi Murri M, Berardi D. Collaborative care for depression in European countries: a systematic review and meta-analysis. Psychosom Res. 2014;77(4):247–63.
16. Coventry P, Lovell K, Dickens C, Bower P, Chew-Graham C, McElvenny D, et al. Integrated primary care for patients with mental and physical multimorbidity: cluster randomised controlled trial of collaborative care for patients with depression comorbid with diabetes or cardiovascular disease. BMJ. 2015;350:h638.
17. Andersson S-O, Ferry S, Mattsson B. Factors associated with consultation length and characteristics of short and long consultations. Scand J Prim Health Care. 1993;11(1):61–7.
18. Campbell MK, Elbourne DR, Altman DG. CONSORT statement: extension to cluster randomised trials. BMJ. 2004;328(7441):702–8.
19. Montgomery SA, Asberg M. A new depression scale designed to be sensitive to change. Br J Psychiatry. 1979;134:382–9.
20. Svanborg P, Asberg M. A new self-rating scale for depression and anxiety states based on the comprehensive psychopathological rating scale. Acta Psychiatr Scand. 1994;89(1):21–8.
21. Arnau RC, Meagher MW, Norris MP, Bramson R. Psychometric evaluation of the Beck depression inventory II with primary care medical patients. Health Psychol. 2001;20(2):112–9.
22. EuroQol Group. EuroQol - a new facility for the measurement of health-related quality of life. Health Policy. 1990;16:199–208.
23. Pellegrin KL, Stuart GW, Maree B, Frueh BC, Ballenger JC. A brief scale for assessing patients' satisfaction with care in outpatient psychiatric services. Psychiatr Serv. 2001;52(6):816–9.
24. Maguire P, Pitceathly C. Key communication skills and how to acquire them. BMJ. 2002;325:697–700.
25. Spitzer RL, Williams JB, Kroenke K, Linzer M, de Gruy FV 3rd, Hahn SR, et al. Utility of a new procedure for diagnosing mental disorders in primary care. The PRIME-MD 1000 study. JAMA. 1994;272:1749–56.
26. Wikberg C, Nejati S, Larsson MEH , Petersson EL, Westman J, Ariai N, et al. Comparison between the Montgomery-Asberg depression rating scale–self and the Beck depression inventory II in primary care. Prim. Care Companion CNS Disord. 2015;17(3):10.
27. Björkelund C, Maun A, Murante AM, Hoffmann K, De Maeseneer J, Farkas-Pall Z. Impact of continuity on quality of primary care: from the perspective of citizens' preferences and multimorbidity - position paper of the European forum for primary care. Qual in prim care. 2013;21(3):193–20.
28. Richards DA, Hill JJ, Gask L, Lovell K, Chew-Graham C, Bower P, et al. Clinical effectiveness of collaborative care for depression in UK primary care (CADET): cluster randomised controlled trial. BMJ. 2013;347:f4913.
29. Huffman JC, Niazi SK, Rundell JR, Sharpe M, Katon WJ. Essential articles on collaborative care models for the treatment of psychiatric disorders in medical settings: a publication by the academy of psychosomatic medicine research and evidence-based practice committee. Psychosomatics. 2014; 55(2):109–22.

13

Clinical drug trials in general practice: how well are external validity issues reported?

Anja Maria Brænd[*], Jørund Straand and Atle Klovning

Abstract

Background: When reading a report of a clinical trial, it should be possible to judge whether the results are relevant for your patients. Issues affecting the external validity or generalizability of a trial should therefore be reported. Our aim was to determine whether articles with published results from a complete cohort of drug trials conducted entirely or partly in general practice reported sufficient information about the trials to consider the external validity.

Methods: A cohort of 196 drug trials in Norwegian general practice was previously identified from the Norwegian Medicines Agency archive with year of application for approval 1998–2007. After comprehensive literature searches, 134 journal articles reporting results published from 2000 to 2015 were identified. In these articles, we considered the reporting of the following issues relevant for external validity: reporting of the clinical setting; selection of patients before inclusion in a trial; reporting of patients' co-morbidity, co-medication or ethnicity; choice of primary outcome; and reporting of adverse events.

Results: Of these 134 articles, only 30 (22%) reported the clinical setting of the trial. The number of patients screened before enrolment was reported in 61 articles (46%). The primary outcome of the trial was a surrogate outcome for 60 trials (45%), a clinical outcome for 39 (29%) and a patient-reported outcome for 25 (19%). Clinical details of adverse events were reported in 124 (93%) articles. Co-morbidity of included participants was reported in 54 trials (40%), co-medication in 27 (20%) and race/ethnicity in 78 (58%).

Conclusions: The clinical setting of the trials, the selection of patients before enrolment, and co-morbidity or co-medication of participants was most commonly not reported, limiting the possibility to consider the generalizability of a trial. It may therefore be difficult for readers to judge whether drug trial results are applicable to clinical decision-making in general practice or when developing clinical guidelines.

Keywords: General practice, Clinical trials, External validity, Applicability, Generalizability, Eligibility determination

Background

When reading a report of a clinical trial, it should be possible to judge whether the results are relevant for the patients in your own practice, namely: *"Can I apply the results of this trial to my patients?"* [1, 2]. The terms external validity, applicability, representativeness, and generalizability are used quite synonymously to denote to which populations or settings the effect of a trial may be generalised or extrapolated [1, 3]. However, this difficult judgement is far too often left for each clinician to decide. By contrast, *"Can I trust the results?"*, is a question of internal validity, where helpful tools have been developed and are commonly used, e.g. The Cochrane Group's Risk of Bias tool [4].

Standards for reporting clinical trials have been developed during the past 20 years, resulting in the CONSORT checklist [5], which is now widely used [6]. However, although there are items in the CONSORT checklist connected to external validity, the main focus is on adequate reporting of trial elements affecting the internal validity of a trial, i.e. the extent to which the design and conduct of a trial eliminates the possibility of bias [5]. The CONSORT extension for pragmatic trials from 2008 elaborates the CONSORT checklist with recommendations for the reporting of pragmatic trials, i.e., trials designed for

* Correspondence: ambraend@medisin.uio.no
Department of General Practice, Institute of Health and Society, Faculty of Medicine, University of Oslo, Postbox 1130 Blindern, N-0318 Oslo, Norway

maximising applicability to usual care settings, thereby complementing the CONSORT statement on external validity issues [7]. The intention of this addition to the CONSORT checklist is to guide authors in reporting factors affecting external validity of trials.

Patients eligible for inclusion in randomised controlled trials (RCTs) are too often not broadly representative of patients encountered in everyday practice [8]. This has been demonstrated for several therapeutic areas, including diabetes [9], chronic obstructive pulmonary disease (COPD) [10], asthma [11], infectious diseases [12], and depression [13]. Patient samples in efficacy or explanatory trials (trials under optimal conditions) are generally more homogenous with less co-morbidity and a lower risk of complications compared with patients included in effectiveness or pragmatic trials (trials under real-world conditions) [14]. Higher-risk patients often account for most of the treatment benefit in trials; therefore, subgroups of patients might have important differences in terms of treatment benefits [15].

Judgements regarding the external validity of a trial depend on the reporting of key characteristics of adequate information regarding participants in the trial, trial settings, the treatments tested and the outcomes assessed [5]. This judgement has been described as a "complex reflection in which prior knowledge, statistical considerations, biological plausibility and eligibility criteria all have place" [16]. Several checklists for considering external validity have been proposed and systematically reviewed [17]. None of the identified checklists were based on empirical data, and those based on literature reviews were not considered to provide a clear connection between the references and checklist items [17]. The authors concluded that there exists no current consensus regarding how to assess external validity [17]. Because external validity depends on the context, there might be inescapable problems with designing a universal checklist [18]. To judge the external validity of a trial, adequate reporting of the setting, intervention and participants is paramount; however, reporting is often insufficient [19, 20].

Our aim was to assess whether articles with published results from a cohort of general practice drug trials gave sufficient information about each trial to consider important aspects of the external validity relevant for general practice. Specifically, the objectives were to assess the reporting of trial settings, the selection of patients, key characteristics of randomised patients, choice of outcome measures, and adverse effects of treatment. We aimed to explore the change in reporting during the time period for these variables. We also present a case study to illustrate clinical characteristics of patients included in the type 2 diabetes trials in the cohort.

Methods

Cohort of general practice drug trials

In Norway, all clinical pharmaceutical trials require approval from the Norwegian Medicines Agency (NoMA), a national regulatory authority for new and established drugs. We hand searched the NoMA paper-based (i.e. not electronic) archive, and identified protocols for trials planned to be conducted in general practice for the 10-year period 1998–2007, before the introduction of a new archive system. Trials were included in the cohort if any of the clinical investigators was a general practitioner (GP). The identification and main characteristics of the trials have been described previously [21]. The trial cohort included 196 trials, of which 189 were industry-initiated and 182 were multinational, with a total planned sample size of over 330,000 patients [21]. The median recruitment target was 673 patients internationally (range 8–31,000). A majority of the 151 trials took place in a combination of general practice and specialist care settings. According to the protocols, the trials were planned to be completed between 1998 and 2012. Diabetes drugs were the most frequent drug group, representing 20% of the trials. We subsequently searched for publications from this cohort of trials in MEDLINE, Embase, and the Cochrane Central Register of Controlled Trials (CENTRAL), and identified that 135 trials had results published in a journal article [22]. The most recent search for publications was performed December 2015; otherwise, there was no exclusion related to publication date. Many trials had several publications, a total of 285 journal articles were connected to the trials, and 134 of these were defined as main journal articles presenting results [22]. In the present paper, we describe how these 134 articles with publication year span of 2000–2015 reported issues relevant for judging external validity. If an issue was not reported in the main article, we checked whether it was reported in an online appendix or in any of the other journal articles we had identified from the same trial.

Data extraction

We developed a data extraction form in a web-based database with written instructions for coding, and then pilot tested it with all three of the present authors.

One author extracted data for all articles regarding the methodological characteristics of each trial. The articles were screened manually for information in the relevant sections; in addition, searches for the relevant search terms were performed using the PDF search option in EndNote X7 bibliographic software. Doubt regarding the coding was resolved by consensus. As it was not feasible for two authors to extract data from all articles, a random sample of 66/134 (49%) trials was selected, data were extracted independently by another author, and kappa statistics for agreement between the two assessors was calculated. We used an Internet based random number generator (www.random.org) to select the random sample based on the trial identification number. Any discrepancies were resolved by discussion and consensus.

We shortened and modified Rothwell's extensive panel of issues potentially affecting external validity for the coding of publication characteristics and methodology (Table 1) [1]. We chose to include the aspects we considered most relevant for general practice, and also feasible for assessment across the wide range of therapeutic areas.

Extracted data included whether the authors reported the clinical setting of the trial, namely whether trial sites were in general practice/family practice/family medicine/ primary care or in hospitals/specialist care. We recorded whether the number of patients screened, i.e., assessed for eligibility before inclusion in the actual trial, was reported. Furthermore, we recorded the numbers of patients who declined, enrolled, and completed the trial.

We determined the primary outcome of the trials as specified in the articles, or, if not specified, we defined the primary outcome as the outcome used in the power calculations, if reported. The primary outcome was classified as clinical, patient-reported, surrogate, costs or other. Clinical outcomes were defined as morbidity or mortality, and measurements of patient survival or function such as incidence of disease or hospitalisation [23]. Patient-reported outcomes included clinical scales (grading of symptoms) and other quantifications of subjective symptoms or complaints. Surrogate outcomes were defined as intermediate outcomes intended to substitute for a clinical endpoint and predict benefit or harm, e.g. HbA1c, cholesterol levels or blood pressure [23]. If several endpoints were mentioned among primary outcomes, we recorded the most clinically relevant outcome. We also recorded whether any of the other presented outcomes were patient-relevant, measured quality of life or costs or if no trial outcomes were in any of the mentioned outcome categories.

For all trials, we recorded whether eligibility criteria (defined as clinical inclusion or exclusion criteria) were reported. We also recorded whether the articles reported the co-morbidity, co-medication, and race/ethnicity of participants.

Table 1 Reporting of major issues that potentially affect external validity according to Rothwell [1]

• Setting of the trial
• Selection of patients
• Characteristics of randomised patients
• Differences between the trial protocol and routine practice
• Outcome measures and follow-up
• Adverse effects of treatment

As a case study, we investigated diabetes trials in more detail because they made up the largest group of tested drugs in the cohort. Specifically, we looked at patient characteristics in RCTs of type 2 diabetes. We recorded details regarding eligibility criteria and the key baseline characteristics of trial participants to discuss in the light of other published data on type 2 diabetes patients in general practice.

For all trials, we recorded whether clinical details of adverse events in the trial were reported.

Statistical analyses

Data were analysed using descriptive statistics. We used chi-square tests for trends in reporting over time during the publication years 2000–2015 [24], with $p < 0.05$ considered as statistically significant. We calculated the kappa measure of agreement between raters, and kappa 0.61–0.8 was considered to represent good agreement [24]. Statistical analyses were performed using IBM SPSS Statistics for Windows (version 24), and chi-square tests for trends were conducted with GraphPad Prism 7.

Results

Of the 134 trials, 125 (93%) were randomised and 101 (75%) were blinded. For 85 trials, information regarding the trial phase [14] was available; six (5%) were phase 2, 55 (41%) were phase 3, and 24 (18%) were phase 4.

Reporting of trial setting

The clinical setting of the trial was described in 30 (22%) of the trials (Table 2). The reporting of setting did not change during the time period (Fig. 1a). The clinical setting was described in a higher proportion of trials with a general practice setting only, 14/29 (48%), compared with trials with a mixed setting, 16/105 (15%) ($p < 0.001$, chi-square test). This was the only variable with a significant difference between reporting for a general practice only vs. a mixed setting.

Reporting of patient selection

The number of patients screened was reported for 61 (46%) trials (Table 2). The proportion of articles reporting the number of screened patients increased during the time period (Fig. 1b). For nine trials, the number of patients completing the trial was not clearly reported; three of these were terminated prematurely, while the others did not clearly report this number. Power or sample size calculations were reported in 97 (72%) trials, whereas no power calculations were reported in 31 (23%); for six (4.5%) trials, we considered this as unclear or irrelevant.

Table 3 shows the reported selection of patients. The mean fraction of enrolled patients completing the trials was 0.83. The mean number needed to be screened to include one participant was 1.94; however, numbers

Table 2 External validity items reported in 134 drug trials in general practice

	Trials reporting data		Change in reporting over time
	n	%	*p*-value*
Total	134	100	
Setting of the trial			
Country	106	79.1	0.12
Clinical setting	30	22.4	0.82
Trial sites	122	91.0	0.05
Number reported	109	81.3	
Names/affiliations listed	55	41.0	
Selection of patients			
Number of patients screened	61	45.5	**0.005**
Number of individuals who declined	24	17.9	0.12
Number of patients enrolled	134	100.0	
Number of patients completed	125	93.3	0.34
Eligibility criteria reported	125	93.3	**0.03**
Characteristics of randomised patients			
Comorbidity of included patients	54	40.3	**0.002**
Co-medication of included patients	27	20.1	**0.002**
Race/ethnicity of included patients	78	58.2	0.05
Outcome measures			
Primary outcome			
clinical	39	29.1	
patient reported	25	18.7	
surrogate	60	44.8	
cost	1	0.7	
other	7	5.2	
not clearly defined	2	1.5	
Surrogate outcomes only[a]	47	35.1	0.72
Adverse effects of treatment			
Details of adverse events	124	92.5	0.20

*Chi-square test for trend in reporting over publication years 2000–2015
[a]Includes primary and all other reported outcomes

available to calculate this were only available for 61 (46%) trials.

A run-in period with active treatment was a part of the trial design in 23 (17%) trials, whereas 95 (71%) did not have a run-in period with active treatment; for 16 (12%) trials, we characterised this to be unclear or irrelevant, e.g. because the trial was an extension of another trial.

Specific eligibility criteria were reported in 93% of the trials (Table 2). The proportion reporting eligibility criteria improved over the time period (Fig. 1c).

Reporting of characteristics of randomised patients

Co-morbidity of trial participants was reported in 54 (40%) trials and co-medication in 27 (20%); the reporting increased over the time period (Table 2, Fig. 1d–f).

In the case study of type 2 diabetes trials, the age groups were restricted to adults over 18 years for 83% of the trials, and 65% restricted participation to patients <80 years (Table 4). No trial excluded female patients, but six (26%) had exclusion criteria related to pregnancy, contraception, and/or lactation. Exclusion criteria related to co-morbidity were reported for 21 (91%) trials; the most common was exclusion of patients with renal dysfunction. Exclusion criteria related to concurrent medication use was reported in 35% of the trials. No trial reported race/ethnicity of patients as an exclusion criterion. Key baseline data of the participants of the trials and reporting of co-morbidity, co-medication or race/ethnicity are shown in Table 4 and compared with other published data regarding patients with type 2 diabetes from a

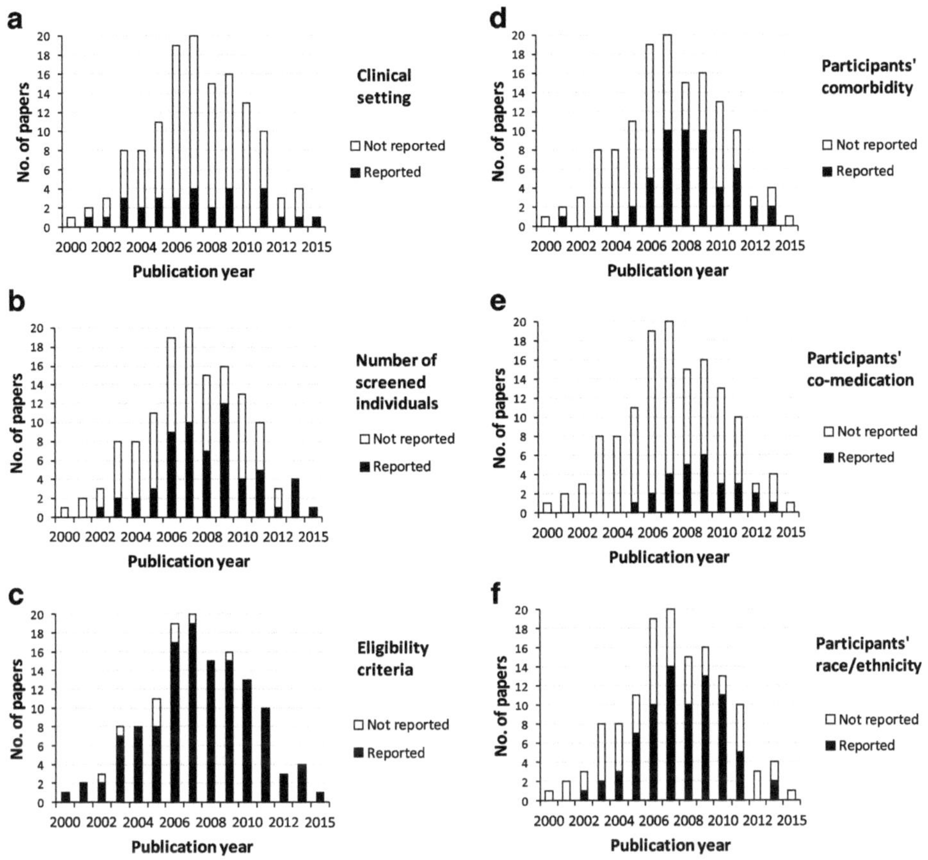

Fig. 1 Reporting of external validity issues in 134 drug trials in general practice published 2000–2015. **a**–**f** shows the development over time of reporting of (**a**) clinical setting, (**b**) screened individuals, (**c**) eligibility criteria, (**d**) participants' co-morbidity, (**e**) co-medication, and (**f**) race/ethnicity

Table 3 Reporting of trial sites, selection of patients, recruitment and completing fractions

	Trials reporting data n (%)	Median[a]	IQR	Min-max	Mean	95% CI
Number of countries	106 (79)	10	7–15	1–45		
Number of trial sites	122 (91)	96	61–171	1–1315		
Number of patients screened	61 (46)	1284	615–2352	14–89,890		
Number of patients enrolled	134 (100)	910	503–1743	13–29,019		
Number of patients completed	125 (93)	648	379–1134	13–25,577		
Recruitment fraction	61 (46)	0.66	0.46–0.83	0.17–1.00	0.64	(0.58–0.70)
Number needed to be screened	61 (46)	1.52	1.20–2.20	1.00–5.84	1.94	(1.64–2.22)
Completing fraction 1	125 (93)	0.83	0.70–0.89	0.19–1.00	0.78	(0.75–0.80)
Completing fraction 2	59 (44)	0.53	0.38–0.70	0.13–0.93	0.53	(0.47–0.58)

Definition of terms:
Recruitment fraction: Proportion of screened people who enrol in the trial (all enrolled/all screened), *Number needed to be screened:* Number of people screened in order to enrol one participant (1/recruitment fraction), *Completing fraction 1:* Proportion of participants who completed the trial (all completed/all enrolled), *Completing fraction 2:* Proportion of screened people who completed the trial (all completed/all screened), *IQR:* Inter-quartile range. *CI:* Confidence interval
[a]Mean not calculated for frequencies because of skewed data

Table 4 Reported eligibility criteria and key baseline characteristics of type 2 diabetes randomised controlled trials ($n = 23$)

Exclusion criteria	Exclusion criteria in total of 23 trials	Baseline data of included patients. Mean (CI)	Data from other population/GP studies for comparison		
			Scotland[a]	Belgium[b]	Norway[c]
Age		58.2 years (56.3–60.1)	66.3	58	62.4
< 18	19				
< 21	1				
< 40	1				
< 65	1				
No lower limit reported	1				
> 70–79	10				
> 80	5				
No upper limit reported	8				
Gender		54.2% male (52.4–56.0)	54.3	51.9	49.9
Females	0				
Pregnancy	3				
Lack of contraception use	3				
Breastfeeding	1				
HbA1c		8.1% (7.85–8.35)	7.4	7.1	7.7
< 6	1				
< 6.5	4				
< 7	8				
< 7.5	5				
No lower limit reported	5				
> 9	2				
> 10–10.9	11				
> 11	4				
> 12	2				
No upper limit reported	4				
BMI		30.6 kg/m^2 (30.1–31.1)	31.4	31	29.7
< 18	1				
< 22–23	4				
> 35	3				
> 40–45	6				
No BMI exclusion criteria reported	14				
Medical comorbidities		7 trials reported participants' comorbidity			
Coronary heart disease	14				
Heart failure	9				
Stroke	4				
Renal dysfunction	17				
Liver dysfunction	14				
Other type of diabetes	13				
Previous or suspected drug intolerance	3				
Other disease	7				
Medication related		5 trials reported participants' co-medication			

Table 4 Reported eligibility criteria and key baseline characteristics of type 2 diabetes randomised controlled trials ($n = 23$) *(Continued)*

Exclusion criteria	Exclusion criteria in total of 23 trials	Baseline data of included patients. Mean (CI)	Data from other population/GP studies for comparison		
			Scotland[a]	Belgium[b]	Norway[c]
Concurrent medication	8				
Race/ethnicity	0	19 trials reported participants' race/ethnicity			

Randomised controlled trials for type 2 diabetes drugs: DPP4-inhibitors ($n = 12$), insulins ($n = 5$), PPAR-agonists ($n = 2$), thiazolidinedones ($n = 2$) and others ($n = 2$). The numbers of trials reporting different key eligibility criteria are presented with mean baseline characteristics of included patients. Baseline characteristics are compared to published data from three population based or general practice studies

Data from other studies:

[a]Scotland: Nationwide diabetes clinical database [9]

[b]Belgium: General practice morbidity registration [26]

[c]Norway: Population based study HUNT-2 [25]

nationwide Scottish cohort [9], a population based Norwegian study (HUNT-2) [25] and a Belgian general practice study [26].

Reporting of outcome measures and follow-up

The primary outcome of the trial was a surrogate outcome in 45% of the trials and a clinical outcome in 29%; 35% of the trials reported a surrogate outcome only, including all secondary outcomes (Table 2). The analyses were done according to the intention-to-treat (ITT) principle in 26 trials (19%), modified ITT analyses were reported in 82 (61%), and no ITT analyses were reported in 17 trials (13%); this was unclear or irrelevant for nine trials (6.7%).

Reporting of adverse effects of treatment

Clinical details of adverse effects of treatment were reported in 93% of the trials (Table 2). Only two articles did not report any numbers of adverse events, while eight reported the numbers without specifying which adverse events the patients had experienced.

The inter-rater reliability for assessing the methodological characteristics of 49% of the randomly selected articles was good, with a mean kappa of 0.70 for all variables.

Discussion

We investigated the reporting of issues relevant for judging the external validity of a 10-year cohort of drug trials conducted in general practice. Important issues potentially affecting external validity were frequently not reported. A minority of the articles reported the clinical setting, the number of patients screened before enrolment and co-medications and co-morbidities.

Setting of the trials

We found that reporting the clinical setting of a trial was frequently omitted because it was only reported in about 20% of the articles, and we did not observe any improvement in this reporting over the time period. The scarce reporting of the clinical setting is inconsistent with the recommendation in the CONSORT criteria [5]. Information about the setting is considered crucial for assessment of the applicability of a trial [1, 7, 16, 27, 28]. Description of the setting and participant eligibility criteria were a collective checklist item in the 2001 version of the CONSORT statement [5]. In the 2010 version, this was split into two sub-items for better interpretation [6]. Both the 2010 version of the CONSORT statement and the CONSORT extension for pragmatic trials were issued during the time period when the articles were published [7]. A study of NICE guidelines aimed at primary care showed that a substantial proportion of relevant recommendations were derived from studies that were not conducted in primary care. The investigators also found surprising difficulty in determining the setting because it was often only vaguely reported, despite the CONSORT guidelines recommendations [29]. Similarly, systematic reviews often do not provide data regarding the clinical setting of trials included, and often do not discuss whether results are applicable for primary care [30]. Moreover, the authors of systematic reviews aimed for primary care should report external validity issues relevant for primary care [30, 31].

Selection of patients: Patient flow

We found that less than half of the articles reported patient selection before randomisation, but this omission decreased during the time period. Compared with similar studies, we found a considerably lower proportion of articles reporting the number of patients screened for eligibility, but a comparable good reporting of participant flow after inclusion. Jones et al. assessed RCTs published in primary care journals 2001–2004 and found that 70% reported the number of individuals assessed by investigators for eligibility, while all reported the actual number recruited [32]. Few of these trials were industry funded, and few were drug trials [32]. In high-impact general medical journals, 52–60% of RCTs published during 1999–2000 and 2004 reported the numbers of patients screened for eligibility [33, 34]. The CONSORT statement recommends reporting of the number of persons assessed for eligibility if available, but this is regarded as less important than the participant flow after inclusion [5, 27]. However, the CONSORT extension for pragmatic trials explicitly recommends reporting of the screening process [7].

Selection of patients: Eligibility criteria

More than 90% of the articles in our cohort of trials reported specific eligibility criteria. The proportion reporting eligibility criteria improved during the time period. Our results are consistent with the findings of van Spall et al.; of RCTs published in major medical journals, they found that 12% of the trials did not report exclusion criteria [35]. Reporting of eligibility criteria has been emphasised as particularly important [1, 7, 16, 28], and it is also one of the CONSORT items, however previously often not reported adequately [5]. Blümle et al. compared the prespecified eligibility criteria in trial protocols submitted to a German ethics committee with the eligibility criteria later presented in journal articles, and they found that trial eligibility criteria were often incompletely or inadequately reported in journal articles [36]. The discrepancies they found might hamper a proper assessment of the applicability of published trial results [36]. In our cohort of trials, we investigated whether eligibility criteria were reported in published articles from the trials only, but did not examine the eligibility criteria reported in the trial protocols.

Characteristics of randomised patients: Multi-morbidity and co-medication

We found that only 40% of articles reported co-morbidity of the participants. This is concerning, as multi-morbidity is common among patients in general practice [37], and is strongly related to adverse drug events [38]. Whether patients with multi-morbidity are included or excluded in a trial should be reported, but is often omitted, even in hypertension trials relevant for general practice populations with a high prevalence of co-morbid conditions [20]. An analysis of published RCTs showed that common medical conditions and commonly prescribed medications were frequent reasons for exclusion, but often poorly justified [35]. Drug trials were more likely than other trials to exclude individuals because of concomitant medication use, co-morbidities or female gender [35]. In a review of methodological papers on the representativeness of RCT samples, patients enrolled in RCTs in cardiology, mental health and oncology generally had fewer co-morbidities than real-world patients [8]. A study of RCTs registered at ClinicalTrials.gov 2014–2015 showed that more than three-quarters of trials for patients with chronic conditions excluded patients with multi-morbidity, suggesting that this remains a highly relevant issue [39].

Only about 20% of articles from our cohort of trials reported concomitant drug use. We find this concerning because polypharmacy is common in general practice. However, the reporting of co-medication improved over time. In clinical practice, dealing with polypharmacy represents a major challenge. Potential interactions between drugs are not typically considered in clinical guidelines, even though potentially serious drug interactions are common when applying several clinical guidelines for frequently co-morbid conditions [40]. GPs find it challenging to treat patients with multi-morbidity using complex medication regimens and disease-specific guidelines that do not consider multi-morbidity [41].

Case: Eligibility criteria and key baseline characteristics in type 2 diabetes trials

Of the diabetes trials in our cohort, none excluded female patients, but co-morbidity or concomitant medication use were frequent reasons for exclusion. Comparing the baseline characteristics of participants in trials included in the present study with cohort studies from Scotland [9], Belgium [26] and Norway [25], participants in the trials were younger than Scottish and Norwegian patients with type 2 diabetes and had a higher baseline HbA1c than patients in all three previous cohort studies. Otherwise, the baseline characteristics were comparable to the population-based data. Saunders et al. found that the external validity of other large diabetes trials was limited compared with the population-based Scottish patient cohort, in particular, trial participants were generally younger than the general patient population [9]. In a U.S. national survey, potential treatment effect modifiers, i.e. specific clinical diseases or conditions with a well-described mechanism for treatment effect modification, were found to be highly prevalent, especially among older adults with type 2 diabetes, with the potential to alter treatment effects in everyday practice compared with clinical trial populations [42]. Only a few articles in our present cohort reported the co-morbidity and co-medication of participants, limiting the assessment of this important aspect.

Outcome measures and follow-up

We found that nearly 50% of the trials had a surrogate outcome as their primary outcome, and more than 30% reported only surrogate outcomes. When a surrogate outcome is the only outcome of a drug trial presented, it is left to the individual clinician or authors of clinical guidelines to judge the clinical benefit of the medication. Our findings are consistent with other studies showing that surrogate outcomes alone often form the basis for drug approval. This was the case for nearly half of all new therapeutic agents approved by the U.S. Food and Drug Administration (FDA) during 2005–2013 [23]. In FDA drug approvals 2003–2013 for drugs used in COPD and diabetes, 78% and 100%, respectively, were based on surrogate outcomes alone, and only 25% of the approvals included a discussion of the scientific rationale for using surrogate outcomes [43]. This is concerning because a surrogate variable might not be a true predictor of the clinical outcome of interest, and might not provide a quantitative measure of clinical benefit that can be directly weighed against adverse events [44]. Sometimes an indirect measurement of an effect with a surrogate outcome is the only feasible possibility in a trial, but this should be justified in each case. We found that most trials presented modified intention-to-treat analyses. This type of analysis represents a post-randomisation exclusion of participants, potentially limiting the external validity [45]. Intention-to-treat analyses are generally recommended as a strategy for RCTs, although a strict intention-to-treat analysis may be difficult to achieve because of missing data or violations of the trial protocol [27]. However, whether the use of modified intention-to-treat analyses actually affects the intervention effect differs between studies [46, 47]. A recent meta-epidemiological study across therapeutic areas found that trials using a modified intention-to-treat strategy generally showed larger intervention effects than trials analysed using intention-to-treat analyses [46].

Adverse events of treatment

As expected, we found that most trials reported adverse events; however, 7% did not report any clinical details of adverse events. Previous studies have shown that adverse events are often inadequately reported in journal articles compared with complete study reports [48]. We could not determine whether this was the case in our present study because we did not have access to the complete study reports. RCTs rarely assess harm as their primary outcome, and systematic reviews frequently report the harmful effects of an intervention inadequately [49]. A balanced reporting of benefits and harms related to an intervention is crucial. Many adverse events are first reported after longer-term use of the intervention than the trial period, which is often relatively short.

Strengths and weaknesses of the present study

In the present study, we included all trials with published results from a complete national cohort of trials planned to be conducted partly in Norwegian general practice; however, there are possible limitations to the identification of the trials in the manual archive search and in the search for publications, as previously described [21, 22].

Several checklists for considering the reporting of aspects relevant for external validity have been proposed. We chose issues judged most relevant and feasible to consider. However, our selection may be discussed. We did not extract data regarding all possible aspects affecting external validity of the trials or all issues listed in Rothwell's framework [1]. This would not be feasible for an entire cohort of trials from many different therapeutic areas. The choice of an active versus non-active comparator is particularly important for the assessment of external validity of a drug trial, and is covered by the domain "Differences between the trial protocol and routine practice" in Rothwell's framework (Table 1) [1]. However, we found this to be beyond the scope of the present article.

Only one author extracted all data. Ideally, two authors should have coded all articles independently. It is therefore likely that some errors may have occurred during data extraction. However, we double-coded a random half to check quality and reliability, and the inter-rater agreement for this proportion was good as assessed by kappa, even though a critical appraisal of reporting involves several assessments. First, screened individuals may not be defined the same way in all articles. Consequently, there has been some room for judgement regarding these data. Further, for adverse events, we used a crude categorisation of reported/not reported. However, reporting of adverse events is not always a yes/no issue [48]. Finally, for surrogate outcomes, there are distinctions between outcomes recommended or not by various drug authorities [50]. However, we have not made distinctions between different surrogate outcomes in this article. Not all trials we assessed were RCTs; therefore, the heterogeneity of our study sample might be another limitation.

Conclusions

We found that important external validity aspects were not always adequately reported in general practice drug trials. Some of these aspects are included in the CONSORT checklist, but despite this, frequently omitted, especially the reporting of clinical settings, but also the selection of patients before inclusion in a trial, which is emphasised in the CONSORT extension for pragmatic trials [7]. By contrast, other issues we consider important for external validity from a primary care viewpoint are lacking in the CONSORT checklist; for example, reporting of co-morbidity and co-medication of participants. These issues were often not reported, but encouragingly, we found that this reporting improved during our study period. Including these items among the reported clinical characteristics of trial participants would improve the assessment of the external validity of a clinical drug trial; therefore, we suggest specifying these issues in future revisions of the CONSORT checklist.

Abbreviations

CENTRAL: Cochrane Central Register of Controlled Trials; CONSORT: Consolidated Standards of Reporting Trials; FDA: US Food and Drug Administration; GP: General practitioner; NoMA: Norwegian Medicines Agency; RCT: Randomised controlled trial

Acknowledgements
We thank Kaspar Buus Jensen for his participation in the initial planning of the study and collection of data from the NoMA archive. We also thank Ingvild Aaløkken, Head of Section for preclinical assessment and clinical trials at NoMA, for support and admission to the NoMA archive during the identification of trials. Rune Jakobsen critically read through the manuscript.

Funding
This study was funded by the Norwegian Research Fund for General Practice. The funding body did not take part in the design of the study or collection, analysis and interpretation of data. The authors alone are responsible for the content and writing of the paper.

Authors' contributions
All authors took part in planning the study and designing the data extraction form. AMB registered data from the publications, performed the statistical analyses and drafted the manuscript. AK extracted data for half the papers for quality check, JS and AK participated in the analyses and interpretation of results and critically revised the manuscript. All authors read and approved the final manuscript and are accountable for all aspects of the work.

Consent for publication
Not applicable.

Competing interests
The authors declare that they have no competing interests.

References
1. Rothwell PM. External validity of randomised controlled trials: "to whom do the results of this trial apply?". Lancet. 2005;365:82–93.
2. Sackett DL, Richardson WS, Rosenberg W, Haynes RB: Evidence-based Medicine. How to Practice and Teach EBM: Churchill Livingstone; 1997.
3. Campbell DT. Factors relevant to the validity of experiments in social settings. Psychol Bull. 1957;54:297–312.
4. Higgins JP, Altman DG, Götzsche PC, Juni P, Moher D, Oxman AD, et al. The Cochrane Collaboration's tool for assessing risk of bias in randomised trials. BMJ. 2011;343:d5928.
5. Altman DG, Schulz KF, Moher D, Egger M, Davidoff F, Elbourne D, et al. The revised CONSORT statement for reporting randomized trials: explanation and elaboration. Ann Intern Med. 2001;134:663–94.
6. Turner L, Shamseer L, Altman Douglas G, Weeks L, Peters J, Kober T, et al. Consolidated standards of reporting trials (CONSORT) and the completeness of reporting of randomised controlled trials (RCTs) published in medical journals. Cochrane Database Syst Rev. 2012;11:MR000030.
7. Zwarenstein M, Treweek S, Gagnier JJ, Altman DG, Tunis S, Haynes B, et al. Improving the reporting of pragmatic trials: an extension of the CONSORT statement. BMJ. 2008;337:a2390.
8. Kennedy-Martin T, Curtis S, Faries D, Robinson S, Johnston JA. Literature review on the representativeness of randomized controlled trial samples and implications for the external validity of trial results. Trials. 2015;16:495.
9. Saunders C, Byrne CD, Guthrie B, Lindsay RS, McKnight JA, Philip S, et al. External validity of randomized controlled trials of glycaemic control and vascular disease: how representative are participants? Diabet Med. 2013;30:300–8.
10. Kruis AL, Stallberg B, Jones RC, Tsiligianni IG, Lisspers K, van der Molen T, et al. Primary care COPD patients compared with large pharmaceutically-sponsored COPD studies: an UNLOCK validation study. PLoS One. 2014;9:e90145.
11. Travers J, Marsh S, Williams M, Weatherall M, Caldwell B, Shirtcliffe P, et al. External validity of randomised controlled trials in asthma: to whom do the results of the trials apply? Thorax. 2007;62:219–33.
12. Falagas ME, Vouloumanou EK, Sgouros K, Athanasiou S, Peppas G, Siempos II. Patients included in randomised controlled trials do not represent those seen in clinical practice: focus on antimicrobial agents. Int J Antimicrob Agents. 2010;36:1–13.
13. Wisniewski SR, Rush AJ, Nierenberg AA, Gaynes BN, Warden D, Luther JF, et al. Can phase III trial results of antidepressant medications be generalized to clinical practice? A STAR*D report. AJ Psychiatry. 2009;166:599–607.
14. Glasgow RE, Lichtenstein E, Marcus AC. Why don't we see more translation of health promotion research to practice? Rethinking the efficacy-to-effectiveness transition. Am J Public Health. 2003;93:1261–7.
15. Kent DM, Nelson J, Dahabreh IJ, Rothwell PM, Altman DG, Hayward RA. Risk and treatment effect heterogeneity: re-analysis of individual participant data from 32 large clinical trials. Int J Epidemiol. 2016;45:2075–88.
16. Dekkers OM, Elm EV, Algra A, Romijn JA, Vandenbroucke JP. How to assess the external validity of therapeutic trials: a conceptual approach. Int J Epidemiol. 2010;39:89–94.
17. Dyrvig AK, Kidholm K, Gerke O, Vondeling H. Checklists for external validity: a systematic review. J Eval Clin Pract. 2014;20:857–64.
18. Atkins D, Chang SM, Gartlehner G, Buckley DI, Whitlock EP, Berliner E, et al. Assessing applicability when comparing medical interventions: AHRQ and the effective health care program. J Clin Epidemiol. 2011;64:1198–207.
19. Pibouleau L, Boutron I, Reeves BC, Nizard R, Ravaud P. Applicability and generalisability of published results of randomised controlled trials and non-randomised studies evaluating four orthopaedic procedures: methodological systematic review. BMJ. 2009;339:b4538.
20. Fortin M, Dionne J, Pinho G, Gignac J, Almirall J, Lapointe L. Randomized controlled trials: do they have external validity for patients with multiple comorbidities? Ann Fam Med. 2006;4:104–8.
21. Braend AM, Jensen KB, Klovning A, Straand J. Clinical drug trials in general practice: a 10-year overview of protocols. Trials. 2013;14:162.
22. Brænd AM, Straand J, Jakobsen RB, Klovning A. Publication and non-publication of drug trial results: a 10-year cohort of trials in Norwegian general practice. BMJ Open. 2016;6:e010535.
23. Downing NS, Aminawung JA, Shah ND, Krumholz HM, Ross JS. Clinical trial evidence supporting FDA approval of novel therapeutic agents, 2005-2012. JAMA. 2014;311:368–77.
24. Altman DG. Practical statistics for medical research. London: Chapman & Hall; 1991.
25. Olsson L, Grill V, Midthjell K, Ahlbom A, Andersson T, Carlsson S. Mortality in adult-onset autoimmune diabetes is associated with poor glycemic control. Results from the HUNT study. Diabetes Care. 2013;36:3971–8.
26. Wami WM, Buntinx F, Bartholomeeusen S, Goderis G, Mathieu C, Aerts M. Influence of chronic comorbidity and medication on the efficacy of treatment in patients with diabetes in general practice. Br J Gen Pract. 2013;63:e267–73.
27. Moher D, Hopewell S, Schulz KF, Montori V, Gøtzsche PC, Devereaux PJ, et al. CONSORT 2010 explanation and elaboration: updated guidelines for reporting parallel group randomised trials. BMJ. 2010;340:c869.
28. Loudon K, Treweek S, Sullivan F, Donnan P, Thorpe KE, Zwarenstein M. The PRECIS-2 tool: designing trials that are fit for purpose. BMJ. 2015;350:h2147.
29. Scullard P, Abdelhamid A, Steel N, Qureshi N. Does the evidence referenced in NICE guidelines reflect a primary care population? Br J Gen Pract. 2011;61:e112–7.
30. Missiou A, Tatsioni A. Systematic reviews do not comment on applicability for primary care. J Clin Epidemiol. 2015;68:1152–60.
31. Nasser M, van Weel C, van Binsbergen JJ, van de Laar FA. Generalizability of systematic reviews of the effectiveness of health care interventions to primary health care: concepts, methods and future research. Fam Pract. 2012;29(Suppl 1):i94–i103.
32. Jones R, Jones RO, McCowan C, Montgomery AA, Fahey T. The external validity of published randomized controlled trials in primary care. BMC Fam Pract. 2009;10:5.
33. Gross CP, Mallory R, Heiat A, Krumholz HM. Reporting the recruitment process in clinical trials: who are these patients and how did they get there? Ann Intern Med. 2002;137:10–6.
34. Toerien M, Brookes ST, Metcalfe C, de Salis I, Tomlin Z, Peters TJ, et al. A review of reporting of participant recruitment and retention in RCTs in six major journals. Trials. 2009;10:52.
35. Van Spall HG, Toren A, Kiss A, Fowler RA. Eligibility criteria of randomized controlled trials published in high-impact general medical journals: a systematic sampling review. JAMA. 2007;297:1233–40.
36. Blumle A, Meerpohl JJ, Rucker G, Antes G, Schumacher M, von Elm E. Reporting of eligibility criteria of randomised trials: cohort study comparing trial protocols with subsequent articles. BMJ. 2011;342:d1828.

37. Barnett K, Mercer SW, Norbury M, Watt G, Wyke S, Guthrie B. Epidemiology of multimorbidity and implications for health care, research, and medical education: a cross-sectional study. Lancet. 2012;380:37–43.
38. Calderon-Larranaga A, Poblador-Plou B, Gonzalez-Rubio F, Gimeno-Feliu LA, Abad-Diez JM, Prados-Torres A. Multimorbidity, polypharmacy, referrals, and adverse drug events: are we doing things well? Br J Gen Pract. 2012;62:e821–6.
39. Buffel du Vaure C, Dechartres A, Battin C, Ravaud P, Boutron I. Exclusion of patients with concomitant chronic conditions in ongoing randomised controlled trials targeting 10 common chronic conditions and registered at ClinicalTrials.gov: a systematic review of registration details. BMJ Open. 2016;6:e012265.
40. Dumbreck S, Flynn A, Nairn M, Wilson M, Treweek S, Mercer SW, et al. Drug-disease and drug-drug interactions: systematic examination of recommendations in 12 UK national clinical guidelines. BMJ. 2015;350:h949.
41. Austad B, Hetlevik I, Mjolstad BP, Helvik AS. Applying clinical guidelines in general practice: a qualitative study of potential complications. BMC Fam Pract. 2016;17:92.
42. Weiss CO, Boyd CM, Wolff JL, Leff B. Prevalence of diabetes treatment effect modifiers: the external validity of trials to older adults. Aging Clin Exp Res. 2012;24:370–6.
43. Yu T, Hsu YJ, Fain KM, Boyd CM, Holbrook JT, Puhan MA. Use of surrogate outcomes in US FDA drug approvals, 2003-2012: a survey. BMJ Open. 2015; 5:e007960.
44. International Conference on Harmonisation of Technical Requirements for Registration of Pharmaceuticals for Human Use. ICH Harmonised Tripartite Guideline: Statistical Principles for Clinical Trials E9. 1998. http://www.ich.org/fileadmin/Public_Web_Site/ICH_Products/Guidelines/Efficacy/E9/Step4/E9_Guideline.pdf. Accessed 31 May 2017.
45. Zwarenstein M. Pragmatic' and 'explanatory' attitudes to randomised trials. J R Soc Med. 2017;110:208–18.
46. Abraha I, Cherubini A, Cozzolino F, De Florio R, Luchetta ML, Rimland JM, et al. Deviation from intention to treat analysis in randomised trials and treatment effect estimates: meta-epidemiological study. BMJ. 2015;350:h2445.
47. Dossing A, Tarp S, Furst DE, Gluud C, Wells GA, Beyene J, et al. Modified intention-to-treat analysis did not bias trial results. J Clin Epidemiol. 2015;72:66–74.
48. Schroll JB, Penninga EI, Gotzsche PC. Assessment of adverse events in protocols, clinical study reports, and published papers of trials of orlistat: a document analysis. PLoS Med. 2016;13:e1002101.
49. Zorzela L, Golder S, Liu Y, Pilkington K, Hartling L, Joffe A, et al. Quality of reporting in systematic reviews of adverse events: systematic review. BMJ. 2014;348:f7668.
50. Institute of Medicine. Evaluation of biomarkers and surrogate endpoints in chronic disease. Washington, DC: The National Academies Press; 2010.

14

Which strategies might improve local primary healthcare in Germany? An explorative study from a local government point of view

Bertolt Kuhn[1*], Kim-Sarah Kleij[1], Sebastian Liersch[1], Jost Steinhäuser[2] and Volker Amelung[1]

Abstract

Background: Facing rising inequities and poorer accessibility of physicians in rural areas, new healthcare delivery structures are being considered to support local healthcare in German communities. To better understand perspectives on and attitudes towards different supplementary models, we examined attitudes among local politicians in the German federal state of Lower Saxony towards the suitability of supplementary care models.

Methods: As part of a cross-sectional study, we surveyed local politicians in Lower Saxony at the local authority and district levels ($n = 449$) by mail questionnaire. We asked for an assessment of four potential supplementary healthcare models at the local level: the use of trained medical assistants, patients' buses, mobile physicians' offices, and telemedicine.

Results: The response rate was 71.0% for mayors ($n = 292$) and 81.6% ($n = 31$) for county administrators. In summary, 72.4% of respondents supported the use of trained medical assistants, 48.9% voted for patients' buses, 22.0% for mobile physicians' offices, and 13.9% for telemedicine. Except for telemedicine, the politicians' approval of the supplementary models in rural areas was higher than in urban areas. The assessment regarding the suitability of each model was not significantly connected with indicators of a positively or negatively assessed local healthcare situation. The analyses showed that the use of trained medical assistants was associated with the positive effects of division of labor and potential to relieve physicians. In contrast, there was skepticism about technical support via telemedicine, mostly due to concerns about its unsuitability for elderly people and the potential lower quality of healthcare delivery.

Conclusion: Local politicians widely accept the use of trained medical assistants, whereas the applicability of technical solutions such as telemedicine is perceived with skepticism. Therefore, the knowledge gap between evidence for and prejudices against telemedicine needs to be addressed more effectively. Reasons for the assessments of the presented models are more likely traceable to personal views than to assessments of the actual estimated local primary care situation.

Keywords: Primary healthcare, Communities, Physician shortage, Supplementary care models, Delegation, Mobility, Telemedicine

* Correspondence: Kuhn.Bertolt@mh-hannover.de
[1]Medical School Hannover, Institute for Epidemiology, Social Medicine and Health Systems Research, OE 5410, Carl-Neuberg-Str. 1, D-30625 Hannover, Germany
Full list of author information is available at the end of the article

Background

In Germany, ambulatory care physicians are traditionally self-employed. However, their distribution is regulated and allocated by the association of statutory health insurance physicians, which is responsible for maintaining a sufficient and high-quality supply of physicians. By federal law, there are different regulations and planning areas for general practitioners and other medical specialists. The distribution aims at achieving a predefined ratio between physicians and the number of people who live in the specific planning area. There is, for example, one full-time working general practitioner (GP) for every 1671 people in a particular planning area [1]. Regions are defined as oversupplied when they have a number of physicians that exceeds the respective reference ratio by more than +10%. In such cases, further settlements of physicians in these areas are blocked. In contrast, physicians are incentivized to settle in regions that are undersupplied. Undersupply is defined as a physician-population ratio below the predefined ratio of −25% for GPs and −50% for specialists [2]. The so-called needs-based planning method was created in the 1990s in response to the increasing number of physicians in Germany, at a time when the buzzword "physician glut" was circulated [3]. Therefore, the spatial planning of physicians mainly aims at equalizing their distribution, with restrictions used to prevent oversupply. However, the planning instruments have turned out to be less suitable for placing new physicians in undersupplied areas. Because physicians can find attractive jobs in cities, in hospitals, or in the non-curative sector, the restrictions on settlements are not forcing doctors to work in rural areas [4].

The distribution of physicians in Germany is not controlled by the type of price competition that would lead to lower incomes for doctors in areas with a high density of providers. Physicians are remunerated according to an official fee scale and receive fixed prices for the provision of individual services. There are separate medical fee scales for patients within the statutory health insurance scheme and those with private health insurance. Fees for privately insured patients are higher; thus, doctors with a higher percentage of private patients usually earn more money [5]. This leads to a politically unintended incentive for physicians to prefer areas with a high share of privately insured people, regardless of the need structure.

At the moment, the supply of healthcare in Germany is still considered good. For a long time, no specific requirements were considered for rural healthcare due to the relatively similar conditions across regions. Compared to other countries, Germany's physician supply and infrastructure are considered to be quite well established. Specialized doctors seem to be acceptably distributed, despite the aforementioned problems and negative developments [6].

Nevertheless, nationwide availability of physician care will be threatened in the future by distinct misalignments between urban and rural areas. Particularly, the following three factors are strengthening the discrepancies between urban and rural areas in Germany:

1. Societal transformation of the doctor's profession. Among physicians, there is a growing desire for flexibility, good working conditions and shorter working hours that will potentially lead to a poorer operational output on the part of an average physician in relation to the population. Instead of being self-employed as rural physician in their own offices, young doctors are increasingly choosing to work for hospitals or as employees in medical service centers in the ambulant sector [7]. These opportunities are mainly located in urban regions.
2. Poorer access to physicians' facilities in rural areas. In rural areas, the travel times for a patient to reach a physician tend to be longer [8]. Often, there is lack of appropriate public transportation. Access to healthcare services is often lower than in urban areas, which leads to challenges for people who are dependent on public transport, especially if they are immobile due to health problems or disabilities [9]. As local transport in rural regions with shrinking populations is limited for economic reasons, problems with access to medical care are increasing in certain regions.
3. Growing number of older people in rural areas. A rising number of older people correlates with an increasing number of people with mobility issues and health problems who need adequate access to medical care [6].

Despite the regulations on physicians' settlements, there is already a considerably lower quantitative physician-population ratio in rural areas [10]. A psychotherapist in the rural district of *Holzminden,* for example, may potentially provide care for 4.4 times as many people as a psychotherapist in the city of *Göttingen* [11]. Regardless of the prevailing opinion that the situation is still acceptable in most areas, the long-term trends are worrying and considerable. Problem-solving approaches require a long lead time before they can have an effect [7]. If too much time elapses without action, there is fear of a downward spiral that will lead to an exodus of rural physicians [10].

Differences in healthcare provision between rural and urban areas are common in Europe, although the extent of the disparity varies from country to country [7, 12].

There are three main strategies with which policy makers can address current and future challenges in response to geographic imbalances in physician supply:

1. Target future physicians: Increase the pool of future physicians who are interested in practicing in underserved regions (e.g., target aspects of medical education).
2. Target current physicians: Maximize the share of current physicians who are willing to practice in underserved areas (e.g., increase the attractiveness of resettling in specific regions through higher wages and subsidies).
3. Do with less: Change existing supply structures to enable more efficient care services so that fewer doctors are required for the delivery of medical services (e.g., implement new service delivery models) [7].

There are rising concerns about finding replacements for retiring physicians and about attracting young physicians to rural areas. Because undergraduate medical studies are usually completed at universities in German cities, students often have little or no contact or practical experience with rural medical care during their education. In addition, training in family medicine is rather unattractive for medical graduates in Germany compared to graduates in other European countries [13, 14]. Particularly for populations in small communities in rural areas, accessibility problems will probably increase due to the reduced number of physicians' offices [15]. In Germany, efforts targeting future and current physicians are typically organized at the national or federal state level. The local level provides a testing ground for new supplementary health care services to tackle specific local needs. If the care supply is going to be more diverse and the situation worse in certain areas, then there is pressure to take specific actions. As a result, new heterogeneous approaches to health service delivery can be tested at the local level in combination with traditional supply models [16]. The main problems seem to be overloaded doctors and access problems for patients. Promising short-term approaches on the local level focus on relieving pressures on physicians by obtaining help from other professional groups, as well as using mobility and telemedicine models to bring patients and doctors together [10].

German communities and municipalities have no direct responsibilities for ensuring that local healthcare is provided by physicians. However, communities and municipalities are affected if the local population faces problems because of insufficient healthcare delivery, long travel times, or other accessibility factors resulting from a local physician shortage [17]. Due to these developments, communities and municipalities are playing a more important role in ensuring local healthcare supplies and satisfying the needs of the population [18]. The municipal governments recognize the specific local conditions and challenges related to healthcare utilization. They are able to support the settlement and distribution of physicians by using different approaches and measures [7]. Models, such as delegation models, new forms of mobility, and telemedicine, are thought to be suitable and are promoted at the federal level [10]. We wanted to know whether these assessments are also reflected at the local level. German municipalities typically make policy decisions by coordinating executive initiatives with the majority of the local council. This process is strongly influenced by the constraint of fiscal consolidation and by the need to avoid resistance from citizen protests [19]. Policy makers are further influenced in decision making by forces such as the opinions of a dominant epistemic social environment or narrative [20]. These aspects, therefore, also contribute to local politicians' assessments of potentially relevant supplement concepts in primary care.

In conclusion, our study aims to investigate local politicians' perspectives on the following questions:

1. What expectations are associated with supplementary care delivery models?
2. Which models are accepted as potentially suitable to ensure healthcare delivery in communities?
3. Are supplementary models more likely to be seen as suitable if local healthcare is assessed as poor?

Methods

Supplementary care models

We surveyed assessments of four supplementary care models considered to be innovative in Germany. The selection of supplementary care concepts was based on models that have been identified as potentially favorable and on concepts for improving outpatient medical care that have been partially implemented by the German council of experts on the assessment of health care developments [10] and current regulatory initiatives. This choice of models was also oriented towards a simultaneously conducted population survey with a similar thematic focus [21]. The following supplementary models complement the existing healthcare supply and do not replace the available infrastructure. They can potentially increase the accessibility of health services and lead to a decrease in the need for home visits by physicians. A visual summary of the supplementary models is given in Fig. 1.

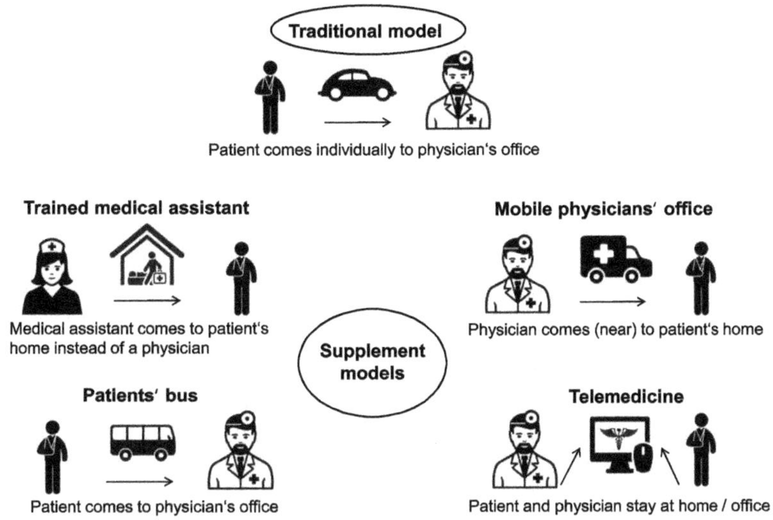

Fig. 1 Basic characteristics of the supplementary models. Icon sources: *Designed by Freepik and distributed by Flaticon.com & Shutterstock*

Trained medical assistant

Models that include the delegation of medical services to qualified non-medical health professionals have been disseminated internationally [6]. The core idea is to allow non-medical healthcare professionals to perform tasks that are traditionally performed by physicians [22]. The desired result is to enable doctors to focus on their original medical activities, which leads to a reduced workforce requirement for physicians [23, 24].

The outpatient healthcare system in Germany is generally centered on physicians, who have a relatively large range of activities. Other healthcare professionals rarely have academic qualifications [1]. From an international point of view, there is currently no standardized way to qualify as a nurse practitioner in Germany. However, German physicians delegate certain activities to other professionals, such as qualified nurses or medical assistants with further education [25]. Since the mid-2000s, delegation models have been implemented in which qualified nurses or medical assistants autonomously perform home visits and some medical activities. This has been done in response to looming supply shortages due to overloaded physicians and due to an increasing need for treatment because of demographic changes and the rising prevalence of chronic diseases [26]. In the remainder of this paper, these additional qualified healthcare staff members are called "trained medical assistants" (TMA).

Patients' bus

A growing problem that impedes access to medical care is the limited public transport in rural areas. Existing public transport services are often aligned with school transport and operate according to school hours and school holidays. Partly, there is a need for alternative modes of transportation to meet the growing need for patient transport to places that provide medical services [27]. Especially in rural areas, people without their own cars or driver's licenses are dependent on appropriate public connections to medical care. Models, which can be summarized under the term "patients' buses", have in common that they provide public transportation from the patient's residence to physicians' offices. A patients' bus can be organized as a demand-based on-call bus or as a scheduled service bus with voluntary or vocational drivers [10].

In the German federal state of Brandenburg, the association of statutory health insurance physicians, in cooperation with the municipalities, developed a project to ensure access to physicians via public transport in one county. Once a week, a minibus brought patients directly from eight districts to different physicians' offices in the center of the neighboring larger city. The traffic connection was arranged according to the doctors' office hours [28].

Mobile physicians' office

Mobile utilities offer a range of physicians' services as a community-based medical supply base. They aim at avoiding regional undersupply; thus, they usually consider specific vulnerable populations (e.g., socially disadvantaged individuals, migrants or older people) [29].

Generally, in Germany, mobile utilities are rarely used to deliver primary healthcare services. In 2013, there was a pilot project in which a utility van was converted into a GP office. Different physicians approached six small communities that lacked an existing GP office [30]. A follow-up project with the same van aims to ensure low-threshold primary care for refugees in the federal state of Schleswig-Holstein [31].

Telemedicine

Telemedical concepts include the provision of healthcare services from a remote location using electronic information and communication technologies [32]. Telemedicine focuses on medical situations in which the personal appearance of the patient in a physician's office is not necessary, e.g., to discuss indications or to obtain a second opinion based on medical findings. In the context of this study, telemedicine is understood in terms of telecare, which means the provision of medical care by a doctor who is at a distance, allowing patients to be treated in their own homes.

Particularly for rural regions, telemedicine is assessed as potentially suitable as a supplementary service model. In these areas, less infrastructure is maintained, and long distances can be bridged spatially with electronic devices [7, 33]. At present, there are approximately 200 pilot projects using telemedicine approaches in the existing German care delivery structures. However, very few tested telemedicine concepts have been transferred to standard care [33].

Questionnaire and survey

We developed an experimental questionnaire (Additional file 1, Additional file 2). Pretests were performed to test the questionnaire's suitability. Therefore, interviews were conducted with representatives of local government associations in the federal state of Lower Saxony (n = 2) and with mayors (n = 5) in neighboring federal states.

In September 2015, a postal survey was conducted. In accordance with the aims of this study, community politicians were questioned regarding three aspects of municipal healthcare:

1. Current local physician supply;
2. Importance of outpatient healthcare for municipalities and assessment of supporting measures;
3. Attitudes towards innovative care models to support outpatient healthcare (trained medical assistants, patients' buses, mobile physicians' offices, and telemedicine).

The study sample consisted of all professional mayors (n = 411) and county administrators (n = 38) in the federal state of Lower Saxony in North-Western Germany (Fig. 2). Lower Saxony is the second largest German state by land area and, with a population of approximately 8 million people, the fourth largest state by number of inhabitants in Germany [34]. The people surveyed were the directly elected policy leaders at the community and county municipal levels.

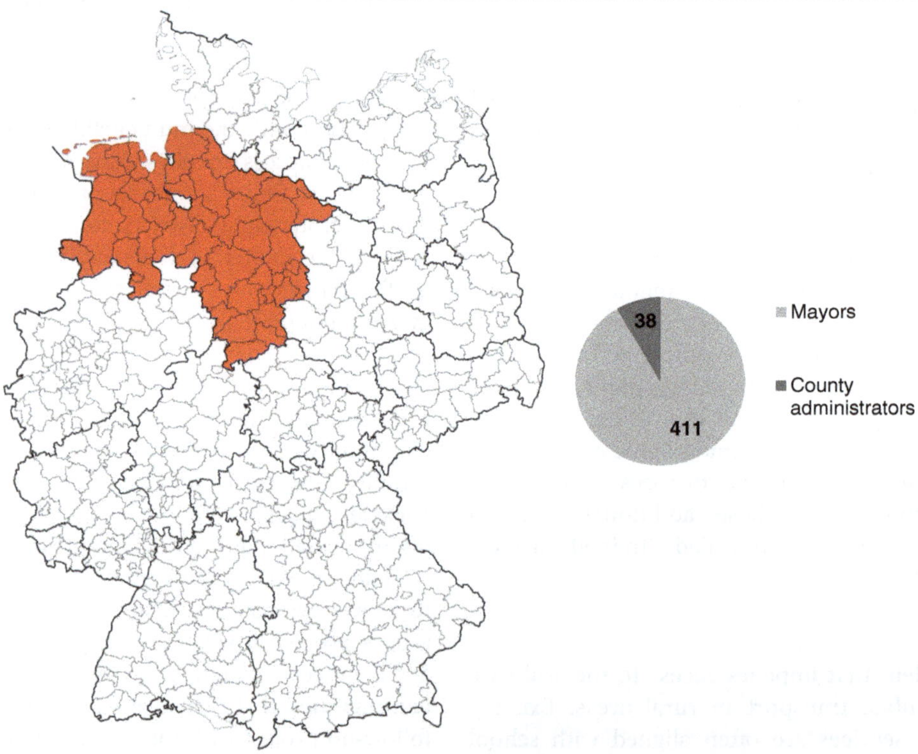

Fig. 2 Study population in Lower Saxony. Map modified from [49]

Data gathered in the study were collected anonymously. We asked about several socio-demographic characteristics of the participating mayors, including age and sex. Due to reasons of anonymization, we did not collect these data from the smaller group of county leaders.

Different classifications and definitions of rural areas are used in the literature [17]. We examined the subjective assessments of the mayors regarding whether their community was located in an urban or densely populated area or a rural area. We were not able to double-check these assessments due to the anonymous character of the survey. In the following, the definition of rural and urban only refers to this subjective classification.

Analysis

The questions were mostly answered on Likert scales that had either four or five options. In addition, the questionnaire included open and semi-open questions. The answers were partly summarized dichotomously (e.g., approval, no approval) for evaluation.

Depending on the level of measurement of the specific variables, we used the Pearson Chi-Square test, the Mann-Whitney U test, Spearman's rank correlation test, and binary logistic regression. A difference at the level of $p < 0.05$ indicates significant results in all performed tests. Shares are given in valid percent. We used SPSS version 23 for the statistical analyses.

We asked the respondents to briefly provide the reasoning behind their given assessments of each supplementary model's suitability. For the categorization, the answers were assigned into three groups according to the related suitability assessment: the 1st group was "positive assessment" (suitable & rather suitable); the 2nd group was "neutral or undecided assessment" (partly / partly); and the 3rd group was "negative assessment" (not suitable & rather not suitable). Next, free text answers were assigned to content categories using MAXQDA version 11 and Microsoft Excel for a basic qualitative evaluation. These categories were defined inductively and revised in the course of the assessment process [34]. Two people performed the categorization parallel to and separately from each other. After discussion, we reached a consensus with a final common category scheme.

Results

The response rate was 70.9% for mayors ($n = 292$) and 81.6% ($n = 31$) for county administrators. The sample was representative of Lower-Saxony with regard to the sex of the mayors and the size of municipality by population classes. A total of 81.3% ($n = 230$) of the participating mayors stated that their community was located in a rural area, which is significantly more than the official spatial distribution in Lower-Saxony, where 57.7% of communities are rural.[1]

Predominantly, the respondents were satisfied with the local outpatient healthcare, and the situation in urban areas was evaluated slightly more positively than that in rural areas ($p < 0.001$) (Fig. 3). The assessment of satisfaction correlated weakly but significantly with the size of the community (Spearman-Rho = 0.17, $p = 0.007$): Mayors of communities with larger populations tended to be more satisfied with the ambulant physician's care.

For each municipality, the inhabitants' ability to access physicians by public transport was assessed differently depending on the spatial location of the respondents: In urban areas, the majority of participants agreed that accessibility was good, whereas in rural areas, most of respondents disagreed (p < 0,001) (Fig. 3).

Asked about possible approaches to improving healthcare delivery, the local politicians evaluated the suitability of the four supplementary models for their respective settings quite differently. In summary, 72.4% of the respondents supported the use of a TMA; 49.4% voted for patients' buses, 22.1% for mobile physicians' offices, and 14.2% for telemedicine (Fig. 4).

The comparison of the mean assessment showed that the presented supplementary models were seen as more suitable in rural communities compared to urban ones, except for telemedicine (TMA: $p = 0.018$; patients' bus: $p = 0.001$; mobile physicians' office: p = 0.001; telemedicine: $p = 0.799$).

We calculated a binary logistic regression model for each of the supplementary models to investigate whether communities with inferior infrastructure and poorer assessments of the actual care situation are more open to the supplementary models (Additional file 3). We used the dichotomized assessments of the suitability of each supplementary model as dependent variables and simultaneously added several covariates and socio-demographic variables to the model. The covariates served as indicators of a more poorly assessed outpatient healthcare situation. As a result, the regression model indicates that the evaluation of the suitability of each supplementary model is not significantly correlated with most of the covariates. The levels of the coefficients of determination of the model range from 0.040 for telemedicine to 0.068 for a TMA (Nagelkerke's R-Squared). Thus, the model fit can be observed as having very low explanatory power for the suitability assessment of the supplementary models.

According to the free text responses, the use of TMAs was often associated with advantages of the division of labor, which could potentially lead to more consultation time for patients and improved availability of home visits. For some respondents, there was also the expectation that a skill transfer from physicians to TMAs could improve the working conditions and satisfaction of both professional groups. Negative arguments were that a

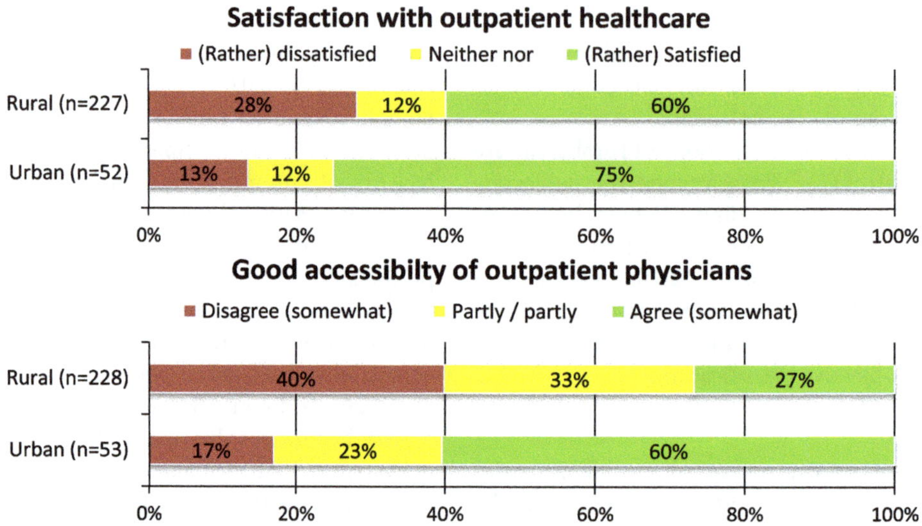

Fig. 3 Satisfaction & assessment of good accessibility regarding outpatient healthcare in urban and rural areas

TMA would not be a substitute for a physician, and some responses expressed a lack of acceptance and trust in a TMA.

The feelings about patients' buses were mixed. The need for public transportation to physicians' practices was noted widely. Some argued that there was no need for buses because of existing public transport. The additional effort required might be too great and not suitable for the respective community structure. On the other hand, some communities reported similar alternative public transport models based on civic engagement, and these were assessed positively.

The need for mobile physicians' offices was predominantly denied. A majority believed that patients' acceptance might be low and that the necessary financial effort would be too high. Furthermore, the driving time required of the physicians, at the expense of treatment time, was remarked on negatively. However, a few respondents thought the model could be suitable in rural areas or specific spatial community situations as a limited workaround.

Telemedicine models were frequently associated with an impersonal treatment model, and there were broad reservations about this approach. Often, it was argued that this model would not be suitable for elderly patients

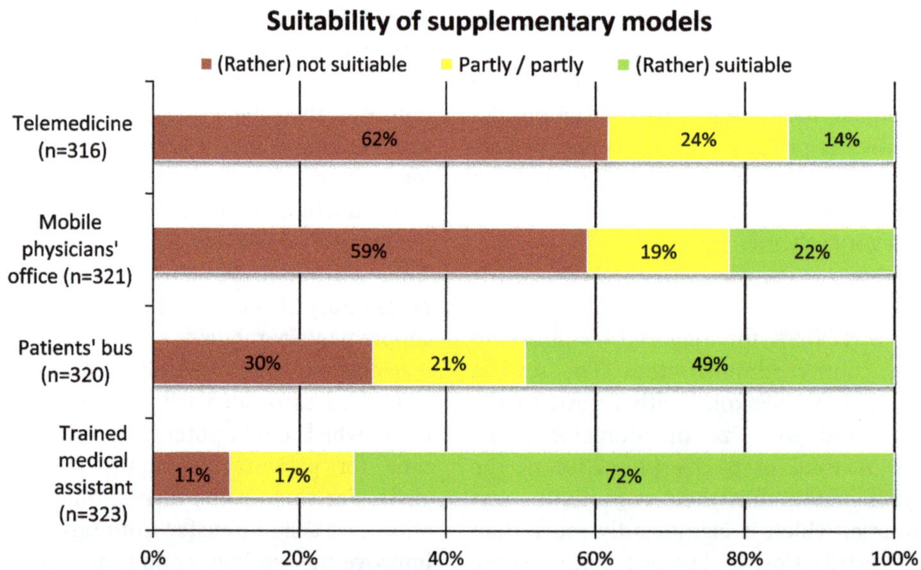

Fig. 4 Summarized assessment of supplementary models in health care

who would be averse to technically supported non-physical contact with doctors. In addition, there were reservations about the availability of the technology and the quality of care. Positive arguments were the possible advantages for certain patient groups, particularly for patients with specific groups of diseases. A few participants argued that telemedicine could represent a model for future generations.

A summary of the main arguments about and associations with the supplementary models is presented in Table 1.

Discussion

In this study, the participants were mostly confident that a TMA would be able to deliver high-quality treatment as part of their responsibilities. The potential relief of doctors through the division or delegation of labor was estimated broadly. The positive assessment of a supporting model with a greater role for TMAs coexists with the rising trend of implementing such models in the German ambulatory healthcare system to support non-medical professions in primary care [35]. In recent years, there have been several projects to expand the scope of activities and responsibilities of non-medical personnel in Germany [26]. The expansion and acceptance among patients of TMAs and nurse practitioners can also be observed in the USA [36] and other countries with highly developed primary care infrastructures [25].

The weak acceptance of technical solutions by the respondents is notable. It was often said that these models would not be suitable for older people. Participants' broad rejection of telemedicine as a complementary care model contrasts with international developments, which promote a greater dissemination of technical solutions and anticipate several advantages, especially for older patients [37, 38]. The expressed skepticism of the survey participants in our study was also observed in patients' surveys [39]. In contrast, consultations between physicians and their patients via telephone or internet devices in order to provide remote healthcare advice are increasingly in demand among patients in comparable European countries such as France, Switzerland and the United Kingdom [40]. Additionally, there is growing evidence in favor of telemedicine regarding clinical outcomes and improved quality of services [41, 42]. A US-American study showed a significant correlation between rising age and an unfavorable attitude towards the use of telemedicine [43]. This corresponds with the often-cited expectations of the municipal leaders that telemedicine would not be suitable for older populations. Rural areas may lack high-speed internet connections, which is an important requirement for the diffusion of telemedicine [7]. Thus, the promotion of fast and reliable communication infrastructure in Germany should be recognized as an important precondition for telemedicine. The results might also be interpreted as reflecting a fear among municipal politicians

Table 1 Summary of categorized arguments about and associations with the supplementary models

Trained medical assistant	Positive	Work-relief for physicians (n = 54)	Improve treatment quality and care (n = 17)	Support for the provision of home visits (n = 12)	Appropriate tasks for delegation (n = 12)	Positive experiences with similar concepts (n = 11)	Remedy for physician shortage (n = 7)
	Negative	Lack of acceptance and trust (n = 10)	Not an adequate substitute for a doctor (n = 7)		No general need (n = 6)	Concerns about treatment quality (n = 5)	
Patients'bus	Positive	Good addition to existing public transport (n = 25)	Similar public transport systems available or planned (n = 21)		Suitable to ensure mobility and accessibility (n = 19)	Suitable supplement for rural and widespread areas (n = 14)	
	Negative	Sufficient mobility offers available (n = 25)	High effort and costs (n = 16)	Not suitable for the specific community and settlement structure (n = 12)	Low demand and utilization projected (n = 6)	Not necessary due to good accessibility or short distances to medical practices (n = 6)	
Mobile physicians'office	Positive	Suitable supplement for rural and widespread areas (n = 16)			Sufficient to secure the supply of medical treatment (n = 7)		
	Negative	Lack of acceptance and trust (n = 39)	Not necessary due to good accessibility or short distances to medical practices (n = 20	Not suitable for the specific community and settlement structure (n = 20)	No general need (n = 15)	Concerns about treatment quality (n = 9)	Inefficient use of doctors due to travel expenses (n = 9)
Telemedicine	Positive	Suitable for specific group of persons (n = 10)		Forward-looking model with potential (n = 7)		Suitable for specific indications (n = 6)	
	Negative	Not suitable for older people (n = 57)	Impersonal type of treatment (n = 33)	Poor availability of necessary technology (n = 29)	Concerns about treatment quality (n = 16)	Lack of acceptance and trust (n = 14)	

that technical instruments will have too much decision-making power at the expense of an accurate personal verification of patients' needs.

Community leaders had different opinions regarding the implementation of transport solutions such as patients' buses intended to transport patients to physicians' offices. It seems to be common sense that physicians' offices are important destinations for public connections. Generally, transport options other than patients' buses seem to be favored. One important aspect of the suitability of patients' buses could be the financial requirements and related municipal involvement.

Mobile physicians' offices were predominantly seen as not suitable; at best, they were seen as the option of last resort for undersupplied communities. There are examples of mobile utilities in other supply areas that have been partly accepted as a way to overcome local supply gaps: e.g., mobile libraries or mobile citizen centers [44]. In medical treatment, there is prevailing skepticism. Often, no need was observed for mobile care solutions, which can perhaps be attributed to a sufficiently dense network of resident doctors in Lower Saxony. According to a study of German medical students, future physicians are potentially quite willing to work in a mobile physician's office [45].

As mentioned above, the Lower Saxony municipal survey collected assessments of supplementary care models, which were also collected in a population survey in Lower Saxony. In both surveys, medical delegation models were relatively frequently accepted as a care option, while a telemedicine treatment contact was mostly not accepted. In the general population, greater acceptance of a mobile doctor's practice compared to a patient's bus was observed [21].

Depending on the need and respective care situation, supplementary care models could be applied individually or in combination. There is not necessarily a trade-off between a TMA and telemedicine. Rather, both, in combination, could support effective healthcare delivery in undersupplied areas [46]. The described models tackle problems of local accessibility in healthcare. However, they do not ensure a sufficient number of doctors. The supplementary models could only help to improve the need-based utilization of physicians if the available physicians are not yet fully occupied. This also applies to delegation models with a TMA, whereby the supervision and cooperation of a physician is necessary, which limits the relief provided to the physician [47].

The binary logistic regression showed little evidence that the supplementary models are more favored if the local physicians' care situation was assessed negatively, with the chosen indicators as covariates. Thus, our model is not appropriate to explain the differences between the overall assessments. This suggests that more than situational and location factors – and not the queried personal opinions and views of the participants – are causing differences in the suitability assessment.

The bivariate analysis of the relation between the spatial classification of the community and the assessed suitability of the supplementary models showed significant differences for the models, with the exception of telemedicine. In multivariate analysis, the spatial classification only had a significant influence on the assessment of the patients' bus model.

Strength and limitations

The study contributes evidence from the local politicians' point of view to current discussions about supplementary models in primary healthcare delivery. This study offers another important perspective – in addition to the patients' perspective – on different innovative approaches. To our knowledge, this survey is the first to focus on the target group of German municipalities and their attitudes towards supplementary models of primary care delivery.

The study's strengths also lie in the high response of more than 70%. Thus, the findings can be considered representative for Lower Saxony. Lower Saxony can be considered representative of the overall German settlement and healthcare supply structure due to its diverse settlement structure, which includes areas that are very rural as well as large centers. The results can therefore be regarded as nationally and internationally transferable.

There are also some limitations that should be considered.

The developed questionnaire was experimental. The supplementary care models were explained in the questionnaire with brief descriptions and illustrating pictures. It remains unclear what additional knowledge the local politicians had about each model and how this potential knowledge influenced their responses. Although the questionnaire was thoroughly tested previously, the descriptions may have been misunderstood by the respondents in some cases.

The opinion of the surveyed respondents towards the supplementary models was assessed on a fundamental level to capture their first impressions of an innovative approach to outpatient care. The analysis shows the expressed basic expectations and reservations of the local authorities. Important aspects, such as financial questions, potential municipal participation, and willingness to pay, were not included in the questionnaire. However, financial aspects certainly matter for a local implementation of supplement concepts and have been partially included in the answers regarding local suitability. In total, the study's findings are not appropriate for use as a political basis of decision-making. For this reason, the results should not be used as arguments for or against the suitability of a model but rather as indications of the personal points of view of local authorities, which contribute to the discussion at the federal level.

Our investigation was based on a cross-sectional study, which has its limitations, such as the selection bias of the respondents. Therefore, the results cannot necessarily be generalized to future sampling.

Conclusions

This study provides information on how local politicians generally contrast different supplement models in primary care and with what arguments and associations the different models are linked. Although these aspects are not usable as broader policy advice, the analysis provides an inventory of existing assumptions and prejudices at the local level, which should be taken into account when implementing supplementary care models.

Although there are significant differences between urban and rural areas, overall, the mayors and county leaders in Lower Saxony are more satisfied than dissatisfied with the local medical care situation.

The survey respondents estimated the practicality of the respective supplementary models very differently. From the politicians' point of view, increased service from non-medical staff such as TMAs is well accepted, and not only in response to a physician shortage. Extended public mobility models that focus on primary care seem to be an important issue for many of those surveyed. For some respondents, patients' buses may be considered a possible useful option, whereas the suitability of mobile physicians' offices is predominantly rejected. The presented telemedicine model has widespread negative associations. If telemedicine approaches are to be implemented, the barriers shown here at the local level should be taken into account.

Currently, for the majority of the population, doctors' offices are still relatively easy to access, for both the urban and rural population. There are usually more barriers to structural changes than to keeping the status quo. The question is whether the assessment of supplementary models will change when the situation worsens in certain areas, as forecasts and social trends predict. Perhaps, the need for physicians must become more severe before the association of statutory health insurance physicians and municipalities will leave the familiar situation behind and try unconventional approaches such as alternative models of access to healthcare.

Endnotes

[1]Spatial classification in accordance with the criterion of population density (<150 inhabitants / square kilometer) [48]

Additional files

Additional file 1: Questionnaire mayors. The translated questionnaire for the survey of mayors in Lower Saxony.

Additional file 2: Questionnaire county administrators. The translated questionnaire for the survey of county administrators in Lower Saxony.

Additional file 3: Binary logistic regression model of the suitability of the supplement models. The regression model investigates possible connections regarding the suitability of supplement models with with indicators of a positively or negatively assessed local healthcare situation.

Abbreviations

GP: General practitioner; TMA: Trained medical assistants

Funding

This study was supported with funds from the General Local Health Insurance Fund (AOK) and the Associations of Statutory Health Insurance Physicians (Kassenärztliche Vereinigung) in Lower Saxony.

Author's contributions

BK designed and conducted the study, collected data, carried out data analyses and wrote the manuscript. KSK assisted in data analysis and revised the manuscript. SL assisted in data analysis and revised the manuscript. JS made substantial contributions to conception of the questionnaire and revised the manuscript. VA coordinated the study and revised the manuscript. All authors read and approved the final manuscript.

Consent for publication

Not applicable

Competing interests

JS is evaluating the use of a mobile physicians' office in Schleswig-Holstein. He has also applied for grants for several research projects that investigate telemedicine approaches. All other authors declare that they have no competing interests.

Author details

[1]Medical School Hannover, Institute for Epidemiology, Social Medicine and Health Systems Research, OE 5410, Carl-Neuberg-Str. 1, D-30625 Hannover, Germany. [2]University Hospital of Schleswig-Holstein, Campus Lübeck, Institute of Family Medicine, Lübeck, Germany.

References

1. Busse R, Blümel M. Germany: health system review. Health Systems in Transition. 2014;16
2. Kühl K. Sicherstellung ambulanter medizinischer Versorgung in ländlichen Regionen. In: Bewältigung medizinischer Unterversorgung am Maßstab und mit den Mitteln des Rechts [ensuring outpatient medical care in rural regions. Management of medical under-supply with regulations and the means of law]. Baden-Baden: Nomos; 2012.
3. Klose J, Uhlemann T, Gutschmidt S: *Ärztemangel - Ärzteschwemme?: Auswirkungen der Altersstruktur von Ärzten auf die vertragsärztliche Versorgung [Physician Glut – Physician Shortage? Impact of the Age Structure of Physicians on Medical Care]*. Bonn; 2003 [WidO].
4. Kopetsch T. *Dem deutschen Gesundheitswesen gehen die Ärzte aus! Studie zur Altersstruktur-und Arztzahlentwicklung [The German Health Care System Is*

Running out of Physicians! A study about the Structure of the Age and Trend of the Number of Physicians]. 5th ed. Berlin: Kassenärztliche Bundesvereinigung [National Association of Statutory Health Insurance Physicians]; 2010.

5. Sundmacher L, Ozegowski S. Regional distribution of physicians: the role of comprehensive private health insurance in Germany. European Journal of Health Economics. 2015;
6. OECD. Health at a glance 2015: OECD indicators. Paris: Organisation for Economic Co-operation and Development; 2015.
7. Ono T, Schoenstein M, Buchan J: *Geographic Imbalances in Doctor Supply and Policy Responses; 2014 [OECD Health Working Papers*, vol. 69].
8. Ozegowski S, Sundmacher L. Understanding the gap between need and utilization in outpatient care - the effect of supply-side determinants on regional inequities. Health Policy. 2014;114:54–63.
9. Hjorthol R. Transport resources, mobility and unmet transport needs in old age. Ageing Soc. 2013;33:1190–211.
10. Gerlach F, Greiner W, Haubitz M, Schaeffer D, Thürmann P, Thüsing G, Wille E: *Bedarfsgerechte Versorgung - Perspektiven für ländliche Regionen und ausgewählte Leistungsbereiche: Gutachten* 2014 *[Needs-based Health Care: Opportunities for Rural Regions and Selected Health Care Sectors. Report 2014].* Bern: Verlag Hans Huber; 2014 *(Sachverständigenrat zur Begutachtung der Entwicklung im Gesundheitswesen [Advisory Council on the Assessment of Developments in the Health Care System]),* vol. 2014].
11. Landesausschuss der Ärzte und Krankenkassen [Federal State Committee of Doctors and Health Funds]: *Bedarfsplanung in der vertragsärztlichen Versorgung - Fortschreibung Nr. 02/2015: II. Allgemeine fachärztliche Versorgung (§ 12 BPL-RL) Fachgruppe Psychotherapeuten [Requirements planning in ambulant care - update No 02/2015: II. General specialist care (§ 12 BPL-RL) Section psychotherapists]*; 2015.
12. World Health Organization (WHO): *Rural poverty and health systems in the WHO European Region*. Kopenhagen; 2010.
13. Sammut MR, Lindh M, Rindlisbacher B. On behalf of EURACT-the European academy of teachers in general practice: funding of vocational training programmes for general practice/family medicine in Europe. European Journal of General Practice. 2009;14:83–8.
14. Flum E, Maagaard R, Godycki-Cwirko M, Scarborough N, Scherpbier N, Ledig T, Roos M, Steinhäuser J: Assessing family medicine trainees – what can we learn from the European neighbours? *GMS Zeitschrift für Medizinische Ausbildung* 2014, 32:Doc21.
15. Giesel F, Köhler K, Nowossadeck E. Alt und immobil auf dem land? Mobilitätseinschränkungen älterer menschen vor dem Hintergrund einer zunehmend problematischen Gesundheitsversorgung in ländlichen Regionen [old and immobile in rural areas? Limited mobility of the elderly in the context of increasingly problematic health care in rural regions]. Bundesgesundheitsblatt. 2013;56:1418–24.
16. Porter ME, Pabo EA, Lee TH. Redesigning primary care: a strategic vision to improve value by organizing around patients' needs. Health Aff. 2013;32:516–25.
17. Weinhold I, Gurtner S. Understanding shortages of sufficient health care in rural areas. Health Policy. 2014;118:201–14.
18. Kenny A, Farmer J, Dickson-Swift V, Hyett N. Community participation for rural health: a review of challenges. Health Expect. 2015;18:1906–17.
19. Bogumil J, Holtkamp L. Kommunalpolitik und Kommunalverwaltung: Eine praxisorientierte Einführung [municipal policy and local government: a practical introduction]. Bonn: Bundeszentrale für politische Bildung [Federal Agency for Civic Education]; 2013.
20. Sutton R. The policy process: an overview. London: Chameleon Press; 1999. [*Working paper / Overseas Development Institute*, vol. 118]
21. Tangermann U, Kleij K, Krauth C, Amelung VE: Sicherstellung der medizinischen Versorgung: Patienten sind offen für Neues [Ensuring medical care – Patients are open-minded]]. *Dtsch Arztebl International* 2016, 113:A-2024.
22. Tsiachristas A, Wallenburg I, Bond CM, Elliot RF, Busse R, van Exel J, Rutten-van Mölken MP, De BA. costs and effects of new professional roles: evidence from a literature review. Health Policy. 2015;119:1176–87.
23. Ono T G. Lafortune G, Schoenstein M: *Health Workforce Planning in OECD Countries: A Review of 26 Projection Models from 18 Countries*. Paris; 2013 [*OECD Health Working Papers*, vol. 62].
24. Bond C, Bruhn H, De BA, van Exel J, Busse R, Sutton M, Elliott R. the iMpact on practice, oUtcomes and costs of new roles for health pROfeSsionals: a study protocol for MUNROS. BMJ Open. 2016;6:e010511.
25. Freund T, Everett C, Griffiths P, Hudon C, Naccarella L, Laurant M. Skill mix, roles and remuneration in the primary care workforce: who are the healthcare professionals in the primary care teams across the world? Int J Nurs Stud. 2015;52:727–43.
26. Schmiedhofer M, Brandner S, Kuhlmey A. Delegation ärztlicher Leistungen an nichtärztliche Fachkräfte: der Versorgungsansatz agneszwei in Brandenburg - eine qualitative Akzeptanzanalyse [delegation of medical treatment to non-physician health care professionals: the medical care structure agneszwei in Brandenburg – a qualitative acceptance analysis]. Gesundheitswesen. 2017;79:453–60.
27. OECD. Ageing and transport: mobility needs and safety issues. Paris; 2001.
28. Misslbeck A: Patientenbus - option gegen Ärztemangel? [patients' bus – option against physician shortage?] *Ärzte Zeitung* 2012.
29. Hämel K, Kutzner J, Vorderwülbecke J. Mobile Versorgungseinrichtungen zur Stärkung der Versorgungssicherheit im ländlichen Raum? Eine Analyse von Konzepten und Implementationsanforderungen [Mobile Health Units: An Analysis of Concepts and Implementation Requirements in Rural Regions]. Gesundheitswesen. 2015;77
30. Schwartze J, Wolf, Rochon, M., K H., Haarbrandt B, Wagner M, Drews M, Fischer T, Hellwig T, Hofmann S, Höft-Budde P, Jäger R, Lorenz S, Naumann R, Plischke M, Reytarowski J, Richter C, Steinbrügge C, Ziegenspeck A, Ingelheim J von, Haux R (Eds): Rollende Arztpraxis - Zwischenfazit eines mobilen Versorgungskonzeptes zur Unterstützung der medizinischen Versorgung in ländlichen Gebieten [Rolling doctor's office - interim conclusion of a mobile care concept to support medical care in rural areas]. Düsseldorf: German Medical Science GMS Publishing House; 2014.
31. Schnack D. Die rollende Arztpraxis jetzt im Einsatz für Flüchtlinge [Rolling doctor's office now in use for refugees]. Ärzte Zeitung. 2015;18
32. Bashshur RL. On the definition and evaluation of telemedicine. Telemedicine journal: the official journal of the American Telemedicine Association. 1995;1:19–30.
33. van den Berg N, Schmidt S, Stentzel U, Mühlan H, Hoffmann W. Telemedizinische Versorgungskonzepte in der regionalen Versorgung ländlicher Gebiete [the integration of telemedicine concepts in the regional care of rural areas]. Bundesgesundheitsblatt. 2015;58:367–73.
34. Mayring P. Qualitative Inhaltsanalyse [qualitative content analyses*]*. In: Flick U, von KE, Steinke I, editors. In *Qualitative Forschung. Ein Handbuch [Qualitative research. A manual]*. Reinbek: Rowohlt Taschenbuch Verlag; 2007. p. 468–75.
35. Urban E, Ose D, Joos S, Szecsenyi J, Miksch A. Technical support and delegation to practice staff - status quo and (possible) future perspectives for primary health care in Germany. BMC medical informatics and decision making. 2012;12:81.
36. Dill M, Pankow S, Erikson C, Shipman S. Survey shows consumers open to a greater role for physician assistants and nurse practitioners. Health Aff. 2013; 32:1135–42.
37. Otto U, Brettenhofer M, Tarnutzer S. Telemedizin in der älteren Bevölkerung [telemedicine in the elderly population]. Ther Umsch. 2015;72:567–75.
38. Cimperman M, Brencic MM, Trkman P, Stanonik, de Leonni M. older Adults' perceptions of home telehealth services. Telemedicine and e-health. 2013; 19:786–90.
39. Bertelsmann Stiftung. Video-Sprechstunden [Video Consultations]. Spotlight Gesundheit. 2015;
40. Simon P. The place of personalised medical e-consultancy in the practice of telemedicine. European Research in Telemedicine. 2015;4:71–80.
41. Wootton R. Twenty years of telemedicine in chronic disease management - an evidence synthesis. J Telemed Telecare. 2012;18:211–20.
42. Moffatt JJ, Eley DS. The reported benefits of telehealth for rural Australians. Aust Health Review. 2010;34:276.
43. Call V, Erickson L, Dailey N, Hicken B, Rupper R, Yorgason J, Bair B. Attitudes toward telemedicine in urban, rural, and highly rural communities. Telemedicine and e-health. 2015;21:644–51.
44. OECD. *Strategies to improve rural service delivery*. Paris: [OECD rural policy reviews]; 2010.
45. Kittel B, Kaczynski A, Bethge S, Mühlbacher A. Was braucht der neue Landarzt? – Ein analytic hierarchy process (AHP) [what does the new country doctor need? – an analytic hierarchy process (AHP)]. Gesundheitsökonomie & Qualitätsmanagement. 2015;20

46. Green L, Savin S, Lu Y. Primary care physician shortages could be eliminated through use of teams, nonphysicians, and electronic communication. Health Aff. 2013;32:11–9.
47. Redaèlli M, Stock S, Simic D, Wilm S: Internationales Literaturreview zur „Effektivität und Effizienz von nicht-ärztlichen Berufen in ambulanten Versorgungskonzepten" [international literature review "effectiveness and efficiency of non-medical professions in ambulatory care concepts"]. Witten; 2009.
48. Bundesinstitut für Bau-, Stadt- und Raumforschung (BBSR)[Federal Institute for Research on Building. Urban Affairs and Spatial Development]: *Indikatoren und Karten zur Raum- und Stadtentwicklung [Indicators and maps for spatial and urban development]. INKAR*. Bonn; 2016.
49. fremantleboy: *Landkreise, Kreise und kreisfreie Städte in Deutschland [Counties, districts and cities in Germany] 2007–07-01 - 2008-07-31: Creative Commons license cc-by-2.5* [https://commons.wikimedia.org/wiki/File:Landkreise,_Kreise_und_kreisfreie_St%C3%A4dte_in_Deutschland_2007-07-01_-_2008-07-31.png

15

An after hours GP clinic in regional Australia: appropriateness of presentations and impact on local emergency department presentations

Kristy Payne[1], Tegan Dutton[1], Kate Weal[2], Maree Earle[2], Ross Wilson[1] and Jannine Bailey[1*]

Abstract

Background: After hours general practice clinics provide medical attention for clients with non-emergency situations but are seeking immediate treatment and unable to wait for a general practitioner during routine opening hours. Evidence on the impact that after hours clinics have on emergency department presentations is equivocal. This study explored outcomes of the Bathurst After Hours General Practice Clinic (BAHGPC). Specifically it examined: clients' perceived urgency of, and satisfaction with their presentation to the BAHGPC; general practitioners' perception of the appropriateness of presentations to the BAHGPC; and whether the frequency of non-urgent and semi-urgent emergency department presentations at Bathurst Base Hospital has changed since the opening of the BAHGPC.

Methods: Clients presenting to the BAHGPC from 01/02/2015 to 30/06/2015 were asked to participate in the client presentation survey and follow-up satisfaction survey. General practitioner surveys were completed for individual clients from 01/12/2014 to 30/06/2015 to document the appropriateness of each presentation. Descriptive statistics are used to describe survey responses. Thematic analysis was applied for qualitative responses. Emergency department presentations were retrieved from the Emergency Department Data Collection. A comparison of presentations in the two years prior and subsequent to the opening of the BAHGPC was conducted using independent T-tests and Chi-square tests to compare mean presentations and proportional data for the different time periods examined.

Results: Most clients (76%) presenting to the BAHGPC classified their visit as essential. General practitioners considered most presentations to be appropriate (87%). Sixty percent (60%) of clients would have gone to the emergency department had the BAHGPC not been operational. Client satisfaction was high and 99% would use the clinic again. A significant reduction in total non-urgent presentations to the Emergency Department occurred in the two years since the opening of the BAHGPC clinic compared to the two years prior (418.5 vs. 245.5; $P < 0.05$).

Conclusions: There was concordance between general practitioners and clients regarding the appropriateness of presentations to the BAHGPC. The findings of this study highlight that after hours general practitioner clinics are an essential service in regional areas and contribute to reducing the burden of non-urgent presentations to the local emergency department.

* Correspondence: jannine.bailey@westernsydney.edu.au
[1]Bathurst Rural Clinical School, School of Medicine, Western Sydney University, Bathurst, NSW, Australia
Full list of author information is available at the end of the article

Background

Acute care services, both in Australia and internationally, are coming under increasing pressure. This is partly due to an increased burden of chronic disease, an ageing population and an overall reduction in general practitioner working hours, particularly in the after hours period [1–3]. In recent years in Australia, the average annual increase in the emergency department (ED) presentation rate [4] has been consistently higher than that of population growth [5]. In addition, it has been estimated that some 10 to 40% of ED presentations represent general practice clients more suited to primary care than acute care [6–11].

This increasing ED workload, and concerns about the appropriateness of some ED presentations, has prompted the implementation of Government initiatives to increase the availability and accessibility of after hours primary care. A recent systematic review [3] identified six models of after hours primary care including minor injury units, walk in centres, telephone triage and advice centres, ambulance officer managed care, the integration of a general practitioner within the ED team, and General Practice (GP) cooperatives. GP cooperatives, otherwise known as after hours GP clinics, provide medical attention for people who are seeking immediate treatment and cannot wait to see their regular general practitioner during their routine opening hours. They are designed to cater for people who do not have an emergency situation, but who would otherwise be likely to access their local ED for treatment due to the perceived urgency of their complaint [2]. International and Australian evidence on the impact of after hours GP clinics on low acuity emergency department presentations is equivocal [3].

One aspect of after hours GP clinics that has received little attention is the appropriateness of presentations to these clinics, both from the client and the general practitioner perspective. Only one study, conducted in the Netherlands, has addressed this and found that up to two-thirds of non-urgent presentations to GP cooperatives were "medically unnecessary" and could have been managed by their regular general practitioner during routine working hours, or could have been managed by the client themselves without professional care [12]. Two key limitations of this study were that the client presentation survey was conducted in the post-consultation period, hence relying on client recall and also leading to low response rates, and the appropriateness of their presentation was judged by two general practitioners retrospectively using only the client survey data. Further examination of after hours GP clinic presentations is therefore warranted to determine whether the presence of after hours GP clinics is providing a suitable alternative to the ED for low acuity clients.

The primary aims of this study, therefore, were to examine (a) the clients' perceived urgency of their presentation to the after hours GP clinic, (b) the general practitioners' perception of the appropriateness of each presentation to the after hours GP clinic, and (c) client satisfaction with the service. A secondary aim was to examine the frequency of semi-urgent and non-urgent presentations to the local ED, and compare data from the two years prior to the opening of the after hours GP clinic, to the two years since its opening.

Methods

Setting

The Bathurst After Hours General Practice Clinic (BAHGPC) is located next door to the Bathurst Base Hospital in the regional town of Bathurst, New South Wales, Australia. It is a bulk-billing, walk-in clinic; meaning that the Australian Government's Medicare benefit covers full payment of the service and there are no out of pocket expenses for clients and no prior appointments can be made. Opening hours are 3 pm to 7 pm on weekends and public holidays (excluding Christmas Day and Good Friday). The clinic is routinely staffed by a receptionist, registered nurse and a general practitioner. The BAHGPC has been in operation since the 1st December 2012 and is the only after hours service in the local area.

Study design

A survey study was conducted using a volunteer sample of participants. All clients who presented to the BAHGPC during the period 1st February 2015 to 30th June 2015 were eligible to participate in the client presentation survey. For presentations where the client was aged 18 years or older, the client was invited to participate. For presentations where the client was under 18 years of age, the client's accompanying parent or guardian was invited to participate and complete the survey on behalf of the client, provided they were themselves aged 18 years or older. Clients were also asked to provide their contact details if they consented to being contacted over the phone for a follow-up satisfaction survey. This information was recorded separately so as to maintain the anonymity of their survey responses. The general practitioner appropriateness of presentation survey was conducted during the period 1st December 2014 to 30th June 2015. All general practitioners at the clinic were encouraged to complete this survey for all client encounters in the study period.

Client presentation survey

The four item, anonymous client survey was administered by the clinic nurse and was completed by all consenting participants prior to their consultation. The survey asked for the clients' reason/s for presenting to the clinic, where they would have sought treatment if the clinic was unavailable at that time, willingness to pay for the clinic, and their health insurance status (Additional file 1).

Client follow-up satisfaction survey

The client follow-up satisfaction survey was conducted over the phone by the BAHGPC administration staff within two weeks following the client's clinic presentation. Verbal consent was obtained from all participants before the survey was administered. Clients were asked to rate how satisfied they were with the outcome of their visit on a scale of 0 (very dissatisfied) to 10 (very satisfied), whether their issue was resolved, whether they would use the clinic again, whether they would recommend the clinic to others, and any additional comments (Additional file 2).

General practitioner appropriateness of presentation survey

The three item general practitioner appropriateness of presentation survey was completed immediately following a client consultation (Additional file 3). General practitioners were asked to classify the appropriateness of the presentation and to rate the appropriateness of the presentation on a scale of 0 (not appropriate) to 5 (absolutely essential). They were also asked to identify the medical outcome identified, which the researchers categorised into one of ten presentation categories, namely: ear, nose and throat; respiratory; genito-urinary; gastrointestinal; neurological; cardiovascular; dermatological; psychological; documentation; and other.

Examination of emergency department presentations

Semi-urgent and non-urgent ED presentations (Australasian triage categories 4 and 5, respectively) at Bathurst Base Hospital were retrieved from the New South Wales Emergency Department Data Collection. Data was extracted for the two years prior to the opening of the BAHGPC (1st December 2010 to 30th November 2012) and the two years subsequent to the opening of the BAHGPC (1st December 2012 to 30th November 2014). Only those presentations occurring between the hours of 12:00 pm Saturday through to 8:00 am Monday were examined. This time frame was chosen as it is during this period that there are no other GP clinics open in the local area (i.e. some GP clinics are open Saturday morning up until 12 pm and reopen on Monday at 8 am) and the only options for clients are the BAHGPC or the local ED. Non-identifiable data retrieved included time of presentation, triage category, age, and sex.

Statistical analysis

Descriptive statistics were used to describe quantitative survey responses and ED presentation data. Independent T-tests were used to compare mean ED presentations during the two time periods examined. Chi-square tests were used to compare proportional data for the different time periods examined. Statistical analyses were conducted using IBM SPSS Statistics (Version 22.0). Statistical significance was set at $P < 0.05$. The qualitative responses on the client follow-up survey were reviewed by two researchers to familiarise themselves with the data. The key themes of positive, negative and neutral service comments were identified and used to categorise the responses.

Results

Presentations to the Bathurst after hours gp clinic

In the first two years of operation (1st December 2012 to 30th November 2014) there were 2125 presentations to the BAHGPC. Of these, 1205 (57%) were female and 920 (43%) were male. During the five month client study period (1st February 2015 to 30th June 2015), there were 827 clinic presentations, of which 62% were female and 38% were male. A total of 219 clients who presented to the clinic during this time frame participated in the client presentation survey. However, 14 were incomplete and not included in the analysis, resulting in a total of 205 surveys; a 25% response rate. The follow-up satisfaction survey was completed by 219 clients, a 26% response rate. During the period 1st December 2014 to 30th June 2015, 452 general practitioner surveys were completed by treating doctors, a response rate of 55%.

Three-quarters of all clients surveyed (76%; 155) deemed their visit to the BAHGPC as essential (Table 1). Sixty per cent (60%; 125) indicated that they would have presented to the ED had the BAHGPC not been operating at the time of their visit, of which 86% (107) classified their visit as essential. A quarter of respondents (27%; 55) indicated they would have waited until the following week to see their own general practitioner rather than present to the ED (Table 1), however 58% (32) of these respondents still deemed their visit as essential. Twenty-eight per cent (28%; 49) of participating clients had a health care card and 44% (75) had private health insurance (Table 1). One-quarter of respondents (25%; 52) reported that they would not use the BAHGPC if they had to pay for the service, i.e. if it was not bulk-billed. Of the clients who said no, only two gave a reason, being: *"Depends on acuity of presentation"*; and *"just in case I didn't have the money at the time"*. Of the 75% that would be willing to pay for the service, 56% (87) would be willing to pay the same amount they currently pay their general practitioner, and 39% (60) would be willing to pay a small co-payment (less than $10). There

Table 1 Client perceptions when presenting at the Bathurst After Hours General Practice Clinic

	Number	Percentage (%)
Main reason for attending the after hours clinic: (*n* = 205)		
Essential visit (had to come)	155	76%
Convenient	18	9%
Couldn't get an appointment with a regular GP	16	8%
Only to get a script (out of my medication)	8	4%
Requested by the hospital ED to attend	1	0%
Requested by the GP to attend	0	0%
Other	7	3%
If the after hours clinic was not operational, the client would: (n = 205)[a]		
Go to the Hospital ED	125	60%
Wait until next week to see the client's own GP	55	27%
Try and consult another GP in town	22	11%
Visit a pharmacist and try to get medication	3	1%
Other	3	1%
If the client had to pay for the clinic, would they use the service: (n = 205)[b]		
Yes:	154	75%
If yes, what is the maximum the client would be willing to pay: (*n* = 154)		
The same amount you would pay at your GP	87	56%
A small co-payment (less than $10)	60	39%
More than you would pay at your GP	4	3%
No response/missing data	3	2%
No	52	25%
Does the client have a health care card: (*n* = 175)		
Yes	49	28%
No	126	72%
Does the client have private health insurance: (*n* = 170)		
Yes	75	44%
No	95	56%

[a]More than one response provided by 3 clients; all responses are included in the analysis
[b]One respondent answered both yes and no; all responses are included in the analysis. Abbreviations: General Practitioner (GP), Emergency Department (ED)

was no significant association between possession of a health care card and willingness to attend the BAHGPC if the client had to pay for the service, i.e., it was not bulk-billed (X^2 1.344, P = 0.246). However, those with private health insurance were significantly more likely to indicate a willingness to attend the BAHGPC if they had to pay for the service (i.e. if it was not bulk-billed), compared to those who did not have private health insurance (X^2 11.926, $P < 0.001$).

From the perspective of the general practitioner, the majority of presentations to the BAHGPC were deemed appropriate (85%; 383) and an additional 2% (7) were considered appropriate *and* needed a referral to the local hospital or ED (Table 2). When queried about how essential the presentations to the BAHGPC were on a scale of 0 to 5 (0 being not appropriate and 5 being absolutely essential), 28% of presentations to the BAHGPC were rated by general practitioners as 5 (absolutely essential), 41% as 4, and 17% as 3 (Table 2). A total of 14% of presentations were rated on the lower end of the scale (0, 1 or 2). The most common presentations recorded by general practitioners were for an ear, nose and throat problem (20%), a dermatological problem (17%) or a respiratory problem (17%) (Table 2).

For the client satisfaction survey, the majority of clients (59%; 129) rated their visit as 10 (very satisfied), and a combined total of 190 (86%) rated their visit as 8, 9 or 10 (Table 3). Seventy-nine per cent (79%; 174) said their health issue was resolved as an outcome of their visit. Of the 45 (21%) issues that were not resolved, within one week of presenting the BAHGPC, 73% (33) saw another GP, 22% (10) went to ED and 9% (4) did not seek additional medical assistance. Ninety-nine per cent (99%; 216) of respondents said that would use the clinic again and 99% (217) would recommend the clinic to someone else (Table 3).

Of the 219 participants that completed the follow-up survey, 162 (74%) provided additional comments about the service when asked. Almost all respondents gave positive comments about the BAHGPC (90%; 147), such as: *"Service is very good and it's wonderful to have in town. Also relieves the Emergency Department. Think it's absolutely marvellous"*, and *"Absolutely excellent service! Nothing worse than having to go to Emergency when "you're not dying". Well-needed service in Bathurst".* Only 5 (3%) respondents gave negative comments about the service which were due to: a lack of equipment, a lack of privacy at reception with personal details being relayed to the client, a long waiting time, and being turned away from the service at 6.45 pm (when the clinic closes at 7 pm). An additional two respondents provided a negative comment about the general practitioner on call, but also said that the BAHGPC was a good service. There were 13 (8%) comments that were neither positive nor negative, for example, *"Would not use the clinic again because have moved to Sydney".*

Some respondents gave recommendations for improvement which included: the clinic being open for longer hours (12), more advertising about the clinic (2), the clinic being connected to an after hours pharmacy (2), having an extra GP at the clinic to decrease waiting times (1), and more infrastructure and equipment (1).

Table 2 General practitioner perceptions of presentations at the Bathurst After Hours General Practice Clinic

	Number	Percentage (%)
Classification of presentations to the Bathurst After Hours GP Clinic: (*n* = 449)		
Consultation was appropriate	383[a]	85%
Consultation was appropriate *and* needed a referral to hospital/ED	7	2%
Consultation was appropriate *and* was requested by clients GP during the week	0	0%
Consultation only for a script	9	2%
Consultation for an administrative reason	10	2%
Consultation for drug-seeker	3	1%
Consultation because it was convenient for the client	29[b]	7%
Other	13	4%
GP perception of appropriateness of presentation: (*n* = 452)		
5 (Absolutely essential)	125	28%
4	186	41%
3	77	17%
2	33	7%
1	17	4%
0 (Not appropriate)	14	3%
Primary reason for presentation: (n = 452)		
Ear, nose and throat	91	20%
Dermatological	77	17%
Respiratory	76	17%
Gastrointestinal	39	9%
Genito-urinary	34	8%
Documentation	20	4%
Neurological	9	2%
Psychological	8	2%
Cardiovascular	3	1%
Other – including dental, injury, immunisation	95	21%

Abbreviations: GP General Practitioner, *ED* Emergency Department
[a]3 responses were also classified as "consultation for an administrative reason"
[b]1 response was also classified as "consultation for drug-seeker" and 1 response was also classified as "consultation for administrative reason"

Presentations to the bathurst base hospital emergency department

Non-urgent and semi-urgent presentations to the Bathurst ED in the two years prior to the BAHGPC opening and in the subsequent two years were compared both in terms of raw numbers and on a population basis (Table 4). There was a significant reduction in non-urgent ED presentations in the two years following the opening of the BAHGPC as compared to the two years prior (418.5 vs 245.5; $P < 0.05$). There was no significant reduction in semi-urgent ED presentations in the same period. On a population basis, in the two years prior to the opening of the BAHGPC non-urgent presentations equated to 1.0% of the Bathurst population (Table 4). This dropped significantly in the two years following the opening of the clinic to 0.6% ($P < 0.05$). There was no significant difference in semi-urgent ED presentations in this period on a population basis.

Non-urgent ED presentations in the two years prior to the opening of the after hours clinic and the two years subsequent to the opening of the clinic were stratified by gender and compared to the number of visits to the after hours clinic in the first two years of operation (Table 4). More males than females presented to the ED with non-urgent complaints during the first two years of the BAHGPC being in operation. In contrast, more females than males attended the BAHGPC in this same period. This difference in proportions was significantly different ($P < 0.05$).

Discussion

After hours GP clinics are intended to relieve pressure on EDs by diverting suitable clients to a primary care alternative. They are designed to cater for people who do not have an emergency situation but who are seeking immediate treatment due to the perceived urgency of their complaint, and are hence unable to wait to see their regular general practitioner during routine opening hours. The primary aim of this study was to examine the appropriateness of presentations to an after hours GP clinic from both the client and the general practitioner perspective and to examine client satisfaction with the clinic. A secondary aim was to examine changes in non-urgent and semi-urgent ED presentations in the two years before, and following, the opening of the after hours clinic.

Clients and doctors can have different perceptions of the level of urgency of a medical complaint, leading to different interpretations of the appropriateness of a presentation to an ED and/or after hours clinic [13, 14]. In this study, we found good concordance between clients and doctors as to the necessity and appropriateness of presentations to the BAHGPC. Seventy-six per cent (76%) of clients deemed their visit as essential whilst general practitioners ranked 87% of presentations as appropriate and 86% as being in the range of moderately to absolutely essential. To our knowledge, only one other study has compared the perceptions of clients and doctors regarding the appropriateness of presentations to an after hours service [12]. They found that nearly two-thirds of non-urgent contacts to an after hours GP cooperative were "medically unnecessary", despite the clients themselves believing their presentation to be urgent, and could have been readily managed by the client or by their regular general practitioner during routine

Table 3 Client satisfaction follow-up survey

	Number	Percentage (%)
Client satisfaction with the visit (*n* = 219)		
10 (very satisfied)	129	59%
9	40	18%
8	21	10%
7	15	7%
6	4	2%
5	8	4%
4	1	0%
3	0	0%
2	0	0%
1	1	0%
0 (very dissatisfied)		
Was the clients issue resolved: (n = 219)		
Yes	174	79%
No	45	21%
Saw another GP within one week of visiting the After Hours clinic (n = 45[a])[b]	33	73%
Went to ED within one week of visiting the After Hours clinic (*n* = 45)[a]	10	22%
Did not anyone else within one week of visiting the After Hours clinic (n = 45)	4	9%
Would the client use the clinic again: (n = 219)		
Yes	216	99%
No	3	1%
Would the client recommend the clinic to someone else: (n = 219)		
Yes	217	99%
No	2	1%

Abbreviations: *GP* General Practitioner, *ED* Emergency Department
[a]2 respondents saw another GP *and* went to ED within one week of visiting the After Hours clinic
[b]The after hours GP routinely encourages clients to make an appointment with their regular GP for the week following the BAHGPC consultation

working hours [12]. The authors suggested that the purpose and intention of the GP cooperative needs to be made clearer to the general public so that they can reduce the number of medically unnecessary contacts that are occurring. In our study, the low percentage of presentations identified by general practitioners on the "not appropriate" end of the scale (14%) suggests that the BAHGPC is being utilised for the purpose of servicing low acuity clients who might otherwise have presented to the ED. As this relatively new service becomes more established in this location it will be important to monitor future trends to ensure the rate of inappropriate presentations to the clinic remains low.

In this regional location, where after hours options are currently limited solely to the BAHGPC, 60% of respondents indicated they would have presented to the local ED had the BAHGPC not been operating on that day. Based on this data alone, we can surmise that the BAHGPC is having a positive impact on reducing unnecessary ED presentations. Certainly, data on ED presentations showed a significant reduction in non-urgent, but not semi-urgent, ED presentations in the two years since the opening of the BAHGPC as compared to the two years prior to this. This trend was maintained even when accounting for population changes that occurred in those time periods. International evidence regarding the impact of after hours clinics on ED presentations is equivocal and differences in health system structures and after hours service delivery make direct comparisons difficult. Australian evidence is limited, but is also equivocal. One urban study of an after hours clinic found a potentially positive impact on unnecessary ED attendances, however they relied solely on client reports of where they would have sought treatment had the after hours clinic not been an option, rather than examining ED presentations directly [15]. In contrast, another urban based study modelled the impact of a hypothetical after hours clinic on ED presentations and concluded that the clinic would be unlikely to produce any remarkable impact on ED presentations [16]. More recently, in a regional location similar to this study, researchers used regression time series analysis to assess the impact of opening an after-hours GP clinic and found a significant reduction in low-urgency ED presentations with the opening of the clinic [17]. Similarly to our study, the above study was conducted in a regional location where after hours options are limited to the clinic and the ED. Unlike the clinic in our study however, their after hours clinic was not a bulk-billing clinic and clients pay to use their service. Notably, in our study three-quarters of respondents indicated a willingness to pay to use the BAHGPC and those with private health insurance were more likely to indicate a willingness to pay.

A significant difference was detected in the proportion of females and males presenting to the BAHGPC versus those presenting to the ED with non-urgent complaints. Females were the majority in after hours clinic presentations whilst males made up the majority in non-urgent ED presentations. This finding concurs with other studies which have also shown that females were more likely to use after hours options than males who tended towards the ED [12, 13, 18]. We did not record gender on either our client presentation survey or the general practitioner appropriateness of presentation survey, so cannot determine from the data if a difference exists between males and females regarding the type of health issue they were presenting to the BAHGPC with. Similarly, no such analysis was possible on the ED data that we retrieved. This represents an avenue for future

Table 4 Emergency Department and After Hours Clinic presentations pre and post commencement of the Clinic

	2 years prior to after hours clinic	2 years subsequent to after hours clinic
Non-urgent and semi-urgent presentations		
Total numbers of people		
Non-urgent presentations (Mean ± SD)	418.5 ± 9.19	245.5 ± 27.58*
Semi-urgent presentations (Mean ± SD)	3984.5 ± 47.38	3931.5 ± 81.32
As a percentage of the Bathurst Population**		
Non-urgent presentations (Mean ± SD)	1.0 ± 0.03	0.6 ± 0.07*
Semi-urgent presentations (Mean ± SD)	9.9 ± 0.05	9.5 ± 0.30
Presentations by gender		
Number (percentage) of non-urgent presentations by gender		
Females	359 (42.9%)	208 (42.4%)
Males	478 (57.1%)	283 (57.6%)
Number (percentage) of after hours clinic presentations by gender***		
Females		1205 (56.7%)
Males		920 (43.2%)

*Indicates value is significantly different ($P < 0.05$) to the corresponding value for the two years prior to the clinic opening
**Source: Australian Bureau of Statistics [19]
***Proportion of females to males significantly different (X^2 41.45; $P < 0.05$) to their respective proportions in non-urgent presentations in the two years following the opening of the clinic

research to determine why males are more likely to present to the ED and examine if their health issues are suitable for treatment at the BAHGPC.

Strengths and limitations

Strengths of this study include that the data regarding client and general practitioner perceptions of the appropriateness and necessity of the presentation were completed at the time of presentation. In the case of the general practitioner assessment of the appropriateness of the presentation, this enabled them to draw on their interaction with the client as part of this process rather than making a retrospective assessment of suitability based on case notes or a client survey, as has been the case in previous research. Another strength is that the clinic examined in this study is a bulk-billing, walk in clinic so there are no apparent access issues for people relating to their socioeconomic status and ability to pay for the service. In addition, it is the only after hours option available in this community, thereby strengthening the conclusions that can be drawn from an examination of ED presentations since the opening of the clinic. It should be acknowledged that there are other factors that can influence ED presentation rate beyond the presence of the BAHGPC alone. However, the absence of other after hours options in this community coupled with the data from this study suggests that the presence of the BAHGPC is having some positive impact on reducing non-urgent ED presentations. Another strength of this study is that we collected both client and general practitioner data regarding the necessity of the presentation. A limitation of this data though is that there was no linkage between the client data and the general practitioner data, therefore we are not able to determine if the participating clients are indeed represented in the general practitioner data. Furthermore, given that clients volunteered to participate and we only obtained a 25% response rate to the client presentation survey, it is possible that the results are not representative of all clients accessing the BAHGPC. Another potential limitation is that the ED presentation data was obtained from 12:00 pm Saturday through to 8:00 am Monday as this is the time-frame over which there are no GP clinics open in Bathurst. However, the BAHGPC is only open for some of these hours (3:00 pm – 7:00 pm Saturday and Sunday). Whilst it is likely that some clients were happy to wait until the BAHGPC was open rather than attend the ED, it is equally as likely that some prospective BAHGPC clients chose to attend the ED rather than wait for the BAHGPC to open. Further research could explore this in greater detail.

Implications

The current research adds to an equivocal evidence base regarding the effectiveness of after hours primary care clinics both nationally and internationally. The positive impact of the after hours clinic seen in this study is likely facilitated by the presence of this bulk-billing, walk in clinic in a regional centre where no other after hours options exist beyond the local ED. This evidence may inform the targeting and implementation of other after hours clinics in similar regional or remote locations to optimise healthcare expenditure on low acuity clients. It is important to note, however, that our findings may not be generalisable to all regions of Australia, particularly metropolitan regions. The current published differences regarding the impact of after hours GP clinics on local ED presentations in Australia may reflect true differences between regions with respect to demand and accessibility. A critical factor at play here could be workforce. Rural and regional areas of Australia, such as Bathurst, are typically identified as areas of general practitioner workforce shortage, as compared to most metropolitan settings which do not bear this label. Hence, the impact of an after hours GP clinic in a rural/regional setting may be more significant in terms of influencing local ED presentations than it would be in metropolitan centres with ample general practitioners and the presence of numerous GP clinics with the capacity to offer after hours services to their clients. Future research could focus on these issues in more depth.

In addition, future research where direct linkage is performed between client perceptions and general practitioner perceptions regarding necessity and appropriateness of a presentation to after hours clinics would add to the evidence base on this topic. Such data can inform client education initiatives to ensure that after hours clinics continue to be used for the purpose for which they were set up – to divert low acuity clients away from the ED – without being burdened by medically unnecessary consultations, borne out of convenience or a clients misguided sense of urgency, that need not have occurred immediately in the after hours period.

Conclusions

The BAHGPC is providing a much needed and appropriately-utilised after hours primary care service to the Bathurst community, that is contributing to reducing the burden of non-urgent presentations to the local ED in this regional centre. The findings highlight the necessity of such a service to rural and regional communities, and regions where there is an identified shortage in the general practitioner workforce, where the impact of demand and accessibility issues is most profound.

Abbreviations

BAHGPC: Bathurst After Hours General Practice Clinic; ED: Emergency department; GP: General practice

Acknowledgements

The authors wish to acknowledge Sarah McKay who assisted with formatting and collation of the manuscript.

Funding

No funding was obtained for this study. The After Hours Services delivered by Marathon Health are funded by the Western NSW Primary Health Network, an Australian Government Initiative.

Authors' contributions

JB, KP, ME, KW, and RW designed the study, collected data and interpreted data. JB, KP and TD analysed the data. JB and TD prepared the manuscript. All authors read and approved the final manuscript.

Ethics approval and consent to participate

Ethics approval to conduct this study was granted by the Western Sydney University Human Research Ethics Committee (Approval #H11011) and the Greater Western Human Research Ethics Committee (LNR 15 GWAHS 38). For general practitioners, consent to participate in the survey was given by their submission of a completed, anonymous survey. For clinic clients, consent to participate in the survey phase was also given by their submission of a completed, anonymous survey. Client consent to be contacted by phone for the follow up survey was also asked at the time of completion of the anonymous survey, and recorded separately so as to maintain the anonymity of the survey responses. Additional verbal consent from all participants in the follow up survey was obtained prior to conducting the survey. Emergency department data was from a Government registry and individual consent was not required to use this non-identifiable data. Consent to access this data was granted by the Greater Western Human Research Ethics Committee as part of their ethics approval process and the data custodians (Population Health Directorate, Western NSW Local Health District) provided the researchers with the dataset for analysis upon presentation of the ethics approval documentation.

Consent for publication

Not applicable.

Competing interests

The authors declare that they have no competing interests.

Author details

[1]Bathurst Rural Clinical School, School of Medicine, Western Sydney University, Bathurst, NSW, Australia. [2]Marathon Health, Bathurst, NSW, Australia.

References

1. Harris MF, Davies PG, Fanaian M, Zwar NA, Liaw ST. Access to same day, next day and after-hours appointments: the views of Australian general practitioners. Aust Health Rev. 2012;36(3):325–30.
2. Carlisle K, Fleming R, Berrigan A. Commissioning for healthcare: a case study of the general practitioners After Hours Program. Aust J Prim Health. 2016; 22(1):22–5.
3. Fry MM. A systematic review of the impact of afterhours care models on emergency departments, ambulance and general practice services. Australas Emerg Nurs J. 2011;14(4):217–25.
4. Australian Institute of Health and Welfare. Emergency department care 2014–15: Australian hospital statistics, Health services series. no. 65 ed. Canberra: AIHW; 2015. p. 9.
5. Australian Bureau of Statistics. 3101.0 - Australian Demographic Statistics, Jun 2015. Canberra: ABS; 2015. [updated 23 March 2016; cited 2017 6 January]; Available from: http://www.abs.gov.au/AUSSTATS/abs@.nsf/allprimarymainfeatures/6CBA90A25BAC951DCA257F7F001CC559?opendocument.
6. Allen PL, Cheek C, Ruigrok M. Rural emergency departments supplement general practice care. Med J Aust. 2015;202(1):17–8.
7. Allen P, Cheek C, Foster S, Ruigrok M, Wilson D, Shires L. Low acuity and general practice-type presentations to emergency departments: a rural perspective. Emerg Med Australas. 2015;27(2):113–8.
8. Thompson MI, Lasserson D, McCann L, Thompson M, Heneghan C. Suitability of emergency department attenders to be assessed in primary care: survey of general practitioner agreement in a random sample of triage records analysed in a service evaluation project. BMJ Open. 2013;3(12): e003612.
9. Cowling TE, Harris MJ, Watt HC, Gibbons DC, Majeed A. Access to general practice and visits to accident and emergency departments in England: cross-sectional analysis of a national patient survey. Br J Gen Pract. 2014; 64(624):e434–9.
10. O'Malley AS. After-hours access to primary care practices linked with lower emergency department use and less unmet medical need. Health Aff. 2013; 32(1):175–83.
11. Nagree Y, Camarda VJ, Fatovich DM, Cameron PA, Dey I, Gosbell AD, et al. Quantifying the proportion of general practice and low-acuity patients in the emergency department. Med J Aust. 2013;198(11):612–5.
12. Keizer E, Smits M, Peters Y, Huibers L, Giesen P, Wensing M. Contacts with out-of-hours primary care for nonurgent problems: patients' beliefs or deficiencies in healthcare? BMC Fam Pract. 2015;16:157.
13. Philips H, Remmen R, De Paepe P, Buylaert W, Van Royen P. Out of hours care: a profile analysis of patients attending the emergency department and the general practitioner on call. BMC Fam Pract. 2010;11:88.

14. Callen JL, Blundell L, Prgomet M. Emergency department use in a rural Australian setting: are the factors prompting attendance appropriate? Aust Health Rev. 2008;32(4):710–20.
15. Haw JE, Perz JM. After Hours General Practice Care: An Investigation of Patient Access Issues to the Nepean After Hours General Practice Clinic. Research Report. Abstract: Western Sydney University 2008.
16. Nagree Y, Ercleve TN, Sprivulis PC. After-hours general practice clinics are unlikely to reduce low acuity patient attendances to metropolitan Perth emergency departments. Aust Health Rreview. 2004;28(3):285–91.
17. Buckley DJ, Curtis PW, McGirr JG. The effect of a general practice after-hours clinic on emergency department presentations: a regression time series analysis. Med J Aust. 2010;192(8):448–51.
18. Smits M, Huibers L, Oude Bos A, Giesen P. Patient satisfaction with out-of-hours GP cooperatives: A longitudinal study. Scand J Prim Health Care. 2012;30(4):206–13.
19. Australian Bureau of Statistics, 3218.0 Regional Population Growth, Australia - Population Estimates by Local Government Area (ASGS 2014), 2004 to 2014 data cube; Retrieved from: http://www.abs.gov.au/AUSSTATS/abs@.nsf/allprimarymainfeatures/6CBA90A25BAC951DCA257F7F001CC559?opendocument.

16

Knowledge, practices and expectations of preventive care: a qualitative study of patients attending government general outpatient clinics in Hong Kong

Denise Y. S. Tam[1*], Yvonne Y. C. Lo[2] and Wendy Tsui[1]

Abstract

Background: Evidence-based preventive care recommendations have been well established, but studies have persistently reported gaps between these recommendations and general practitioners' practices in providing preventive care. Many studies have explored factors that affect the delivery of preventive care from the perspectives of the practitioners, but relatively few have evaluated the patients' point of view. The purpose of this study was to explore patients' understanding of preventive care, the actions they were taking in terms of preventive health and their expectations from family doctors in providing preventive care.

Methods: A qualitative study was conducted based on one-on-one in-depth interviews. Twenty-eight patients without chronic illnesses were purposively recruited from government general outpatient clinics in Hong Kong. The interviews took place between November 2013 and February 2014.

Results: The participants' knowledge of preventive care was limited, and their preventive practices were mostly restricted to healthy lifestyle practices. They rarely obtained individualised preventive care advice from doctors. Screening investigations were initiated after symptoms had already occurred, and the decision of what to check was arbitrary. Few of the participants knew what they wanted from their doctors in terms of preventive care.

Conclusions: These findings show significant gaps between evidence-based preventive recommendations and patients' current knowledge and practice, and show the need for a wider spectrum of preventive care education and reliable sources to provide individualised and affordable preventive assessment and screening services. Most importantly, primary care providers must take a more proactive role to provide preventive services.

Keywords: Primary health care, Prevention, Patients' perspective

Background

Preventive care is an important component of family medicine. Family doctors are in a unique position to assess, educate and counsel individuals to improve their general health status, facilitate screening and prevent the onset of disease [1]. However, overseas studies have persistently reported gaps between evidence-based recommendations and general practitioners' practices in providing preventive care [2, 3]. The 2004 Commonwealth Fund International Health Policy Survey examined the experiences of thousands of adults in Australia, Canada, New Zealand, the United Kingdom and the United States and found an overall lack of emphasis on prevention in primary care practice [3].

Similar shortcomings were noted in a study conducted in government general outpatient clinics in Hong Kong [4]. Overall, few health promotion activities were offered, and significantly more lifestyle counselling was geared for patients with chronic diseases in whom the undesirable damage from risky behaviour had already occurred. Similar deficiencies were noted in the private health care

* Correspondence: denise_tam@yahoo.com
[1]Department of Family Medicine and Primary Healthcare, Hong Kong West Cluster, Hospital Authority, North Wing, Room 601, 6/F, Tsan Yuk Hospital, 30 Hospital Road, Hong Kong, Hong Kong

sector. A local audit of the practice of anticipatory care in a private outpatient clinic showed that even after interventions, most preventive categories, including immunisation, cancer screening and elderly functional assessment, failed to meet the target standards [5].

Hong Kong has no structured population-based health screening program. Some patients schedule check-ups via commercially available packages that offer screening investigations. Why do patients choose such services? Is it for preventive purposes? How do they choose where to go and for what to screen? Assessment of patients' attitudes and current behaviour in terms of screening is important to understand their preventive care needs.

Various studies have explored factors that affect the delivery of preventive care. Many were conducted from the perspectives and experiences of the practitioners [6–10]. In contrast, studies that directly evaluate patients' perspectives are comparatively limited [11–15].

In 2012, the Primary Care Office released a reference framework for preventive care for adults in the primary care setting in Hong Kong [16]. This framework provided evidence-based recommendations in areas like vaccination, practice of healthy lifestyles, dental health, chronic illness screening, cancer screening, functional disability assessment, mental disorder screening, polypharmacy and adverse drug reaction screening and social support assessment. However, despite the availability of this comprehensive framework, little is known about local patients' views and beliefs regarding preventive care, their current health-seeking behaviour regarding prevention and their expectations of preventive care from their primary care doctors. In family medicine, in which a collaborative care model is emphasised, it is crucial to understand patients' knowledge, current practices and expectations to facilitate delivery of quality preventive care.

The objectives of this study were:

- To examine the participants' understanding about preventive care;
- To explore participants' current preventive practices;
- To examine participants' attitudes regarding commercial screening packages, their reasons for choosing particular services and the extent to which such screening was carried out; and
- To elucidate participants' expectations of primary care doctors in providing preventive services.

Methods

This study was approved by the Institutional Review Board of The University of Hong Kong/Hospital Authority Hong Kong West Cluster. All subjects gave informed consent to participate.

Study design

We chose a qualitative method for this study because little was known about the study topic. Also, an exploratory approach was useful for evaluation of perceptions and expectations. Through this approach, we wished to capture the participants' understanding, contexts and reasons associated with their preventive care experiences and expectations. Qualitative study can be done in the form of individual interviews or focus-group interviews. We believed that one-on-one interviews were a better option for our study because they would likely touch upon sensitive issues such as personal medical history and financial status.

Sample and data collection

The study sample was drawn from two government general outpatient clinics in Hong Kong. Patients without chronic diseases were included because we were especially interested in primary prevention and secondary prevention in terms of screening. The following inclusion and exclusion criteria were applied. Patients were recruited if they were older than 18 years of age and were willing to participate in the study. Patients were excluded if they had any chronic illness or a hearing problem; were unable to communicate in Cantonese; were mentally incapacitated, rendering participation in the study inappropriate (e.g., mental retardation or dementia); or refused to participate in the study.

As a qualitative study, the sample size was not predetermined. Participants were purposively sampled to ensure, as far as possible, an even representation of the various sex and age categories (18 to 29 years, 30 to 39 years, 40 to 49 years, 50 to 59 years and 60 years and above).

We gave potential participants an information sheet that explained the aims of the study. All participants were asked to sign a written consent form before enrolment. A $50 (Hong Kong dollars) supermarket coupon was issued to each participant as an incentive to take part in the study.

We interviewed all participants individually in a quiet room to ensure confidentiality. Basic demographic data were collected, and the interviews were semi-structured and guided by pre-set questions (Table 1). The questions were developed based on the study objectives and were pilot tested on two subjects to ensure the clarity and understandability of each question. The lead investigator (DT) conducted all interviews between November 2013 and February 2014. All interviews were audiotaped and transcribed verbatim. Data collection was continued until thematic saturation was reached, as agreed by the first and second coders after review of the raw data.

Table 1 Interview guide

1. What is preventive care? Would you give some examples?
If the respondent could not answer at all, give hints: Smoking cessation and regular exercise are both examples of effective preventive measures, can you think of others?
2. Have you intentionally done something to improve your own health or to screen for disease?
If yes: what have you done?
If no: Why not?
3. Where did you get the health information concerning preventive care?
Aside from the mentioned sources, where else would do you prefer to obtain such information?
4. Have you ever had physical check-up?
If yes: Under what circumstance was it done? How did you choose where to go for the check-up? How did you choose what to do for the check-up? What did the check-up include? Was a doctor available to explain the result? If no: Why not? If you were to have physical check-up, how would you choose what to do? Where to go?
5. How do you think of commercially available check-up packages?
6. Do you have a doctor that you regularly attend? Have you ever discussed with this doctor anything in terms of preventive care? If yes, what have you discussed before? If no, why not?
7. If given the opportunity, what would you want to discuss with your doctor in terms of preventive care?

Table 2 Participant Characteristics

Marital status	Household income	Education	Health insurance	Has a family doctor?
Single	4	Tertiary	No	No
Married	6	Secondary	Yes	Yes
Married	4	Secondary	Yes	No
Married	5	Secondary	Yes	Yes
Widowed	6	Secondary	No	No
Married	6	Secondary	Yes	No
Single	2	Secondary	No	No
Single	4	Tertiary	No	No
Married	2	Secondary	Yes	No
Married	2	Primary	Previously	Yes
Single	3	Tertiary	Yes	Don't know
Married	2	Secondary	Previously	No
Single	2	Tertiary	No	No
Single	3	Tertiary	Yes	Yes
Single	5	Tertiary	Yes	No
Single	3	Secondary	Yes	No
Married	5	Tertiary	Yes	No
Widowed	1	Primary	Yes	No
Single	5	Tertiary	Yes	Yes
Single	2	Tertiary	No	No
Married	1	Secondary	Yes	Yes
Married	5	Tertiary	Yes	No
Single	3	Tertiary	Yes	No
Married	4	Secondary	Yes	Yes
Divorced	3	Secondary	No	Yes
Single	2	Tertiary	Yes	No
Married	1	Secondary	Yes	No
Married	5	Tertiary	No	No

Key: Monthly income (Hong Kong Dollars): 6: Refused to answer; 5: ≥$40,000; 4: $30,000- < $40,000; 3: $20,000- < $30,000; 2: $10,000- < $20,000; 1: <$10,000

Analysis

The data were analysed by a content analysis approach in a stepwise manner. The qualitative research program N Vivo 10 was used to enhance the accuracy of the coding process. The lead investigator (DT) carried out the coding. First, the audiotapes were reviewed, and the transcripts were read. The content of each transcript was then coded from key words and phrases. Similar codes were grouped into categories. New categories were added and adjusted as appropriate for an ongoing, non-linear analysis, and themes were generated. To avoid bias in the coding process, the second investigator (YL) independently coded a sample of the transcripts. The two coders discussed and compared their findings at different stages to ensure consensus in coding and theme identification. There were no disagreements in coding for which a consensus could not be reached. Representative quotations were selected to exemplify the findings.

Results

Participant characteristics

We interviewed 28 participants, whose characteristics are shown in Table 2. We purposefully selected participants to provide equal representations of various age groups and sexes. Most participants had secondary or higher education. We included participants with and without medical insurance coverage and with and without a family doctor.

Understanding of preventive care

Only a quarter of the participants could accurately define preventive care as taking actions to maintain health before the onset of disease. Four participants believed that to take action shortly after symptoms occurred also counted as preventive measures. The remaining participants could not tell specifically the purpose of preventive care. When probed they were only able to give examples of practices that they believed would keep one healthy. One participant mentioned that preventive care was needed when one was old but did not elaborate on the reasons that elderly people need preventive practices. Diet control (20 participants), exercise (15 participants) and hygienic measures (11 participants) were the most commonly mentioned preventive methods. Other methods included screening tests (7 participants), maintaining good mental health (6 participants), getting sufficient rest (6 participants), taking supplements or health products (5 participants), avoiding smoking or drinking (4 participants) and keeping warm (4 participants). Some participants mentioned specific evidence-based methods such as receiving vaccinations (3 participants) and checking cervical smears (2 participants).

The participants' preventive health concepts were mixed with ideas from traditional Chinese medicine and alternative medicine. For example, whilst participants understood that getting enough rest might enhance their health, one participant chose to sleep before a certain time in the evening to allow the body to remove 'toxins' effectively, according to Chinese Medicine theory:

> *'To sleep early can enhance your body's efficiency in removing toxins. For example, our liver starts to remove toxins after 11 o'clock at night.'* (Subject 11)

The emphasis on the intake of Chinese herbal soups and proprietary Chinese medicine are also examples of cultural influence on health beliefs:

> *'For preventive care, our family makes herbal soup once in a while.'* (Subject 17)

> *'I think prevention is when we use proprietary Chinese medicine to protect our liver and kidneys... I am referring to those over-the-counter medications that we can buy at Mannings or Watsons (local pharmacy chains). I think this is what preventive care is about.'* (Subject 20)

The participants' concepts of what it means to eat well might also be influenced by alternative medicine. For example, one participant mentioned that one should choose less 'acidic' fluid for drinking:

> *'Our family knows that mineral water is better than distilled water. This is because mineral water is less acidic. I think women should limit their intake of acidic fluid.'* (Subject 14)

Sources of preventive information

The participants' knowledge of preventive care comes from a variety of sources. More than half of the participants obtained preventive information from the television or the Internet. Television sources included television programs, news and government-funded advertisements. Internet sources included websites or Internet forums. Only two participants specified the use of government health-related websites. Other information channels included health pamphlets distributed from hospitals and clinics and health talks held at elderly centres, community centres, schools and libraries. In addition, about one third of the participants relied upon their friends and/or family as sources of preventive information. One patient expressed that he would depend on his own instincts. Only one participant referred to a health care professional for preventive advice.

Almost all participants believed that the availability of preventive care information was adequate. However, some of them recognised a lack of individualised advice:

> *'Everyone's condition is different. Some preventive measures may apply to certain individuals only, but not to me...'* (Subject 15)

At the same time, some participants were uncertain about the accuracy of the available information:

> *'The information delivered through television or newspaper is nothing new, but sometimes I wonder if all the information delivered is true.'* (Subject 17)

Current behaviour and attitudes regarding screening

Most participants had negative feelings towards commercial screening packages and took a rather passive role in initiating such check-ups. They generally lacked confidence in these packages, regarding them as overpriced, profit-driven, excessive and unreliable. One patient also expressed the concern that screening in itself might produce false reassurances and thus perpetuate one's unhealthy lifestyle.

Amongst our participants, primary care doctors had little role in initiating screening tests; only one participant completed a check-up as suggested by his doctor. Whilst some participants had initiated screening tests with the primary aim of understanding their own body condition and to prevent the onset of illnesses, about the same number of participants sought check-ups because symptoms already existed or because of past illnesses. When participants were feeling well, they generally did not see the need for screening. This perception was universal across both genders and different age groups.

> *'I know I may go for [a physical examination], but I do not have much concern because there is no sign to show that anything is going wrong in my body; therefore, I did not go.'* (Subject 5)

> *'The first time I went was because I had discomfort.'* (Subject 10)

> *'I did not perceive the urgency. When I feel well, I would not do anything.'* (Subject 19)

When they went for screening, the participants had a vague idea of what should be checked. In general, they believed that older people warranted more thorough check-ups and that older people should be screened for chronic illnesses like hypertension, diabetes and heart diseases. Apart from that, the participants' beliefs about testing needs were quite arbitrary and were often related to their self-perceived health risks, which might or might not be based on medical grounds.

> *'I would like to see if there is a chance of getting cancer or to check for HIV or hepatitis B. (Why do you want to check for such things?) Because those are more significant diseases.'* (Subject 7)

> *'(What would you screen for when you go for a health check?) I think there is a greater urgency to examine the colon because it is an urban disease...more young people and increasing numbers of people are getting colon diseases, I think this is why examining the colon is a more popular option. Other [physical examinations] may examine the bones and the eyes, so far I don't think I have needs in these areas...other check-ups may examine the lungs, I think I am ok in this area...mainly, I would like to screen the parts that I worry about the most.'* (Subject 2)

Cost was another significant influence on behaviour related to preventive care. Regardless of their level of perceived health risks, participants might be reluctant to participate in screening because of the cost. The participants sometimes chose a particular health check package simply because it was the cheapest.

The participants had a superficial idea of what constitutes a quality screening service. Most looked for 'reputable places' or 'big centres' to ensure the quality of their health check; for 'reputable places', participants generally referred to places that were recommended by friends or relatives.

> *'(How do you choose where to go?) Ask my friends, because I have no clue, see where they think is good for check-up then I would choose that place.'* (Subject 10)

> *'Bigger centres are more reliable, more credible... because as a company they need to run their business; they would not want to ruin their own brand name.'* (Subject 16)

> *'...Depends on where others have visited, which place offered more comprehensive and detailed examination...and which place had better feedback...'* (Subject 19)

Expectations on primary care doctors in terms of preventive advice

Experience

Few participants stated that their doctors had given them preventive advice.

Perceived barriers

When asked why they had not asked their doctors for preventive care advice, most participants expressed that their doctors were too busy. This perception was shared amongst participants of various sex and age groups.

> *'I felt that he was very busy, I would not talk about these things (preventive information) for no reason and then demand that my doctor reply to me.'* (Subject 3)

> *'There is no reason to talk about such things (preventive advice)...It would hinder the next patient from seeing the doctor. We should have empathy; the doctor was busy, and there was no reason for us to talk about these and that...this is meaningless.'* (Subject 6)

> *'There were only few minutes in the consultation, nothing more could be said.'* (Subject 9)

> *'My doctor had many patients lining up to see him, I had to wait 1 to 2 hours every time, I did not want to hinder his work.'* (Subject 14)

It was obvious that anticipatory care was considered 'inappropriate' in a busy clinic. Most participants perceived the presenting illness as the main agenda of the consultation. If they did not have symptoms, the patients would not consult a doctor solely for anticipatory advice.

> *'Everybody is like this...you consult a doctor when you are sick, you would not go to a doctor for prevention.'* (Subject 10)

> *'Seeing a doctor is mainly for treating your disease.'* (Subject 11)

A lack of initiation by the doctor was another barrier. Some participants expected their doctor to be the one who initiated preventive care in a consultation.

> *'It was over 20 years...I felt that if I have been with this doctor for so long and he knew my record, he should have told me if there was anything I needed to know or do about disease prevention...but he never said anything.'* (Subject 14)

A lack of patient awareness of the importance of preventive care was another barrier.

'...I was not aware that I should ask about prevention.' (Subject 8)

'I don't know how to ask people about these things, I felt I was being passive...I hope someone could tell me and then I would learn about it; otherwise, I would remain ignorant about it (preventive care).' (Subject 12)

Expectations

When asked about what they would like to ask their primary care doctors concerning anticipatory care, more than one third of participants stated that they would like to obtain advice on current symptoms or past illnesses. One third of participants did not know what to ask or had nothing to ask. Less than one third of participants could raise specific questions related to prevention. Specifically, these participants were interested in learning about their current health status, determining whether they need a physical examination or where they should go to get one, and acquiring age-specific health advice and other dietary advice.

Discussion

We found that the participants' knowledge of preventive care was limited and that their preventive practices largely focused on healthy lifestyle practices. They rarely obtained first-hand or individualised preventive care advice from doctors, and they lacked the means to evaluate the heath information they received from other sources. Screening tests were initiated after symptoms had already occurred, and the decision of what to check was arbitrary. When given the opportunity, less than one third of the participants knew what they wanted to ask their doctors in terms of prevention. Perceived barriers to seeking preventive advice from doctors include an excessive focus on presenting illnesses, a lack of doctor initiative, a lack of awareness of the importance of prevention and time pressure.

Our participants' preventive knowledge and behaviour focused largely on lifestyle practices, which is in line with the results of a local study that explored patients' attitudes about health and self-care [17]. This local study found that patients' self-care referred mostly to diet and exercise and included massage, Tai chi, herbal remedies, dietary supplements and vitamins and traditional 'food therapies' such as certain types of soups. Our participants also mentioned the use of Chinese herbal therapies, supplements and 'keeping warm' as preventive methods; such practices are in line with the context of our local Chinese culture. The lack of awareness and low uptake of evidence-based recommendations for adult vaccination and cancer screening were in line with the findings from the 2012 local census, which found that only 5.7% of Hong Kong adults had received a flu vaccination within the past year and that only 6.8% of women had undergone a cervical smear within the past 3 years [18]. Certain preventive care domains such as functional disability assessment were barely mentioned by the participants. Such findings reveal significant discrepancies between the health recommendations and actual practices. One explanation might be insufficient health literacy. There is consistent evidence that people's level of health literacy is associated with their health behaviour [19]. A local study explored the relationship between health literacy and health behaviour in Chinese parents with preschool children regarding the prevention of seasonal influenza. It found that Hong Kong parents had inadequate knowledge and that their reported preventive behaviour did not concur with their actual health practices [20]. A study on the development of a Health Empowerment Programme to improve the health of working poor families in Hong Kong is currently underway, and health literacy is one of its intervention components [21]. This study may shed light on strategies that may improve one's health practices and enhance disease prevention.

A Hong Kong survey of the public's perception of primary health care and their expectations of related services reported that 75.5% of subjects either agreed or strongly agreed that primary care doctors should provide preventive care [22]. However, for various reasons, very few participants in our study received or sought anticipatory care from primary care doctors. First, compared to medical staff, patients tend to assign higher priority to acute or minor conditions than to preventive check-ups for chronic conditions [23]. This lack of patient concern might lead to doctors' lack of initiative to provide anticipatory care. Existing studies of doctors' points of view have also reported patient resistance as one of the most common barriers to the provision of health-promoting activities [6–8, 10].

Second, some patients did not actively seek anticipatory care during consultation because they did not know what to ask. Our findings show that, when given the opportunity, few participants could raise questions related to prevention. Patients may not know what preventive measures were relevant to them, which may prevent them from seeking preventive care from their family doctors [11]. This finding highlights the importance of family doctors in initiating anticipatory advice.

Third, time pressure was another barrier. Our participants generally believed that doctors were too busy to give anticipatory advice. The existing literature on doctors' perceptions also reported a lack of time as a major barrier to the delivery of preventive care [6–8, 10]. In Hong Kong, the average duration of a consultation in a government clinic is about 6 to 7 min. One study in the

United States suggested that simply providing the grade A preventive care recommendations of the US Task Force would require a primary care doctor 2 h per day in a typical practice of 2500 patients [24]. Previous studies had indicated that a shorter consultation time was associated with fewer preventive activities [25] and that a longer consultation time was associated with increased performance of preventive activities [26].

Fourth, we found that participants had a low level of perceived health risk in the absence of symptoms. They considered health as the absence of symptoms and commonly believed that healthy people did not need to consult a doctor [17]. The classic Health Belief Model proposed that although a person may perceive himself or herself as being susceptible to illness, action to reduce that risk will not be taken unless a cue to action is present [27]. Our findings suggest that asymptomatic patients generally do not perceive the need for prevention. Therefore, they could not be expected to take the lead in terms of preventive care.

Finally, we were worried to see that even if the subjects participated in health screening, they tended not to seek professional advice beforehand. It would be problematic if patients were left to their own discretions in terms of health screening, because their choices are often arbitrary and may not fit their specific medical needs. Also, a study on preventive services offered by private hospitals in Hong Kong showed that not all evidence-based preventive activities were being offered and that many unproven or even possibly harmful services were provided [28]. In our study, only one participant was concerned about false reassurance as a result of negative screening results; none of the others raise any issues about the possibility of harm from inappropriate screening. This finding again could be related to the participants' insufficient level of health literacy.

This study is first of its kind to explore the views and behaviour of local patients regarding preventive care. The qualitative approach of this in-depth interview is appropriate, and the results derived are informative. We believe that many of the findings regarding the participants' beliefs and attitudes might not be easily elicited with quantitative research methods.

Our study is not without limitations. The two government general outpatient clinics used for patient recruitment were not randomly selected, and both are located on Hong Kong Island, which is generally more affluent than other parts of Hong Kong. However, our sampling frame did include patients of both genders and various ages and socio-economic statuses. Patients who do not speak Cantonese were also under-represented. These patients comprise a small proportion of the Hong Kong population and may not have the same access to health care services as their Chinese-speaking counterparts. Because our participants were recruited from public general outpatient clinics, their views and attitudes may differ from those who only attend private doctors for their health problems. Nevertheless, the aim of this study, as with all other qualitative studies, was not to bring about findings to represent the general population, but to determine themes related to preventive care issues.

Our study has highlighted deficiencies that must be addressed to facilitate better delivery of preventive care amongst patients who attend public general outpatient clinics.

There is a need for a wider spectrum of preventive care education that is not limited to the promotion of a healthy lifestyle and that also includes evidence-based cancer screening, cardiovascular disease screening, functional assessment and other aspects as outlined in the Primary Care Office preventive care framework. At the time this manuscript was written, the Hong Kong government had launched an age-based colorectal cancer screening program. The effect of this program on patients' preventive care awareness and practices is yet to be determined. There is also a need for reliable sources – governmental, non-governmental or private – to provide affordable and individualised assessment, preventive advice and screening services so that asymptomatic patients may become better aware of their potential health risks and take appropriate action. The relationship between preventive care and the level of health literacy in Hong Kong also requires further exploration. Primary care doctors should be more proactive in initiating anticipatory care, and their role in providing primary preventive care should be further promoted in the community. In view of limited consultation times, some possible solutions include the use of computer-generated prevention summaries and reminders [29] and the recruitment of practice nurses to provide preventive care assessment.

Conclusions

Preventive care is an important component of family medicine. This study identified gaps between local evidence-based preventive recommendations and the participants' current knowledge and practices. Our findings indicate a need for a wider spectrum of preventive care education and reliable sources to provide individualised and affordable preventive assessment, counselling and screening services. Most importantly, primary care doctors must take a more proactive role in advocating for and providing preventive care services.

Acknowledgements

Ms. Lisa Luk provided professional assistance in transcribing the audio recordings of the interviews.

Funding
This study was funded by the Hong Kong College of Family Physicians Trainee Research Fund. The funding body did not participate in the design of the study, the collection, analysis and interpretation of data, or in writing the manuscript.

Authors' contributions
DT conducted the interviews. DT and YL analysed the data. DT, YL and WT interpreted the data and contributed to writing the manuscript. All authors read and approved the final manuscript.

Competing interests
The authors declare that they have no competing interests.

Author details
[1]Department of Family Medicine and Primary Healthcare, Hong Kong West Cluster, Hospital Authority, North Wing, Room 601, 6/F, Tsan Yuk Hospital, 30 Hospital Road, Hong Kong, Hong Kong. [2]Wellness Family Medical Practice, Room 605, Hang Seng Tsim Sha Tsui Building, 18 Carnarvon Road, Hong Kong, Hong Kong.

References

1. The Royal Australian College of General Practitioners "Green book" Project Advisory Committee. Putting prevention into practice: guidelines for the implementation of prevention in the general practice setting. South Melbourne: The RACGP, 2006.
2. Hensrud D. Clinical preventive medicine in primary care: background and practice: 1. Rationale and current preventive practices. Mayo Clin Proc. 2000; 75:165–72.
3. Schoen C, Osborn R, Huynh PT, et al. Primary care and health system performance: adults' experiences in five countries. Health Aff [Internet]. 2004. Available from: http://www.commonwealthfund.org/usr_doc/W4-487Schoen.pdf. [cited 2018 April 30].
4. Pei GK, Chem B, Hedley AJ, et al. Preventive health measures and counseling in government outpatient clinics. Hong Kong Practitioner. 1991; 13:1838–53.
5. Chiu B. Audit on the practice of anticipatory care. Hong Kong Practitioner. 2008;30:177–84.
6. Cornuz J, Ghali WA, Di Carlantonio D, et al. Physicians' attitudes towards prevention: importance of intervention-specific barriers and physicians' health habits. Fam Pract. 2000;17(6):535–40.
7. Lambe B, Collins C. A qualitative study of lifestyle counseling in general practice in Ireland. Fam Pract. 2010;27:219–23.
8. Walter U, Flick U, Neuber A, et al. Putting prevention into practice: qualitative study of factors that inhibit and promote preventive care by general practitioners, with a focus on elderly patients. BMC Fam Pract. 2010;11:68.
9. Drewes YM, Koenen JM, de Ruijter W, et al. GPs' perspectives on preventive care for older people: a focus group study. Br J Gen Pract. 2012;62(604): e765–72.
10. Geense W, van de Glind I, Visscher T, et al. Barrier, facilitators and attitudes influencing health promotion activities in general practice: an explorative pilot study. BMC Fam Pract. 2013;14:20.
11. Mazza D, Shand LK, Warren N, et al. General practice and preventive health care: a view through the eyes of community members. Med J Aust. 2011; 195(4):180–3.
12. Brotons C, Bulc M, Sammut MR, et al. Attitudes towards preventive services and lifestyle: the view of primary care patients in Europe. The EUROPREVIEW patient study. Fam Pract. 2012;29:i168–76.
13. Lu S, Harris MF. Prevention of diabetes and heart disease. Patient perceptions on risk, risk assessment and the role of their GP in preventive care. Aust Fam Physician. 2013;42(5):328–31.
14. Tan D, Zwar NA, Dennis SM, et al. Weight management in general practice: what do patients want? Med J Aust. 2006;185(2):73–5.
15. Codori A, Peterson G, Miglioretti D, et al. Health beliefs and endoscopic screening for colorectal cancer: potential for cancer prevention. Prev Med. 2001;33:128–36.
16. Primary Care Office: Hong Kong reference framework for preventive care for older adults in primary care settings [Internet]. Hong Kong: Primary Care Office; 2012. Available from: https://www.pco.gov.hk/english/resource/files/ref_framework_adults.pdf. [Cited 2013 28 July].
17. Mercer SW, Griffiths SM, Lam CLK, et al. Incentives and barriers to adopting the family doctor model in Hong Kong: an in-depth qualitative study of the views, knowledge, and attitudes of patients. Hong Kong Med J. 2011;17:25–7.
18. Centre for Health Protection of the Department of Health: Statistics on behavioural risk factors. [Internet]. Hong Kong: The Behavioural Risk Factor Surveillance System (BRFSS), The Surveillance and Epidemiology Branch. Available from: http://www.chp.gov.hk/en/behavioural/10/280.html. [Cited 2013 July 28].
19. von Wagner C, Knight K, Steptoe A et al. Functional health literacy and health-promoting behaviour in an national sample of British adults. J Epidem Comm Health. 2007;61(12):1086–90.
20. Lam W, Dawson A, Fowler C. The health literacy of Hong Kong Chinese parents with preschool children in seasonal influenza prevention: a multiple case study at household level. PLoS ONE [Internet]. 2015;10(12):e0143844. Available from: http://journals.plos.org/plosone/article?id=10.1371/journal.pone.0143844. [cited 2017 February 6].
21. Fung CS, Yu EY, Guo VY, et al. Development of a health empowerment programme to improve the health of working poor families: protocol for a prospective cohort study in Hong Kong [Internet]. BMJ Open. 2016;6(2): e010015. Available from: http://bmjopen.bmj.com/content/6/2/e010015?utm_source=trendmd&utm_medium=cpc&utm_campaign=bmjopen&trendmdtrendmdshared=1&utm_content=Journalcontent&utm_term=TrendMDPhase4.
22. Research committees, The Hong College of Family Physicians. What sort of Primary Healthcare Service does the Public want? The Hong Kong Practitioner. 2008;30:24–28.
23. Arvidsson E, Andre M, Borgquist L, et al. Setting priorities in primary health care – on whose conditions? A questionnaire study. BMC Fam Pract. 2012; 13:114.
24. Yarnall KS, Pollak KI, Ostbye T, et al. Primary care: is there enough time for prevention? Am J Public Health. 2003;93:635–41.
25. Gelly J, Le Bel J, Aubin-Auger I, et al. Profile of French general practitioners providing opportunistic primary preventive care – an observational cross-sectional multicentre study. Fam Pract. 2014;31(4):445–52.
26. Frank O, Litt J, Beilby J. Preventive activities during consultations in general practices. Aust Fam Physician. 2005;34:508–12.
27. Rosenstock I. The health belief model and preventive health behavior. Health Education & Behavior [Internet]. 1974;2:354–386. Available from: http://journals.sagepub.com/doi/pdf/10.1177/109019817400200405. [cited 2013 August 30].
28. Dickinson JA, Chee S. Preventive services advertised to the public by private hospitals in Hong Kong. Hong Kong Med J. 2000;6(4):415–22.
29. Frank OR, Stocks NP, Aylward P. Patient acceptance and perceived utility of pre-consultation preventive summaries and reminders in general practices; pilot study. BMC Fam Pract. 2011;12:40.

Analytical typology of multiprofessional primary care models

Damien Contandriopoulos[1*], Mélanie Perroux[2], Aurore Cockenpot[2], Arnaud Duhoux[2] and Emmanuelle Jean[3]

Abstract

Background: There is only limited evidence to support care redefinition and role optimization processes needed for scaling up of a stronger primary care capacity.

Methods: Data collection was based on a keyword search in MEDLINE, EMBASE and CINAHL databases. Three thousand, two hundred and twenty-nine documents were identified, 1851 met our inclusion criteria, 71 were retained for full-text assessment and 52 included in the final selection. The analysis process was done in four steps. In the end, the elements that were identified as particularly central to the process of transforming primary care provision were used as the basis of two typologies.

Results: The first typology is based on two structural dimensions that characterize promising multiprofessional primary care teams. The first is the degree to which the division of tasks in the team was formalized. The second dimension is the centrality and autonomy of nurses in the care model. The second typology offers a refined definition of comprehensiveness of care and its relationship with the optimization of professional roles.

Conclusions: The literature we analyzed suggests there are several plausible avenues for coherently articulating the relationships between patients, professionals, and care pathways. The expertise, preferences, and numbers of available human resources will determine the plausibility that a model will be a coherent response that is appropriate to the needs and environmental constraints (funding models, insurance, etc.). The typologies developed can help assess existing care models analytically or evaluatively and to propose, prospectively, some optimal operational parameters for primary care provision.

Keywords: Primary health care, Comprehensive health care, Nursing care, Health services research

Background

Demographic changes, technological developments, and fiscal constraints are jeopardising the sustainability of health systems. Technical innovations and rapid growth in the intensity of care being provided are exerting significant pressure on available resources [1, 2]. Likewise, data on demographic changes and healthcare expenditures suggest that continued reliance on current healthcare provision models to address population health needs is likely to put enormous pressure on public finances [3]. Evidence suggests that public health systems need to change significantly to preserve their capacity to maintain universal access to healthcare [4, 5]. Capacity strengthening in primary care provision is widely considered to be an approach with the potential to simultaneously reinforce health system sustainability and accessibility, continuity of care, and ultimately population health [2, 5–10].

In this study, primary care is defined according to the terminology of the Institute of Medicine, as *"the provision of integrated, accessible healthcare services by clinicians who are accountable for addressing a large majority of personal healthcare needs, developing a sustained partnership with patients, and practicing in the context of family and community"* [6]. It is interesting to note that this definition does not focus on the types of clinicians who are providing care. Rather, it emphasizes the nature of the response being provided to meet the needs.

To address the above-cited challenges, there is growing evidence not only that health systems need to evolve

* Correspondence: damien1@uvic.ca
[1]School of Nursing, University of Victoria, PO Box 1700, STN CSC, Victoria, British-Columbia V8W 2Y2, Canada

to reinforce the provision of primary care, but that, in fact, the nature of that care itself will need to change [11–16]. In particular, professional teams need to move toward more collaboration and a broadening of fields of practice [17–19]. Numerous convergent data suggest that one possible progression would be to expand the interdisciplinary composition of primary care teams, the scope of practice of non-physician team members, and their intersectoral action [20–26]. In particular, greater use of an extended scope of nursing practice is likely to enhance both accessibility of care and efficiency of service delivery [12, 27–32]. Likewise, the care on offer should evolve to encompass a wider basket of services, less intensive and more appropriate interventions as well as more interventions targeting the determinants of health [1, 2, 4, 5, 16, 33–40]. Such a shift toward increased prevention and interventions that are more intersectoral has a better chance of curbing the growing burden of chronic disease management [22, 41].

However, there is little data available on the operational characteristics of care provision models that would be most promising to move in that direction. Generally speaking, the available literature indicates there are several plausible avenues to improve service provision performance, and that their relative merits are contingent on several clinical, organizational, and systemic factors. Against this backdrop, we conducted a realist review of the literature, grounded in a logic analysis approach, with the aim of producing conceptual tools to support the transformation of primary care models. Inductive analysis of the selected publications led to the development of two typologies. These typologies allow us to assess existing care models analytically or evaluatively and to propose, prospectively, some optimal operational parameters for primary care provision.

Methods

Logic analysis and realist review

To better understand the characteristics of high-performing multiprofessional primary care teams, we adopted a methodology based on two complementary approaches: Pawson and colleagues' work on the realist review approach [42–45], and the work of Brousselle and colleagues on logic analysis, and more specifically, on reverse logic analysis [46].

The logic analysis approach was developed in the context of evaluating complex interventions. The underlying principle is to interpret the available scientific data with a view to understanding the causal processes that explain the outcomes of the intervention under study. Reverse logic analysis, on the other hand, is a prospective approach in which scientific data are used to identify the conditions and operational mechanisms of an intervention that would make it possible to achieve predetermined objectives.

The principle underlying realist review is conceptually very similar. It is based on the idea that systematic literature review methods developed for studying the effectiveness of clinical interventions are not appropriate for analyzing complex interventions [43]. In the latter case, a "generative" approach [45] is needed that incorporates existing knowledge, either to propose new plausible interventions or to adjust existing interventions. This type of knowledge synthesis generates theoretical propositions regarding the intervention's functioning.

The method used here, inspired by these two sources, draws from reverse logic analysis the notion of a relatively systematic synthesis of available knowledge and then incorporating this knowledge into efforts aimed at pre-determined objectives. From a realist review, we derive the notion of an approach that is more generative than summative, in which the data are interpreted inductively to propose recommendations for practice.

This work is part of a larger research project and will serve as a conceptual framework for analyzing practice in the pilot sites studied in this project [47].

Analytical model

The objective of the present study was to better understand the structural characteristics and operational processes of high-performing multiprofessional primary care teams. We used primarily Donabedian's conceptual framework [48] to categorize the information gleaned from the articles analyzed and to identify the causal links among: 1) the structures of primary care provision models, 2) the processes of care provision and management, and 3) the outcomes produced.

Definition of performance

To normatively assess the desirability of care provision models, we used a definition of performance inspired by the work of Shortell and colleagues [49]. This definition conceives of performance as combining four components: 1) accessibility; 2) quality of care; 3) efficiency; and 4) collective learning capacities [47]. Accessibility is defined, based on Donabedian [48, 50], as the fit between structures of production, on the one hand, and society's needs and their geographic distribution, on the other.

The definition of quality used here is based on an adaptation of the work done by the teams of Pineault, Beaulieu, and Haggerty [51–54] on operationalizing the measurement of primary care quality. Quality of care is defined as the combination of technical quality, continuity, and comprehensiveness. Technical quality is made up of three components: the quality of the act itself, the appropriateness of care, and the quality of communication. Continuity is defined, based on the work of Haggerty et al. [53], as the fact that a patient is treated by the same professional or the same team over time (relational continuity) and that services are harmoniously integrated with each other (management continuity). We interpret harmonious integration of care as occurring on two levels. On the one hand, care and services should be organized in such a way that medical care, nursing care, social services, curative practices, and preventive practices are harmoniously linked, sustained over time, and optimal (horizontal integration), and, on the other hand, that there are linkages between the different service levels (vertical integration) [54–56]. Finally, comprehensiveness refers to a care structure's ability to respond in an integrated manner to all of a patient's needs. Comprehensiveness encompasses two dimensions that make up the scope of patient management: taking into account all of a patient's needs (whole person focus) and providing a complete basket of services (scope of services) [53].

Efficiency is defined here, based on A Brousselle, J Lachaine and AP Contandriopoulos [57], as the ratio between quality of care and resource use. This definition corresponds to technical efficiency, which is aimed at minimizing costs for any given outcome.

Finally, to implement organizational, administrative, and clinical practices that will foster the efficient production of good-quality services adapted to patients' preferences, teams and organizations must have a strong learning capacity. Learning capacity here refers to the organization's collective capacity to adapt and to assimilate new learning and new practices [49]. This requires a collective commitment to identifying and resolving problems [58, 59].

Documentary search strategy

In a first step, we conducted a keyword search on MEDLINE that was subsequently adapted to the EMBASE and CINAHL databases (see endnote[1]). To be considered eligible, articles had to have been published in either English or French in peer-reviewed journals after 1999 and be focused on an intervention carried out in an Organisation for Economic Co-operation and Development (OECD) country. That search identified 3204 references, of which 1826 met our inclusion criteria.

In addition to the results of the keyword search in clinical databases we included articles known to the researchers and results from online search engines. Some documents cited in the bibliographies of the articles retained were also added. This approach was inspired by the work of Greenhalgh and colleagues [60, 61]. These deliberative approaches identified an additional 25 articles.

The second step was to sort the articles based on the criterion of relevance to our objective of better understanding the structural characteristics and operational processes of high-performing multiprofessional primary care teams. This initial sorting was based on titles and abstracts. We retained only articles documenting primary care provision by multiprofessional teams in which nurses played a significant role. Articles dealing with services provided in hospital or that did not pertain to a general primary care clientele were excluded (e.g. emergency services, ambulatory care, rehabilitation). At the end of this step, 65 of the 1826 articles identified by keywords and 6 of the 25 articles from other sources were retained for full-text analysis. Three of the authors (DC, AC, and MP) subsequently read the full text of the selected articles and discussed the relevance of each article. In the end, 52 articles were retained for analysis. Figure 1 provides a flow diagram of the process [62].

Analysis process

The analysis process was done in four steps. First, the articles retained for analysis were positioned according to their main contribution(s) according to a structure–process–outcomes grid. In a second step, numerous subcategories were inductively identified based on elements discussed in the articles. For example, many articles discussed the process of redefining professional roles [63], which was identified as a sub-category of processes. Likewise, the literature we examined included several analyses of the effects of primary care provision structures on certain clinical outcomes [41, 64, 65]. The work of categorizing and inductively identifying subcategories was conducted in parallel by each of the three readers. The classification exercise primarily served as a basis for discussing the presumed or tested causal links between the categories and sub-categories identified.

In a third step, the three readers organized a group discussion on the subcategory tree structure and the presumed causal links. The starting point for discussion

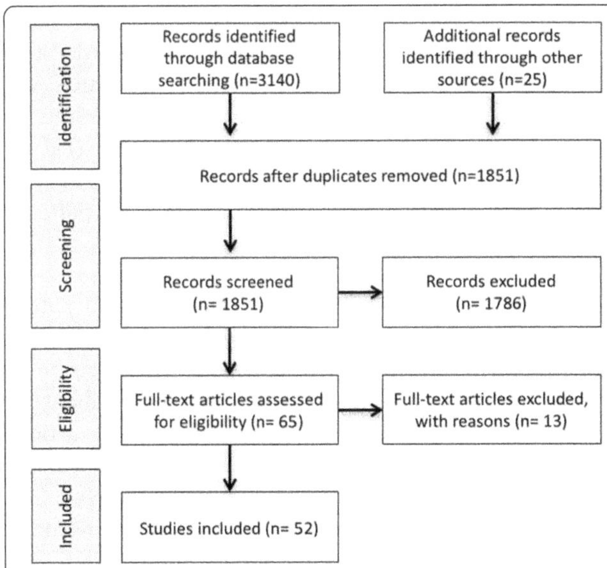

Fig. 1 PRISMA 2009 Flow Diagram

was a series of iteratively produced causal models in the form of diagrams linking the subcategories among themselves. As soon as a satisfactory causal model was stabilized, the discussion turned toward identifying the conceptual tools needed to envision how existing primary care models might be modified to become higher-performing models, as defined above.

From this step, the group discussion then focused on elements that stood out as being particularly central to the process of transforming the primary care service offer. The elements that were found to be essential were specifically the links of accountability between care teams and the patient populations under their responsibility, the continuity and comprehensiveness of service provision, the operational efficiency of the model, the care pathways involved in the teams' different methods of patient management, team composition, and especially the process of redefining professional roles and the scope of practice of non-physician professionals.

Finally, in a fourth step, the elements that were identified as particularly central to the process of transforming primary care provision were compared among themselves, which led progressively to the development of the typologies presented in the following section. As such, the typologies are not a synthesis of the causal models identified, but rather are "generative" models, in the sense of Pawson [45], that are useful for reflecting on the plausible characteristics of high-performing primary care models.

Results and discussion

Care team structure

The literature analysis identified two structural dimensions to characterize multiprofessional primary care teams. The first was the degree to which the division of tasks in the team was formalized. At one extreme were formal approaches based on explicit procedures that specified which service would be provided by which professional, to which patient, and at what point in time. At the other extreme were organic approaches based on mutually adjustable mechanisms, where professionals adapted to structural circumstances and to patients' characteristics in deciding on care processes.

The second dimension was the centrality and autonomy of nurses—regardless of their exact title or level of training—in the care model. Some models were based primarily on nurses as the front-line professionals, while others were based mainly on physicians. In the articles analyzed, we did not find any primary care models based on professionals other than physicians or nurses. The two structuring dimensions can be used to construct a matrix divided into quadrants and to devise four ideal types of primary care models (see Fig. 2).

Formalized model with medical hub

The formalized model with a medical hub is probably the dominant model in OECD countries [66]. In this model, a group of physicians jointly manages a panel of patients. Here the core professional is a physician, who establishes the care plan in the initial consultation and determines the diagnosis and treatment plan. Subsequently, depending on the patient's needs, the physician may refer the patient for further follow-up in what we here call "modules" of non-medical treatment (e.g. psychological, metabolic disease, or nutritional problems). These modules, centred around a specialized or disciplinary practice, include technical acts and patient education, and offer relatively autonomous follow-up by non-physician professionals of certain common problems or problems specific to chronic diseases. When the professionals in charge of service provision in these modules are nurses, they generally work in areas of specialization (e.g. diabetes, asthma, mental health, pregnancy care). For example, once a physician has diagnosed and created a treatment plan for a diabetic patient, that patient can be regularly followed by a nurse specialized in that disease. Often, that nurse will be autonomously responsible for adjusting the patient's medication and assessing the progress of the disease. In most cases, there are a certain number of patient management protocols stipulating the point at which the patient should be seen again by the physician, such as an annual physical exam or every second visit. When the patient's health status changes, he or she is referred back to the physician.

Formalized model with nursing hub

The formalized model with nursing hub differs from the preceding model in that the core professional is a nurse, generally a primary healthcare nurse practitioner (PHCNP). This form represents one of the possible operationalizations of a *nurse-led clinic*, such as exists in Ontario or in the United States [67–69]. We consider this model formalized because, as in the medical model described above, the PHCNP determines the diagnosis and establishes the treatment plan and, for some of their needs, refers patients to the same types of care modules described above. However, the particular feature of this model is that one of the PHCNP's options is to refer the patient to a physician. For instance, the PHCNP looks after patients' needs that fall within the PHCNP's field of practice and set of skills. Patients whose needs are more complex or who require a treatment or diagnostic test that requires a physician's intervention are referred to physicians.

We will return to these points, but in both these formalized models, the main challenge is to ensure the best possible flow for patients among the different resources within the team, especially for patients with multimorbidities. This is a horizontal integration challenge.

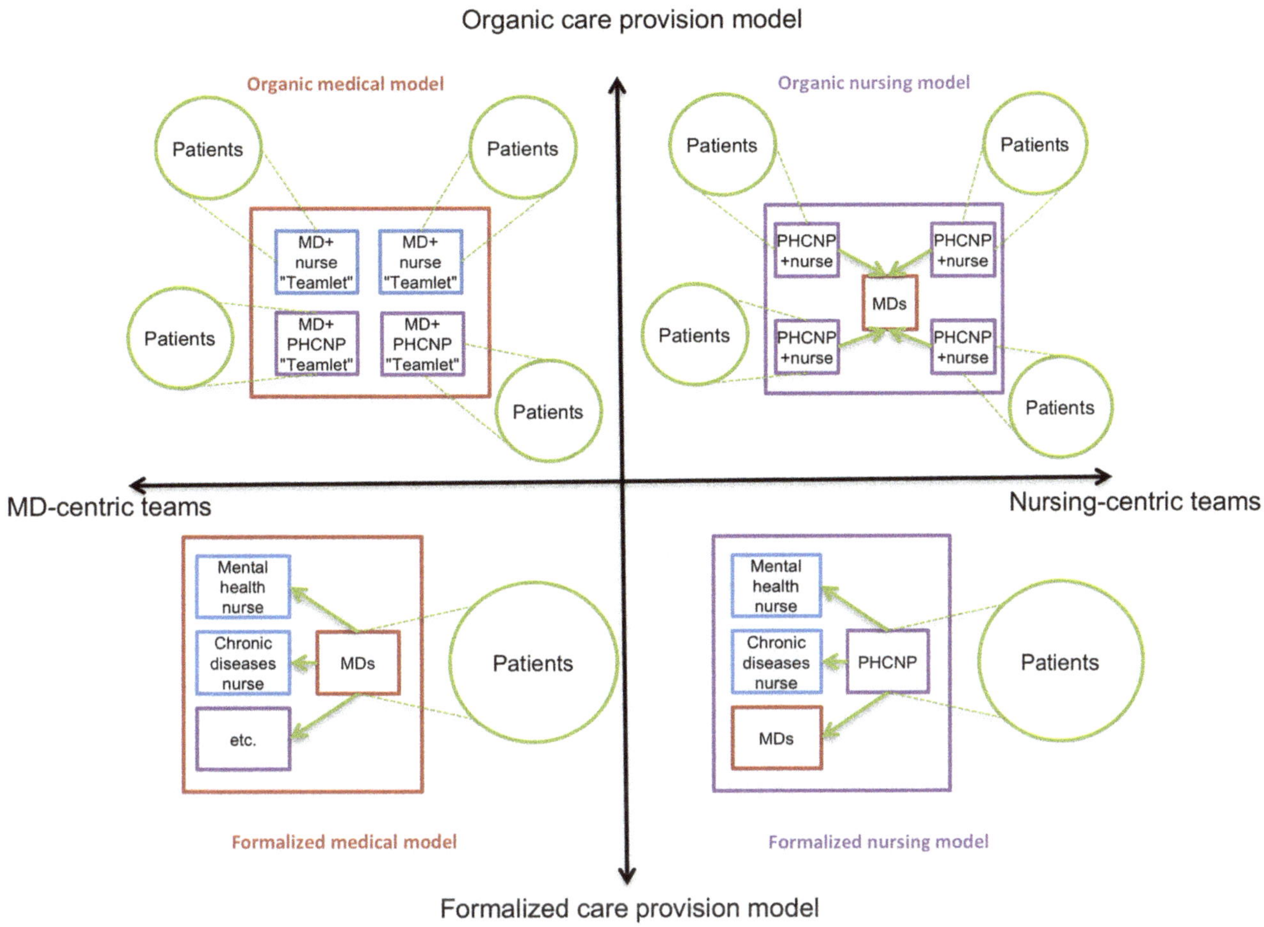

Fig. 2 Two dimensional typology of primary care models

Organic model with medical hub

In comparison with the two preceding models that both have formal procedures for referring patients within the team, organic models are based on the comprehensive management of all needs by small multidisciplinary teams. What characterizes organic models is that service provision is based on micro-teams—an approach much publicized by the Veteran's Health Administration (VHA) system in the U.S. under the name "teamlets" [70]. In a medical-hub model, for example, physician–nurse duos, or physician–NP–nurse trios, or other combinations of two to four professionals work closely together in a joint patient management model [28, 71]. This means patients being followed by a micro-team will see one, two or all of the professionals in the team at each visit, based on flexible parameters. In terms of comprehensiveness of care, each micro-team can handle a wide range of primary care needs. Patient pathways are less fragmented than in the two preceding models. Roles are less formally defined in micro-teams, and professionals decide who will see which patient for what service and at what time by mutual accommodation according to the circumstances. The patient panels for each team might be constituted randomly depending on team availability, but in a same group, there can also be micro-teams working in specific areas (e.g. perinatal care, pediatrics, geriatrics, etc.).

Organic model with nursing hub

Lastly, the organic model with a nursing hub, the most hypothetical of the four models, is also based on micro-teams; here, however, the centre of gravity is a PHNCP working jointly with other professionals. This is another possible form of *nurse-led clinic*. When a patient's needs require medical expertise, nursing micro-teams will call on one or more physicians, who either belong to the clinic or who are outside the clinic and with whom there are partnership arrangements. The level of collaboration between the PHCNP and the nurses depends on which acts are legally reserved, and practice overlaps are self-regulated in each micro-team. What distinguishes this model from the formalized nursing-hub model is the integrated and joint management of a panel of patients by a micro-team of professionals whose centre of gravity is a PHCNP.

Theoretically, the main challenge of organic models is to optimize the process by which every professional in each micro-team is being used to their fullest capacity. The risks are that subsidiarity in task definition might not be pushed as far as it could go and that the range of services might be limited, especially in the organic nursing-hub model.

Care comprehensiveness and role structuring

The second conceptual tool developed from our literature review have to do with the comprehensiveness of care offered, how work and patient management are organized within the team, and the collaboration processes upon which this management is based. In practice, the scope of services actually offered in a primary care vary significantly. In many care models comprehensiveness of care is suboptimal in relation to what is suggested in the literature [54]. The "one problem per visit" model of some walk-in clinics is an extreme example of this situation, as is the practice of refusing to manage certain clienteles (more serious mental health problems, dual diagnoses involving mental health and addiction, etc.).

Referring back to the dimensions set out in the performance model presented above, we recall that comprehensiveness of care consists, on the one hand, of responding to the full set of patients' needs (*whole person focus*) and, on the other, of offering a complete basket of services (*scope of services*). Our analysis of the literature has led us to refine this definition.

First, the consideration of all needs must be conceptualized at the population level rather than at the individual level. A care team that only looks after young patients without any complex needs could easily meet all their needs but would not, in our view, be providing comprehensive care. Here we conceptualize the notion of responding to all needs in relation to the needs of the population to whom care is being provided and with no exclusion criteria being applied.

Second, we conceptualize the offer of a complete basket of services in terms of the complexity of care provided. By defining primary care as a response to "a large majority of personal healthcare needs" [6] we are in fact relying on a definition of comprehensive primary care. There are, implicitly, more specialized services that require expertise, a technical platform, or specific resources that fall within the purview of specialized or hospital medicine. In this respect, offering a complete basket of services also means ensuring that primary care teams manage the full complexity of common care delivery and do not refer their patients unnecessarily or too readily to specialized services.

Given the two dimensions of comprehensiveness we have defined, this concept can be visualized as a square in which the horizontal sides represent all population needs, while the vertical sides represent complexity of care (Fig. 3).

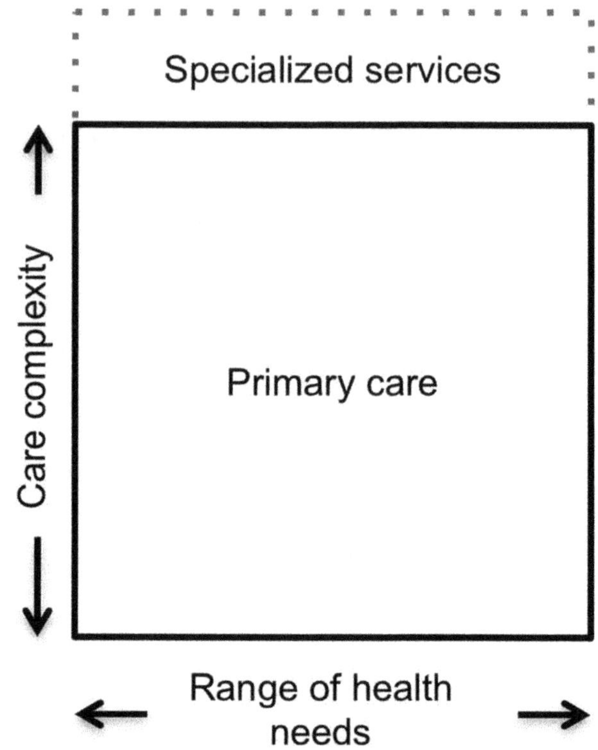

Fig. 3 Conceptualization of care comprehensiveness and professional roles

Applying the typology to primary care comprehensiveness

In our view, this comprehensiveness typology is useful on two levels. Firstly, it can be used to visually represent the actual comprehensiveness of care provided by a team as compared to a normative ideal of the optimal comprehensiveness. By comparing the services actually provided by a team against what is done in other teams or what the scientific literature identifies as best practices, it is possible to characterize certain models as offering a limited comprehensiveness. Thus, in Fig. 4 models A and B some zones in the optimal primary care square are empty, whereas ideally they should all be filled.

At a second level, this typology can be used to conceptualize the role of each professional or of each professional group in the provision of comprehensive care. We use the term role to describe the services a health professional actually performs owing to the available resources, skills, knowledge, patients needs and preferences and so forth [72]. The typology makes it possible not only to visualize the relative contributions of each professional group to the services provided, but to discern how the sharing of roles and responsibilities is structured in relation to the two dimensions of range of needs and complexity of care. As a tool for transforming practice, the aim of this typology is to maximize potential comprehensiveness by linking role definition with available professional resources.

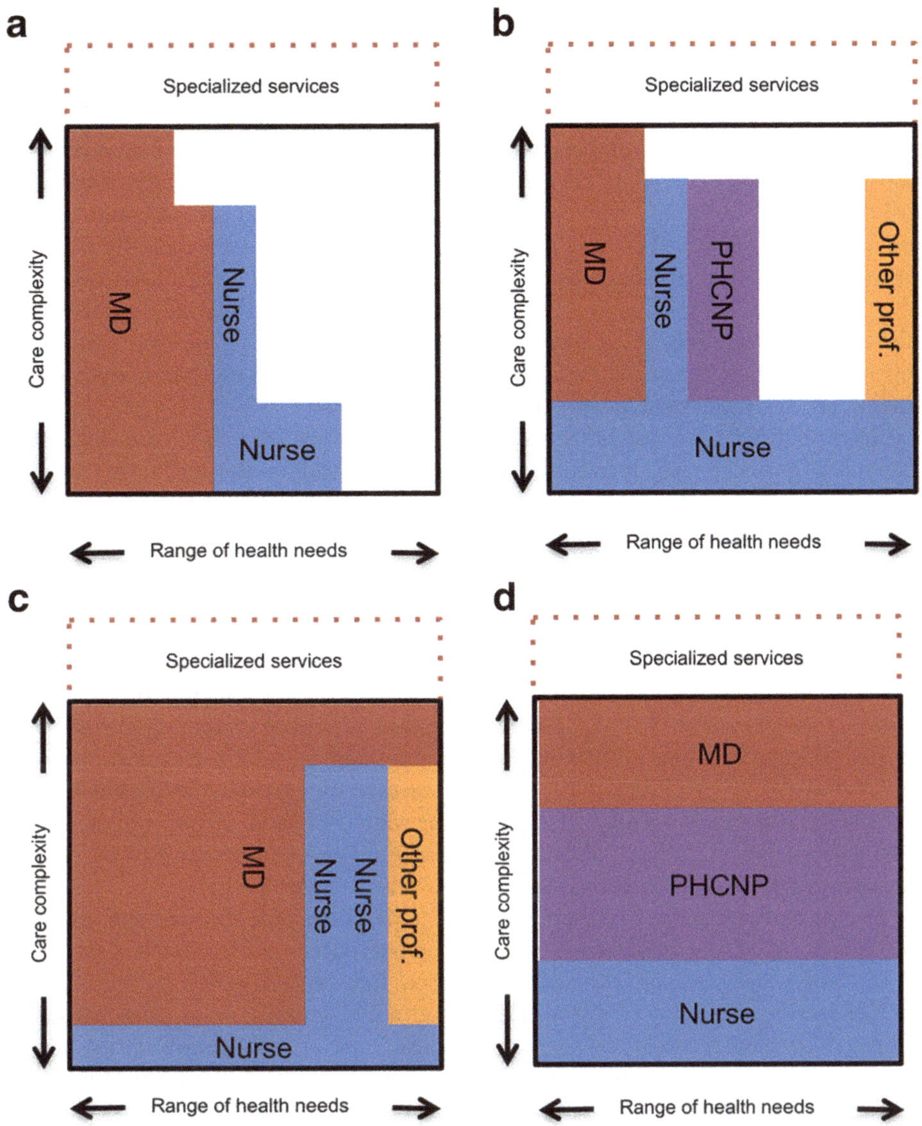

Fig. 4 Illustration of four hypothetical primary care models: **a** and **b** are examples of models with limited scope while **c** and **d** are examples of models providing a full scope of services

In Fig. 4, the two hypothetical models presented, A and B, do not cover all needs (limited scope). Model A, in the top left quadrant, for example, is a primarily medical model with limited scope and limited complexity. In such a model, it quickly becomes impossible for patients to be followed for complex problems and for health problems not handled by this team. Model B, in the upper right quadrant, is a second model, this time multiprofessional, of limited comprehensiveness. In this hypothetical team, there is a response to the full scope of needs, but for several types of care and services, that response is only for problems of low complexity. For example, a patient with a routine mental health problem such as anxiety would be seen by a nurse who, rather than setting up a regular follow-up within the team, would probably refer the patient to psychological resources in another care structure.

Conversely, the two hypothetical models C and D cover the entire scope of primary care. Model C, in the lower left quadrant, is primarily medical, while Model D, in the lower right quadrant, is primarily a nursing model. In both cases, these models incorporate the idea—based on the principle of subsidiarity—that low-complexity care is assigned to nurses. It would be possible, however, to imagine models that also incorporate this principle using other professionals for certain services. Models C and D differ, though, in how their role definitions are structured. Model C is based on tasks being shared according to what we described earlier as non-physician patient management modules. It is possible to imagine that all patients are seen initially by a nurse, who performs a first needs assessment, after which patients are followed and treated by a physician. However, still in this model, for certain visits or certain patients who come for a specific type of follow-up, the care could be provided by non-physician professionals. In our view, it is plausible to hypothesize that the models described as formalized in the structural typology presented in the preceding section would be represented by a more vertical division of roles when visualized using the present model.

In contrast, Model D is based on tasks being shared according to complexity. All patients, whatever their needs or their characteristics, are followed by a nurse for the simple aspects, and by a PHCNP for most other needs. The physician, in the role of primary care "specialist", sees only those patients with complex needs. The representation is simplified, but it is conceivable that, depending on the nature of the care and needs, the horizontal cut-offs would vary according to types of needs. We believe it is plausible to hypothesize that the models in which professionals are divided horizontally are more consistent with a structure considered organic in the typology presented in the preceding section, with less formalized boundaries and greater recourse to clinical judgment and mutual accommodation to manage overlaps.

Obviously such a representation remains very schematic and could never adequately convey all the sophistication of actual service provision by primary care teams. Nevertheless, we believe this conceptualization is interesting in that it incorporates the concept of role definition as a parameter of comprehensiveness optimization. As observed in the introduction, high-performing primary care models will move toward broader coverage of needs and a redrawing of professional boundaries. In operationalizing the decisions needed to make these transitions successfully, it is thus important that both these processes be considered together.

Expansion and extension of roles

As stated in the introduction, one of the main challenges facing most health systems today is how to enlarge the contribution of primary care in the total healthcare services offer. Based on the two dimensions of the care comprehensiveness typology, this would involve, on the one hand, increasing the range of population needs for which primary care teams would be responsible and the level of complexity of care provided in primary care. In the diagram we have proposed (see Fig. 2), this mean drawing a large square, i.e., the normative definition of what constitutes primary care.

On the other hand, it is also important to ensure that most teams develop collaboration practices and roles that enable them, in practice, to actually cover all those needs. On our proposed diagram, this would mean filling all the space in the square, i.e., aligning the operationalization of professional roles with the response to needs.

However, while our proposed care comprehensiveness typology is useful for thinking about the different performance components of primary care models in an integrated way (such as accessibility and quality) it does not take efficiency into account. For example, a primary care team relying exclusively on physicians that would cover the full range of needs and all complexity of care (a full red square) would be perfectly adequate in terms of comprehensiveness, but would probably, in most countries, be characterized by an excessively high per-patient cost.

Analysis of the literature suggests, not surprisingly, that expanding the primary care services offer while maintaining or improving efficiency calls for greater use of multiprofessional teams. In reflecting on the growth of nursing practice, Richards et al. [73] recommend differentiating between *expanding* and *extending* practice. Building on their idea, we address this issue from a broader interprofessionnal perspective.

Expanding the practice of non-physician professionals essentially means retaining current professional roles but increasing the number of non-physicians in the teams to increase the intensity of treatment or quantity of services provided. Expanding non-physician practice—in particular, nursing—can improve physician productivity or team productivity as a whole.

Extending practice, on the other hand, means that non-physician professionals develop new areas of practice that would allow them, for example, to manage certain clienteles or certain visits more autonomously, based on a substitution rationale [29]. Such practice extension can take the form of increasing the complexity of care provided by non-physician professionals (vertical extension in our diagram), or of broadening the range of needs covered (horizontal extension in our diagram). In all cases, what characterizes the notion of extension is that non-physician professionals' roles transcend established professional boundaries.

From a logical standpoint, some combination of expansion and extension of practice would likely be needed to increase the space allocated to primary care in the overall healthcare services offer while improving health system efficiency. The data we analyzed, however, offer no indication of what proportions of the two avenues constitute the optimal response. According to the data available in the literature, the choice is made idiosyncratically, primarily based on the professional and financial resources available. The real impact on efficiency of combining the expansion and extension of non-physician professionals' practice will depend, in each case, on how consistently roles are defined and operationalized in practice [74].

Conclusions

Referring back to the original objective of the present literature review, which was to understand the structural characteristics and operational processes of high-performing multiprofessional primary care teams, our analytical review of the literature leads us to four conclusions.

First, developing a coherent response to the challenges facing health systems today will require a rethinking of both the structural aspects of accountability for patient management (who is responsible for following which patients, and for what care?) and the redefinition of professional roles that this entails. As indicated by our proposed typology of structural characteristics of primary care models, there are several plausible avenues for articulating the relationships between patients, professionals, and care pathways. We found no solid evidence upon which to determine whether one or another of the quadrants of our typology is more promising in terms of performance. Our interpretation is that there is probably a contingency relationship between these structural parameters [75] and performance. In other words, for a primary care team's operational performance, what counts is that the model uses available resources coherently. In particular, the expertise, preferences, and level of available human resources will determine the plausibility that a model will be a coherent response that is appropriate to the needs and environmental constraints (funding models, insurance, etc.).

Second, even though it is heuristically interesting to differentiate among the various dimensions of primary care performance, in reflecting on their operationalization it is clear that they are strongly interrelated. For example, according to the model developed here, improving accessibility involves ensuring that primary care models cover the full range of health needs. When care models cover only a portion of needs (limited scope and/or complexity), this means in practice that certain health problems or clienteles are being under-served. There is therefore a direct logical link between this situation and problems of accessibility and care continuity. When specific populations are excluded (such as homeless persons, patients with a dual diagnosis of mental health disorder and addiction, or immigrants—three cases of populations often under-served by the dominant care models), the problem is felt at the intersection of comprehensiveness and accessibility. For specific health problems (such as HIV, hepatitis C, mental health disorders, or when rapid access is required for semi-urgent acute problems), patients often have to contend with being treated in silos, in which different teams, in different healthcare structures, each manage just one part of the problem. In this case, poor comprehensiveness presents significant challenges for care continuity. In this respect, our comprehensiveness typology can be useful for rethinking several different dimensions of primary care performance in a more integrated manner.

Third the literature we analyzed included many analyses of the challenges involved in transforming care structures and practice models [63, 76–80]. Managing change processes and redefining roles require skills and resources that are not always available on the ground. In the performance model we have used, these elements are included in the notion of learning capacity. Learning capacity is both a result of performance and, at the same time, an essential condition for achieving positive results in terms of accessibility, efficiency, and quality [49]. Learning capacity is required for teams to be able to better manage complexity [81] and adapt to the frequent changes occurring in today's health systems [82–84]. Some authors posit that learning capacity is very closely linked with success or failure in the implementation of innovations [85], and even with organizational survival. As such, our research team is continuing to work on identifying how collective learning capacity is manifested in the transformation of care provision models.

In closing, as mentioned earlier, the literature we reviewed does not allow us to form any simple or reliable judgment on the structural characteristics or operational processes of primary care teams. Our anticipation of this outcome explains the choice of approach used here. In effect, the type of literature review conducted here makes it possible, up to a certain point, to bypass this limitation by connecting available knowledge in a generative way. The proposed typologies are generative, in that they allow us to consider how several structuring performance parameters of primary care models might fit together. Ultimately, what matters is that care models are developed in which resources, structures, professional roles, care pathways, and population needs come together in a coherent whole. We believe the models proposed in this article are useful tools to this end.

Endnotes

[1]An optimized search strategy was developed for each database. As an example, the CINHAL one could be summarized as: [primary health care OR ambulatory care OR family practice OR community health services OR group practice OR patient centred medical home OR walk-in centre] **AND** [nurse led OR nurse-managed centres OR advanced nursing practice OR registered nurses OR nurse practitioners OR nursing role] **AND** [quality of health care OR health service accessibility OR organizational efficiency OR multidisciplinary care team OR interprofessional relations OR model of care OR delivery model].

Abbreviations
OECD: Organisation for Economic Co-operation and Development; PHCNP: Primary healthcare nurse practitioner; VHA: Veteran's Health Administration

Acknowledgements
Donna Rilley edited the manuscript.

Funding
This work was supported by the Canadian Institutes of Health Research (grant number MOP136851). Damien Contandriopoulos also benefited from a CIHR Applied Public Health research chair (www.pocosa.ca).

Authors' contributions
The project was led by DC. AC was responsible for most data collection. Data analysis was shared by DC, MP and AC. First draft was co-written by DC, MP and AC. AD and EJ were involved in the drafting of the final article. All authors read and approved the final manuscript.

Consent for publication
Not applicable.

Competing interests
The authors declare that they have no competing interests.

Author details
[1]School of Nursing, University of Victoria, PO Box 1700, STN CSC, Victoria, British-Columbia V8W 2Y2, Canada. [2]Faculty of Nursing, Université de Montréal, C.P. 6128 succ. Centre-ville, Montréal, Québec H3C 3J7, Canada. [3]School of Nursing, Université du Québec à Rimouski, 300, allée des Ursulines, C. P. 3300, succ. A, Rimouski, Québec G5L 3A1, Canada.

References
1. Commission on Social Determinants of Health. Achieving health equity: from root causes to fair outcomes. Interim statement. Geneva: World Health Organization; 2007.
2. Rittenhouse DR, Shortell SM, Fisher ES. Primary care and accountable care – two essential elements of delivery-system reform. N Engl J Med. 2009; 361(24):2301–3.
3. Clavet N-J, Duclos J-Y, Fortin B, Marchand S, Michaud P-C. Les dépenses en santé du gouvernement du Québec, 2013-2030 : projections et déterminants. Montreal: CIRANO Scientific Series; 2013. p. 2013s–45.
4. Ham C, Dixon A, Brooke B. Transforming the delivery of health and social care: the case for fundamental change. London: King's Fund; 2012.
5. Starfield B, Yushi L, Macinko J. Contribution of primary care to health systems and health. Milbank Q. 2005;83(3):457–502.
6. Donaldson MS, Yordy KD, Lohr KN, Vanselow NA. Primary care: America's health in a new era (committee on the future of primary care, Institute of Medicine). Washington, DC: National Academies Press; 1996.
7. Feachem RG, Sekhri NK, White KL, Dixon J, Berwick DM, Enthoven AC. Getting more for their dollar: a comparison of the NHS with California's Kaiser Permanente. BMJ. 2002;324(7330):135–43.
8. Haggerty J, Pineault R, Beaulieu M-D, Brunelle Y, Gauthier J, Goulet F, Rodrigue J. Practice features associated with patient-reported accessibility, continuity, and coordination of primary health care. Ann Fam Med. 2008; 6(2):116–23.
9. Hutchison B. From hall to now: reflections on Canadian Medicare from a primary care perspective. In: Emmett hall memorial lecture. Vancouver: Canadian Association for Health Services and Policy Research (CAHSPR); 2013.
10. Macinko J, Starfield B, Shi L. The contribution of primary care systems to health outcomes within Organization for Economic Cooperation and Development (OECD) countries, 1970–1998. Health Serv Res. 2003;38(3):831–65.
11. Christensen CM, Grossman JH, Hwang J. The innovator's prescription: a disruptive solution for health care. New York: Mc Graw Hill; 2009.
12. Laurant MG, Hermens RP, Braspenning JC, Akkermans RP, Sibbald B, Grol RP. An overview of patients' preference for, and satisfaction with, care provided by general practitioners and nurse practitioners. J Clin Nurs. 2008;17(20):2690–8.
13. Naylor M, Kurtzman ET. The role of nurse practitioners in reinventing primary care. Health Aff. 2010;29(5):893–9.
14. Sibbald B, Laurant M, Scott A. Changing task profiles. In: Saltman RB, Rico A, Boerma W, editors. Primary care in the driver's seat? Organizational reform in European primary care. Berkshire: Open University Press; 2006. p. 149–64.
15. Commission on the Reform of Ontario's Public Services. Public services for Ontarians: a path to sustainability and excellence. Chapter 5: health. Toronto: Ontario Ministry of Finance; 2012.
16. Marmot M. Achieving health equity: from root causes to fair outcomes. Lancet. 2007;370:1153–63.
17. Bodenheimer TS, Smith MD. Primary care: proposed solutions to the physician shortage without training more physicians. Health Aff. 2013;32(11):1881–6.
18. Lavis JN, Boyko JA. Evidence brief: strengthening primary health care in Canada. Hamilton: McMaster Health Forum; 2009.
19. Delamaire M-L, Lafortune G. Nurses in advanced roles: a description and evaluation of experiences in 12 developed countries. In: OECD health working papers no 54. Paris: OECD Publishing; 2010.
20. Bailey P, Jones L, Way D. Family physician/nurse practitioner: stories of collaboration. J Adv Nurs. 2006;53(4):381–91.
21. Bamford D, Griffin M. A case study into operational team-working within a UK hospital. Int J Oper Prod Man. 2008;28(3):215–37.
22. Litaker D, Mion L, Kippes C, Mehta N, Froliks J. Physician-nurse practitioner teams in chronic disease management: the impact on costs, clinical effectiveness, and patients' perception of care. J Interprof Care. 2003;17(3):223–37.
23. Hasselback P, Saunders D, Dastmalchian A, Alibhai A, Boudreau R, Chreim S. The Taber integrated primary care project: turning vision into reality. Ottawa: Canadian Health Services Research Foundation; 2003.
24. Bonsall K, Cheater FM. What is the impact of advanced primary care nursing roles on patients, nurses and their colleagues? A literature review. Int J Nurs Stud. 2008;45(7):1090–102.
25. Baker GR, MacIntosh-Murray A, Porcellato C, Dionne L, Stelmacovich K, Karen B. High performing healthcare systems: delivering quality by design. Toronto: Longwoods Publishing Corporation; 2008.
26. Doherty RB, Crowley RA. Health and public Committee of the American College of physicians. Principles supporting dynamic clinical care teams: an American College of Physicians position paper. Ann Int Med. 2013; 159(9):620–6.
27. Reay T, Patterson EM, Halma L, Steed WN. Introducing a nurse practitioner: experiences in a rural Alberta family practice clinic. Can J Rural Med. 2006; 11(2):101–7.
28. DiCenso A, Matthews S. Report of the nurse practitioner integration task team submitted to the Ontario minister of health and long-term care. Ministry of Health and Long-Term Care: Toronto; 2007.
29. Laurant MG, Reeves D, Hermens R, Braspenning J, Grol R, Sibbald B. Substitution of doctors by nurses in primary care. In: Cochrane database Syst rev, vol. 2; 2005. p. CD001271.
30. Martin-Misener R, Downe-Wamboldt B, Cain E, Girouard M. Cost effectiveness and outcomes of a nurse practitioner-paramedic-family physician model of care: the long and Brier Islands study. Prim Health Care Res Dev. 2009;10(1):14–25.
31. Richardson G, Maynard A, Cullum N, Kindig D. Skill mix changes: substitution or service development? Health Policy. 1998;45:119–32.
32. Thille P, Rowan MS. The role of nurse practitioners in the delivery of primary health care: a literature review. In: Unpublished report submitted to Health Canada; 2008.
33. Grady D, Redberg RF. Less ss more: how less health care can result in better health. Arch Intern Med. 2010;170(9):749–50.
34. Krogsbøll LT, Jørgensen KJ, Grønhøj Larsen C, Gøtzsche PC. General health checks for reducing illness and mortality. In: Cochrane database systematic rev; 2012. p. CD009009.

35. Krogsbøll LT, Jørgensen KJ, Grønhøj Larsen C, Gøtzsche PC. General health checks in adults for reducing morbidity and mortality from disease: Cochrane systematic review and meta-analysis. BMJ. 2012;345:e7191.
36. Fisher ES, Bynum JP, Skinner JS. Slowing the growth of health care costs — lessons from regional variation. N England J Med. 2009;360(9):849–52.
37. Hadler NM. Worried sick: a prescription for health in an overtreated America. Chapel-Hill: The University of North Carolina Press; 2008.
38. Cassels A. Seeking sickness: medical screening and the misguided hunt for disease. Vancouver: Greystone Books; 2012.
39. Moseley JB, O'Malley K, Petersen NJ, Menke TJ, Brody BA, Kuykendall DH, Hollingsworth JC, Ashton CM, Wray NP. A controlled trial of arthroscopic surgery for osteoarthritis of the knee. N England J Med. 2002;347(2):81–8.
40. Wright CJ, Chambers GK, Robens-Paradise Y. Evaluation of indications for and outcomes of elective surgery. CMAJ. 2002;167(5):461–6.
41. Griffiths P, Maben J, Murrells T. Organisational quality, nurse staffing and the quality of chronic disease management in primary care: observational study using routinely collected data. Int J Nurs Stud. 2011;48(10):1199–210.
42. Pawson R, Tilley N. Realistic evaluation. London: SAGE Publications; 1997.
43. Pawson R, Greenhalgh T, Harvey G, Walshe K. Realist review–a new method of systematic review designed for complex policy interventions. J Health Serv Res Policy. 2005;10(Suppl. 1):21–34.
44. Pawson R. Evidence-based policy: a realist perpective. London: SAGE Publications; 2006.
45. Pawson R. Evidence-based policy: the promise of `realist synthesis. Evaluation. 2002;8(3):340–58.
46. Brousselle A, Champagne F. Program theory evaluation: logic analysis. Eval Prog Plan. 2011;34(1):69–78.
47. Contandriopoulos D, Duhoux A, Roy B, Amar M, Bonin J-P, Da Silva RB, Brault I, Dallaire C, Dubois C-A, Girard F. Integrated primary care teams (IPCT) pilot project in Quebec: a protocol paper. BMJ Open. 2015;5(12): e010559.
48. Donabedian A. The quality of care. How can it be assessed? JAMA. 1988; 206(12):1743–8.
49. Shortell SM, Schmittdiel J, Wang MC, Li R, Gillies RR, Casalino LP, Bodenheimer T, Rundall TG. An empirical assessment of high-performing medical groups: results from a national study. Med Care Res Rev. 2005;62(4):407–34.
50. Wilson K, Rosenberg MW. Accessibility and the Canadian health care system: squaring perceptions and realities. Health Policy. 2004;67:137–48.
51. Beaulieu M-D, Haggerty JL, Beaulieu C, Bouharaoui F, Lévesque J-F, Pineault R, Burge F, Santor DA. Interpersonal communication from the patient perspective: comparison of primary healthcare evaluation instruments. Healthc Policy. 2011;7(Special issue):108–23.
52. Haggerty JL, Burge F, Beaulieu M-D, Pineault R, Beaulieu C, Lévesque J-F, Santor DA, Gass D, Lawson B. Validation of instruments to evaluate primary healthcare from the patient perspective: overview of the method. Healthc Policy. 2011;7(Special issue):31–46.
53. Haggerty JL, Burge F, Lévesque J-F, Gass D, Pineault R, Beaulieu M-D, Santor D. Operational definitions of attributes of primary health care: consensus among Canadian experts. Ann Fam Med. 2007;5(4):336–44.
54. Pineault R, Lévesque J-F, Roberge D, Hamel M, Couture A. Primary care services organisational models and the population's care experience. Centre de recherche de l'Hôpital Charles LeMoyne: Longueuil; 2008.
55. Pineault R. Accessibility and continuity of care: a study of primary healthcare in Québec. Research report presented to the Canadian Institutes of Health Research (CIHR) and the Canadian health services research Fondation (CFSRF). Centre de recherche de l'Hôpital Charles Lemoyne: Longueuil; 2008.
56. Waddington C, Egge D. Integrated health services– what and why? Technical brief no.1, 2008. Geneva: World Health Organization; 2008.
57. Brousselle A, Lachaine J, Contandriopoulos AP. L'évaluation économique. In: Brousselle A, Champagne F, Contandriopoulos AP, Hartz Z, editors. Concepts et méthodes d'évaluation des interventions. Montreal: Presses de l'Université de Montréal; 2009. p. 199–235.
58. Decuyper S, Dochy F, Van den Bossche P. Grasping the dynamic complexity of team learning: an integrative model for effective team learning in organisations. Educ Res Rev. 2010;5(2):111–33.
59. Raes E, Boon A, Kyndt E, Dochy F. Measuring team learning behaviours through observing verbal team interaction. J Workplace Learning. 2015; 27(7):476–500.
60. Greenhalgh T, Robert G, Macfarlane F, Bate P, Kyriakidou O. Diffusion of innovations in service orgrnizations: systematic review and recommendations. Milbank Q. 2004;82(4):581–629.
61. Greenhalgh T, Robert G, Macfarlane F, Bate P, Kyriakidou O, Peacock R. Storylines of research in diffusion of innovation: a meta-narrative approach to systematic review. Soc Sci Med. 2005;61(2):417–30.
62. Moher D, Liberati A, Tetzlaff J, Altman DG, The PRISMA Group. Preferred reporting items for systematic reviews and meta-analyses: the PRISMA statement. PLoS Med. 2009;6(7):e1000097.
63. Rosen R, Mountford L. Developing and supporting extended nursing roles: the challenges of NHS walk-in centres. J Adv Nurs. 2002;39(3):241–8.
64. Iglesias B, Ramos F, Serrano B, Fàbregas M, Sánchez C, García MJ, Cebrian HM, Aragonés R, Casajuana J, Esgueva N. A randomized controlled trial of nurses vs. doctors in the resolution of acute disease of low complexity in primary care. J Adv Nurs. 2013;69(11):2446–57.
65. Venning P, Durie A, Roland M, Roberts C, Leese B. Randomised controlled trial comparing cost effectiveness of general practitioners and nurse practitioners in primary care. BMJ. 2000;320(7241):1048–53.
66. Contandriopoulos D, Brousselle A, Breton M, Sansgter-Gormley E, Kilpatrick K, Dubois C-A, Brault I, Perroux M. Nurse practitioners, canaries in the mine of primary care reform. Health Policy. 2016;120(6):682–9.
67. Heale R, Butcher M. Canada's first nurse practitioner-led clinic: a case study in healthcare innovation. Nurs Leadersh. 2010;23(3):21–9.
68. Martínez-González NA, Djalali S, Tandjung R, Huber-Geismann F, Markun S, Wensing M, Rosemann T. Substitution of physicians by nurses in primary care: a systematic review and meta-analysis. BMC Health Serv Res. 2014; 14(1):214.
69. Wong FKY, Chung LCY. Establishing a definition for a nurse-led clinic: structure, process, and outcome. J Adv Nurs. 2006;53(3):358–69.
70. Rosland A-M, Nelson K, Sun H, Dolan ED, Maynard C, Bryson C, Stark R, Shear JM, Kerr E, Fihn SD, et al. The patient-centred medical home in the veterans health administration. Am J Manag Care. 2013;19(7):e263–72.
71. Bush NJ, Watters T. The emerging role of the oncology nurse practitioner: a collaborative model within the private practice setting. Oncol Nurs Forum. 2001;28(9):1425–31.
72. Nelson S, Turnbull J, Bainbridge L, Caulfield T, Hudon G, Kendel D, Mowat D, Nasmith L, Postl B, Shamian J, et al. Optimizing scopes of practice: new models of care for a new health care system. Report of the expert panel appointed by the Canadian academy of health sciences. Ottawa: Canadian Academy of Health Sciences; 2014.
73. Richards A, Carley J, Jenkins-Clarke S, Richards DA. Skill mix between nurses and doctors working in primary care-delegation or allocation: a review of the literature. Int J Nurs Stud. 2000;37(3):185–97.
74. Liu N, D'Aunno T. The productivity and cost-efficiency of models for involving nurse practitioners in primary care: a perspective from queueing analysis. Health Serv Res. 2012;47(2):594–613.
75. Donaldson L. The normal science of structural contingency theory. In: Clegg SR, Hardy C, Nord WR, editors. Handbook of organization studies. Thousand Oaks: SAGE Publications; 1996. p. 57–76.
76. Ainsworth B, Hayward S. Developing an innovative model of care for nurse-led walk-in centres in the ACT. Aust Nurs J. 2010;18(4):28–31.
77. Heale R. Overcoming barriers to practice: a nurse practitioner-led model. J Am Acad of Nurse Pract. 2012;24(6):358–63.
78. Hoff T. Medical home implementation: a sensemaking taxonomy of hard and soft best practices. Milbank Q. 2013;91(4):771–810.
79. Krothe JS, Flynn B, Ray D, Goodwin S. Community development through faculty practice in a rural nurse-managed clinic. Public Health Nurs. 2000;17(4):264–72.
80. Tuepker A, Kansagara D, Skaperdas E, Nicolaidis C, Joos S, Alperin M, Hickam D. "We've not gotten even close to what we want to do": a qualitative study of early patient-centred medical home implementation. J Gen Intern Med. 2014;29(Suppl. 2):S614–22.
81. McGrath RG. Exploratory learning, innovative capacity and managerial oversight. Acad of Manage J. 1991;44:118–31.
82. Antonacopoulou EP, Sheaffer Z. Learning in crisis rethinking the relationship between organizational learning and crisis management. J Manage Inquiry. 2014;23(1):5–21.
83. Balasubramanian BA, Cohen DJ, Davis MM, Gunn R, Dickinson LM, Miller WL, Crabtree BF, Stange KC. Learning evaluation: blending quality improvement and implementation research methods to study healthcare innovations. Implementation Sci. 2015;10(31):1.
84. Engler ES, Jones SL, Van de Ven AH. Organizing healthcare for changing markets: the case of Ascension health. J Organ Design. 2013;2(3):3–15.
85. Jiménez-Jiménez D, Sanz-Valle R. Innovation, organizational learning, and performance. J Bus Res. 2011;64(4):408–17.

Enhancing delivery of osteoarthritis care in the general practice consultation: evaluation of a behaviour change intervention

Mark Porcheret*, Chris Main, Peter Croft and Krysia Dziedzic

Abstract

Background: Professionally-focussed behaviour change intervention (BCI) workshops were utilised in the Management of OsteoArthritis in Consultations (MOSAICS) trial investigating the feasibility of implementing the National Institute for Health and Care Excellence (NICE) Osteoarthritis (OA) Guideline in general practice. The workshops aimed to implement the general practitioner (GP) component of the trial intervention: an enhanced consultation for patients presenting with possible OA. This study presents an evaluation of the BCI workshops on GP competency in conducting these enhanced consultations.

Methods: A before-and-after evaluation of the workshops, delivered to GPs participating in the intervention arm of the MOSAICS trial, using video-recorded GP consultations with simulated OA patients. GPs attended four workshops, which had been developed using an implementation framework. Videos were undertaken at three time-points (before workshops and at one- and five-months after) and were assessed by independent observers, blinded to time points, for GP competency in undertaking 14 predetermined consultation tasks.

Results: Videos of 15 GPs were assessed. GP competency increased from a median of seven consultation tasks undertaken by each GP at baseline to 11 at both time-points after the workshops. Specific tasks which were undertaken more frequently after the workshops related to explaining that OA is treatable and not inevitably progressive, eliciting and addressing patient expectations of the consultation, and providing written OA information. However, the use of the word "osteoarthritis" in giving the diagnosis of OA was not enhanced by the workshops.

Conclusions: BCI workshops can enhance GP competency in undertaking consultations for OA. Further initiatives to implement the NICE OA Guideline and enhance the care of people with OA in primary care can be informed by the content and delivery of the workshops evaluated in this study.

Keywords: Osteoarthritis, Primary care, Consultations, Behaviour change, Implementation, Simulated patients, Evaluation, Video-recording

* Correspondence: m.porcheret@keele.ac.uk
Arthritis Research UK Primary Care Centre, Research Institute for Primary Care & Health Sciences, Keele University, Staffordshire ST5 5BG, UK

Background

Osteoarthritis (OA) is a highly prevalent long-term condition in older adults for which extensive recommendations on assessment and treatment have been published [1–5]. It is predominantly managed in primary care, notably in the UK in general practice, but surveys of care, and interviews with patients and professionals, indicate that management of OA in general practice is suboptimal [6–8].

One aspect of suboptimal OA care is the conduct by general practitioners (GPs) of consultations for older patients presenting with peripheral joint pain, those likely to have OA. Evidence suggests that elements of the consultation could be improved, including: making the diagnosis of OA clinically; providing accurate information about the condition and on prognosis; promoting and supporting the use of non-pharmacological treatments; and adopting a patient-centred approach [9–11].

In the UK the National Institute for Health and Care Excellence (NICE) recommends that: OA should be diagnosed clinically; a holistic assessment should be undertaken; OA self-management should be supported; core treatments should be information, advice on activity and exercise and, if relevant, interventions to achieve weight loss; non-pharmacological and pharmacological treatments, and referral for consideration of joint should be used as additional treatment options [3, 12]. To implement these recommendations in UK general practice they would need to be acted on by GPs – to whom the majority of people with possible OA first present. Given current evidence of suboptimal GP consultations for OA, implementation of NICE OA guidance would need to include activities to enhance GP OA consultations.

This approach was taken in the Management of OsteoArthritis in Consultations (MOSAICS) trial, a cluster randomised trial to investigate the impact of implementing the 2008 NICE OA Guideline [13]. The trial intervention was a "model OA consultation" delivered by intervention arm practices to patients aged 45 years and over presenting to their GP with peripheral joint pain. This consisted of an OA Guidebook, an "enhanced initial OA consultation" with the GP, and a nurse-led OA clinic. A behaviour change intervention (BCI) was developed, and delivered as a series of BCI workshops, to implement the delivery of the "enhanced initial OA consultation" by GPs in intervention arm practices [14].

When evaluating the impact of behaviour change interventions, direct measurement of the intended behaviour, such as GP performance in day-to-day clinical practice, is recommended wherever possible, but indirect proxy measures are available when this is not practical [15]. Such proxy measures include the use of patient report, analysis of medical record entries, and the use of video-recorded consultations with simulated patients to measure competency – what someone is capable of doing in "controlled representations of professional practice" [16]. In the context of the MOSAICS trial it was not practical to directly measure GP performance in delivering the "enhanced initial OA consultation" – due to the logistics of recording such consultations in day-to-day practice – and a proxy measure was chosen.

This study aimed to evaluate the success of BCI workshops to implement delivery by GPs of the "enhanced initial OA consultation" by measuring workshop impact on GP competency to conduct these consultations using video-recorded consultations with simulated patients.

Methods

Design

A before-and-after evaluation of BCI workshops (for simplicity henceforth referred to as "the workshops") was conducted using paired data on video-recorded consultations between GPs and simulated patients presenting with joint pain. GPs were video-recorded at their practices at three time-points: baseline before the workshops, and 1 month and 5 months after the workshops.

Setting and participants

The study took place in four UK general practices which were participating in the intervention arm of the MOSAICS trial. All GPs working in these practices were invited to attend the workshops on OA management and delivery of the "enhanced initial OA consultation". Eligible GPs for this study were those working in one of the practices and who had a video-recorded consultation at each time-point.

The workshops

The development of the content and style of the workshops has been described in detail elsewhere [14]. In brief they were developed using an implementation of change model [17], presented the GPs with a "concrete proposal for change" [17], addressed "determinants of change" identified using the Theoretical Domains Framework [18], and incorporated systematically selected behaviour change techniques [19]. They consisted of four workshops, which used a mixture of didactic and interactive sessions, were learner-centred and facilitated by local opinion leaders, principally addressed identified knowledge and skills gaps relevant to delivery of OA consultations, and were mainly delivered at the GP practices. Full details are given in Additional file 1 using the Guideline for Reporting Evidence-based practice Educational interventions and Teaching (GREET) checklist [20].

Video-recorded consultation data capture

Five simulators, who each portrayed a simulated patient with a different "story", were recruited and trained for the study. At each time-point a research nurse and simulated patient attended the practice and GPs were invited, during an organised break in morning surgery, to undertake a simulated consultation (one at each time-point). At baseline (before the workshops) GPs were instructed to undertake the consultation as they would normally do, at the two later time-points (after the workshops) they were asked to undertake the consultation as promoted in the workshops. At each time-point the simulated patient, and so the scenario he or she presented, was new to the GPs, so providing a proxy for a new patient first presenting with a new problem (see Additional file 2).

Assessment of video-recorded consultations

Videos were assessed for the presence of 14 predetermined OA consultation tasks. The tasks were the elements of the "enhanced initial OA consultation" which had been identified from a consensus study [21] as key elements of an initial consultation between a GP and an older adult presenting with peripheral joint pain (Table 1).

Videos were assessed by four trained assessors (GPs who were all independent of the MOSAICS trial), using a rating tool whose validity, and reliability in use, had been established (for details of assessor training, and validity and reliability testing see Additional file 3). Assessors were instructed to decide for each video and for each task whether the task had been undertaken or not, i.e. a binary assessment of "task present" or "task not present". Each assessor was randomly allocated a set of trial GPs' videos, (those of three or four GPs) and they assessed in random order all the videos of each of their allocated GPs, blinded to time-point.

Table 1 Osteoarthritis (OA) consultation tasks assessed in the video-recorded consultations between GPs and simulated patients

Giving the diagnosis	
1.1	The GP elicits the patient's ideas or worries or concerns about what they think is the matter with them, or the cause of their problem
1.2	The GP tells the patient the problem is due to OA, the word osteoarthritis needs to be used
Explaining the diagnosis	
2.1	The GP elicits what the patient knows or understands about OA, the word osteoarthritis needs to be used
2.2	The GP tells the patient that OA does not always / inevitably get worse, the word osteoarthritis does NOT need to be used
2.3	The GP tells the patient that OA is treatable: that there are things which can be done to help, the word osteoarthritis does NOT need to be used
Addressing expectations	
3.1	The GP elicits the specific expectation(s) the patient has of the GP about the problem
3.2	The GP responds to the patient's specific expectations (as noted at 3.1)
Providing analgesia	
4.1	The GP elicits what the patient has tried or is trying for the problem
4.2	The GP advises about, or prescribes for, pain relief
Promoting self-management	
5.1	The GP elicits what the patient has tried or is trying for the problem, other than for the pain
5.2	The GP tells the patient that exercise(s) or physical activity is beneficial for patients with OA or for the patient's problem
5.3	The GP tells the patient that losing weight, or not being overweight, is beneficial for patients with OA or for the patient's problem
Promoting self-management support	
6.1	The GP offers, or gives, the patient general written information on OA
6.2	The GP offers, or gives, the patient an appointment with a practice nurse to help with OA

Analysis

Duration of videotaped consultations was calculated in minutes, and paired *t* tests were used to compare duration at baseline with that at one- and five-months.

We sought to measure both the competence of an individual GP in conducting an entire consultation, and the extent to which an individual task was undertaken by all the GPs at a given time-point. Two summary measures were therefore defined:

1. GP competency score: the number of tasks assessed as present in each video.
2. Task delivery score: the number of videos at a given time-point in which the task was assessed as present.

GP competency score was determined for each GP at each time-point. For each time-point median, interquartile range and range of competency scores across all GPs were calculated. Wilcoxon matched pairs signed-rank sum test [22] was used to compare median GP competency score at baseline with that at one- and five-months.

Task delivery score was calculated for each consultation task at each time-point and McNemar test with continuity correction (2-sided) [23] was used to compare scores at baseline with those at one- and five-months.

Results

Thirty-one GPs in total were eligible to take part from the practices participating in the MOSAICS trial. All were invited to attend the workshops and be video-recorded. Baseline videos were obtained for 24 GPs. Of these, there were 15 GPs who had a video suitable for analysis from all three time-points (baseline plus two follow-ups), resulting in a total of 45 videos assessed and used for the main analysis (full details given in Fig. 1 (participant recruitment flowchart)). Of the 15 GPs, 12 had attended all the workshops, two GPs two of the three workshops and one GP none.

Mean duration of all videos was 14.46 min (range of 8.80 to 26.93 min) with no difference in duration at the three time-points (paired t test: baseline v one-month, $p = 0.28$: baseline v five-months, $p = 0.63$; one-month v five-months, $p = 0.13$).

GP competency score increased after the workshops from median of seven consultation tasks undertaken before the workshops to 11 at both one-month and five-months after (Wilcoxon signed-rank test: one-month v baseline, $p = 0.001$; five-months v baseline, $p = 0.001$), see Table 2 for full details.

Task delivery score was high at baseline for two tasks (eliciting what the patient is trying for pain, and advising or prescribing analgesia) which were present in all baseline videos. The score for six other tasks increased after the workshops at one-month (McNemar test: one-month v baseline, $p < 0.05$), with the increase for three of these tasks sustained at five-months (McNemar test: five-month v baseline, $p < 0.05$), see Table 3 for full details.

The task delivery score for "Giving the diagnosis of OA using the word "osteoarthritis"" decreased non-significantly after the workshops (Table 3), an unexpected finding given this task was a key focus of the workshops. Further analysis determined that the reason for the low task delivery scores after the workshops was that the diagnosis was often given using the word "arthritis", and not "osteoarthritis" (see Additional file 4).

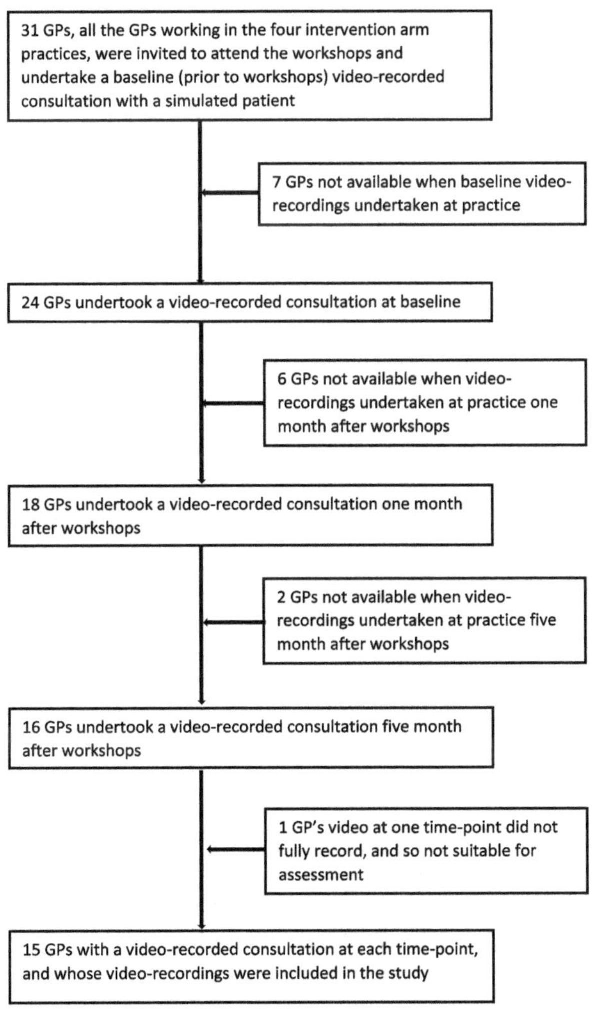

Fig. 1 Participant recruitment flowchart

Discussion

This study has demonstrated that GP competency for undertaking consultations for OA can be significantly increased by workshops. After the workshops, GPs were undertaking a median of 11 of 14 pre-determined OA consultation tasks in each consultation, and nine of the tasks were being undertaken by at least 80% of GPs at each consultation. Six tasks increased in frequency from baseline and were those relating to: giving more positive explanations about OA, eliciting and addressing patient expectations about the consultation, offering written information, and, in the context of the MOSAICS trial, offering a follow-up in a nurse-led OA clinic. Tasks relating to managing pain and advising on exercise were undertaken by nearly all GPs at baseline and continued to be so after the workshops, but those relating to eliciting patient ideas about their problem, their understanding of OA, and their prior use of non-pharmacological treatments were not increased by the workshops and were variably undertaken by the GPs.

Despite being a specific focus of the workshops, using the word "osteoarthritis" when giving the diagnosis of OA did not increase after the workshops, with OA often being referred to as "arthritis". This finding aligns with

Table 2 Median, interquartile range and range of GP competency scores by time-point

	Baseline	1 month after workshops	5 months after workshops
Median	7	11*	11*
Interquartile range	5–9	10–12	10–11
Range	5–11	8–14	7–13

*Wilcoxon signed-rank test: one-month v baseline, $p = 0.001$; five-months v baseline, $p = 0.001$

Table 3 Task delivery score by consultation task by time-point and comparison of one- and five-months with baseline

Consultation task	Task delivery score			Change in task delivery scores, *p* values from McNemar test	
	Baseline	1 month after	5 months after	1 month v baseline	5 months v baseline
Eliciting ideas about problem	11	11	8	0.62	0.45
Giving the diagnosis of OA, using the word "osteoarthritis"	10	6	9	0.22	1.00
Eliciting understanding of OA	1	2	4	1.00	0.37
Explaining that OA does not get inevitably worse	4	13	14	0.01	0.01
Explaining that OA is treatable	9	15	14	0.04	0.13
Eliciting expectations of the consultation	6	14	11	0.01	0.13
Addressing expectations	6	13	11	0.02	0.13
Eliciting what the patient is trying for pain	15	15	14	-[a]	1.00
Advising or prescribing analgesia	15	14	15	1.00	-[a]
Eliciting what the patient is trying for the problem other analgesia	6	9	3	0.51	0.45
Advising that exercise is beneficial	12	15	15	0.25	0.25
Advising that weight loss is beneficial	10	6	11	0.13	1.00
Offering general written info	4	14	14	0.004	0.004
Offering a nurse appointment to help with the problem	0	15	15	0.000	0.000

[a]McNemar Test not computable

the conclusion from a recent observational study on real-life consultations for OA that there is much confusion as to how to portray and explain OA in the general practice consultation [10]. The average duration of the video-recorded consultations was longer than GP consultations in day-to-day practice, and may reflect the effect of being observed, but the increase in competency was not associated with longer consultations. This is an important finding for generalisability and implementation of the optimal consultation.

To our knowledge this is the first study which has evaluated the effect of a behaviour change intervention to optimise GP consultations for OA on clinical practice. Other studies on primary care management of OA have evaluated the effect of standardised consultations [24], interactive peer-group training [25] and a training course about OA care [26] on patient outcomes but not clinical practice. Studies which have evaluated the effect of workshops using a similar approach to skills training for GPs as used in this study, those based on the "context-bound" skills training method [27] (a method which focuses on the management of the clinical problem and not simply the uptake of specific communication skills), have shown that this approach can significantly enhance clinical practice in consultations for other conditions [28, 29].

Study strengths included the robust assessment methodology used, with each assessor viewing all the videos of an individual GP in random order and blinded to time-point, and the establishment of validity and reliability of use of the video rating tool. All bar one of the GPs included in the evaluation had attended two or more workshops.

Study limitations included the use of a non-randomised before and after design to evaluate the workshops, but the logistics of embedding the study in the intervention arm practices of the MOSAICS trial precluded randomising GPs to training or not training, as all needed to be trained to deliver the trial intervention. In addition resources precluded undertaking video-recorded consultations with control arm practices. However, the use of paired before and after observations enabled us to control for the effect of GP characteristics differing between time-points. A possible limitation is that in two practices not all the GPs invited to attend the training were included in this study as not all had a full set of video-consultations. This could have resulted in selection bias in that those included might not have been typical of all GPs from these practices. The GPs who were included might have been more committed to the study, in that they undertook all the videos, and so may have been more motivated to enhance their clinical practice. However, two of the 11 GPs included from these practices were only "partially trained" and one not trained at all, suggesting that even among the included GPs there was a range of commitment to the study. Furthermore, whether GPs had a full set of videos for assessment, or not, was due to whether they were working in the practice on the days the videos were undertaken and not solely to their commitment to the study: the research nurse endeavoured to video all GPs who were present in the surgery at the time of the video sessions. Another possible limitation, with the use of repeat video-recorded consultations to evaluate the workshops, is that of a learning effect from previously undertaking the consultation. We addressed this by using different simulated patients with different scenarios at each of the three time-points.

The finding that the workshops increased GP competency for OA consultations should be generalisable to GPs as a whole: although the GPs in this study were those in practices which had signed up to participating in the MOSAICS trial, and so may have differed from GPs as a whole, their reported views and practice at baseline on OA management were similar to those reported by GPs more generally [30, 31]. Although the findings are for GP competency for OA consultations, and not performance, the consultations with simulated patients were made as real and naturalistic as possible by undertaking them in the GPs' own surgeries and by having detailed and realistic patient scenarios and biographies (see Additional file 2). The use of the workshops, in the specific manner in which they were delivered in this study, to enhance other GPs' clinical practice for OA may not be feasible across the health service as a whole: the workshops were quite labour-intensive to deliver and required GPs to commit considerable time to attendance. In the UK NICE has recently updated its guidance on the care of people with OA [32] and, given current evidence on the management of OA in general practice in the UK, implementation of its recommendations will require GP consultations for OA to be optimised. The evidence from this study, on how to enhance GP competency for such consultations, will contribute to developing training resources for more general use, evidenced by its use in the development of written [33] and on-line [34] educational material for UK GPs and in underpinning OA implementation projects in UK regionally and in Europe. One issue that the detailed information from the current study will enable us to reflect on and consider is whether the content and delivery of training can be streamlined and made more efficient for general use without reducing its effectiveness in changing GP behaviour.

Further research is needed on how to help GPs better communicate with patients about OA, both in terms of what to call it, which was not resolved by this study, and of how to explain what it is. The latter can build on the approach taken in this study which led to GPs giving more positive OA explanations, namely that OA is treatable and is not inevitably progressive.

Conclusions

In summary, this before and after study has demonstrated that GP competency in undertaking consultations for OA can be enhanced. The workshops evaluated in this study to enhance competence can inform development of future generalised initiatives to enhance OA care in general practice.

Additional files

Additional file 1: GREET 2015 checklist for the behaviour change intervention workshops.

Additional file 2: Development of simulated patient scenarios and biographies (a description of their development and a synopsis of the six scenarios developed), and arrangements for undertaking video-recorded simulated patient consultations.

Additional file 3: Validity, and reliability in use, of the video rating tool - methodology and results of establishing validity and reliability of the video rating tool.

Additional file 4: Further analysis of task delivery score for "Giving the diagnosis of OA using the word "osteoarthritis – methodology" and results of further analysis undertaken".

Abbreviations

BCI: Behaviour change intervention; GP: General practitioner; MOSAICS trial: Management of OsteoArthritis in Consultations trial; NICE: National Institute for Health and Care Excellence; OA: Osteoarthritis; UK: United Kingdom

Acknowledgements

We would like to thank the following who have contributed to the work presented in this article: the GPs in the four intervention practices of the MOSAICS trial who attended the workshops and agreed to undertake repeated video-recorded consultations; Richard Hayward, John Edwards, Simon Somerville and Claire Burton for agreeing to be assessors for the videos; Doreen Briggs, Tim Briggs, Jean Clarke, Bernard Moss and Sheila Moss who acted as simulated patients for the videos; Kelvin Jordan for help with statistical analysis; Ashley Ford for technical help with the videos;. June Handy, Chan Vohora and Angela Pushpa-Rajah who helped organise the set-up and delivery of the workshops and video sessions; members of the MOSAICS trial research team, especially Emma Healey, Vince Cooper and Zoe Paskins who helped develop and deliver the training workshops.

Funding

This paper presents independent research commissioned by the UK National Institute for Health Research (NIHR) Programme Grant (RP-PG-0407-10386). This research was also commissioned by the Arthritis Research UK Centre in Primary Care grant (Grant Number 18139). KD and MP are supported by the UK NIHR Collaborations for Leadership in Applied Health Research and Care West Midlands. KD is part-funded by a Knowledge Mobilisation Research Fellowship (KMRF-2014-03-002) from the NIHR. MP was supported by an NIHR In-Practice Fellowship. The views expressed in this paper are those of the author(s) and not necessarily those of the National Health Service, the NIHR or the Department of Health.

Authors' contributions

MP developed the methodology, organised data collection and assessment of the videos, undertook the data analysis and drafted the manuscript. CM, PC and KD participated in developing the methodology, analysing data, and drafting the manuscript. All authors read and approved the final manuscript.

Competing interests

The authors declare that they have no competing interests.

References

1. Thomas E, Peat G, Croft P. Defining and mapping the person with osteoarthritis for population studies and public health. Rheumatology (Oxford). 2014;53(2):338–45.
2. Jordan KP, Joud A, Bergknut C, Croft P, Edwards JJ, Peat G, et al. International comparisons of the consultation prevalence of musculoskeletal conditions using population-based healthcare data from England and Sweden. Ann Rheum Dis. 2014;73(1):212–8.
3. Conaghan PG, Dickson J, Grant RL, Guideline DG. Care and management of osteoarthritis in adults: summary of NICE guidance. BMJ. 2008;336(7642):502–3.
4. Zhang W, Doherty M, Arden N, Bannwarth B, Bijlsma J, Gunther KP, et al. EULAR evidence based recommendations for the management of hip osteoarthritis: report of a task force of the EULAR standing Committee for International Clinical Studies Including Therapeutics (ESCISIT). Ann Rheum Dis. 2005;64(5):669–81.
5. Jordan KM, Arden NK, Doherty M, Bannwarth B, Bijlsma JW, Dieppe P, et al. EULAR recommendations 2003: an evidence based approach to the management of knee osteoarthritis: report of a task force of the standing Committee for International Clinical Studies Including Therapeutic Trials (ESCISIT). Ann Rheum Dis. 2003;62(12):1145–55.
6. Steel N, Hardcastle AC, Clark A, Mounce LT, Bachmann MO, Richards SH, et al. Self-reported quality of care for older adults from 2004 to 2011: a cohort study. Age Ageing. 2014;43(5):716–20.
7. Porcheret M, Jordan K, Jinks C, Croft P. Primary care rheumatology society. Primary care treatment of knee pain–a survey in older adults. Rheumatology (Oxford). 2007;46(11):1694–700.
8. Jinks C, Ong BN, Richardson JC. A mixed methods study to investigate needs assessment for knee pain and disability. Population and individual perspectives. BMC Musculoskelet Disord. 2007;8:59.
9. Paskins Z, Sanders T, Hassell AB. Comparison of patient experiences of the osteoarthritis consultation with GP attitudes and beliefs to OA: a narrative review. BMC Fam Pract. 2014;15:46.
10. Paskins Z, Sanders T, Croft PR, Hassell AB. The identity crisis of osteoarthritis in general practice: a qualitative study using video-stimulated recall. Ann Fam Med. 2015;13(6):537–44.
11. Coxon D, Frisher M, Jinks C, Jordan K, Paskins Z, Peat G. The relative importance of perceived doctor's attitude on the decision to consult for symptomatic osteoarthritis: a choice-based conjoint analysis study. BMJ Open. 2015;5(10):e009625,2015–009625.
12. NICE Pathway for the Management of Osteoarthritis. Available at: https://pathways.nice.org.uk/pathways/osteoarthritis. Accessed 30 Jan 2018.
13. Dziedzic KS, Healey EL, Porcheret M, Ong B, Main CJ, Jordan KP, et al. Implementing the NICE osteoarthritis guidelines: a mixed methods study and cluster randomised trial of a model osteoarthritis consultation in primary care - the management of OsteoArthritis in consultations (MOSAICS) study protocol. Implement Sci. 2014;9(1):95.
14. Porcheret M, Main C, Croft P, McKinley R, Hassell A, Dziedzic K. Development of a behaviour change intervention: a case study on the practical application of theory. Implement Sci. 2014;9(1):42.
15. Hrisos S, Eccles M, Francis J, Dickinson H, Kaner E, Beyer F, et al. Are there valid proxy measures of clinical behaviour? A systematic review. Implement Sci. 2009;4(1):37.
16. Rethans JJ, Norcini JJ, Baron-Maldonado M, Blackmore D, Jolly BC, LaDuca T, et al. The relationship between competence and performance: implications for assessing practice performance. Med Educ. 2002;36(10):901–9.
17. Grol R, Wensing M, Eccles M. Improving patient care: the implementation of change in Clinical Practice. 2005.
18. Michie S, Johnston M, Abraham C, Lawton R, Parker D, Walker A, et al. Making psychological theory useful for implementing evidence based practice: a consensus approach. Qual Saf. Health Care. 2005;14(1):26–33.
19. Michie S, Johnston M, Francis J, Hardeman W, Eccles M. From theory to intervention: mapping theoretically derived Behavioural determinants to behaviour change techniques. Appl Psychol. 2008;57(4):660–80.
20. Phillips A, Lewis L, McEvoy M, Galipeau J, Glasziou P, Moher D, et al. Development and validation of the guideline for reporting evidence-based practice educational interventions and teaching (GREET). BMC Med. Educ. 2016;16:237.
21. Porcheret M, Grime J, Main C, Dziedzic K. Developing a model osteoarthritis consultation: a Delphi consensus exercise. BMC Musculoskelet Disord. 2013;14:25.
22. Altman DG. Practical statistics for medical research. 1st ed. London: Chapman and Hall; 1991.
23. Siegel S, Castellan N. Nonparametric statistics for behavioural sciences. 2nd ed. New York: McGraw-Hill Book Company; 1988.
24. Ravaud P, Flipo RM, Boutron I, Roy C, Mahmoudi A, Giraudeau B, et al. ARTIST (osteoarthritis intervention standardized) study of standardised consultation versus usual care for patients with osteoarthritis of the knee in primary care in France: pragmatic randomised controlled trial. BMJ. 2009;338:b421.
25. Rosemann T, Joos S, Laux G, Gensichen J, Szecsenyi J. Case management of arthritis patients in primary care: a cluster-randomized controlled trial. Arthritis Rheum. 2007;57(8):1390–7.
26. Chassany O, Boureau F, Liard F, Bertin P, Serrie A, Ferran P, et al. Effects of training on general practitioners' management of pain in osteoarthritis: a randomized multicenter study. J Rheumatol. 2006;33(9):1827–34.
27. Rollnick S, Kinnersley P, Butler C. Context-bound communication skills training: development of a new method. Med Educ. 2002;36(4):377–83.
28. Rollnick S, Seale C, Kinnersley P, Rees M, Butler C, Hood K. Developing a new line of patter: can doctors change their consultations for sore throat? Med Educ. 2002;36(7):678–81.
29. Cals JW, Scheppers NA, Hopstaken RM, Hood K, Dinant GJ, Goettsch H, et al. Evidence based management of acute bronchitis; sustained competence of enhanced communication skills acquisition in general practice. Patient Educ Couns. 2007;68(3):270–8.
30. Kingsbury SR, Conaghan PG. Current osteoarthritis treatment, prescribing influences and barriers to implementation in primary care. Prim Health Care Res Dev. 2012;13(4):373–81.
31. Cottrell E, Roddy E, Foster NE. The attitudes, beliefs and behaviours of GPs regarding exercise for chronic knee pain: a systematic review. BMC Fam Pract. 2010;11:4. 2296-11-4
32. Osteoarthritis. Care and management in adults. Available at: http://guidance.nice.org.uk/CG177/NICEGuidance/pdf/English. Accessed 16 June 2014.
33. Osteoarthritis: a modern approach to diagnosis and management. Available at: http://www.arthritisresearchuk.org/health-professionals-and-students/reports/hands-on/hands-on-autumn-2011.aspx. Accessed 16 June 2014.
34. Musculoskeletal Care (osteoarthritis module). Available at: http://elearning.rcgp.org.uk/course/info.php?popup=0&id=206. Accessed 30 Jan 2018.

19

Is problem alcohol use being detected and treated in Irish general practice?

Andrew O'Regan[1*], Walter Cullen[2], Louise Hickey[1], David Meagher[1] and Ailish Hannigan[1]

Abstract

Background: The pattern of alcohol consumption in Ireland has serious societal and health consequences. General practice is well placed to screen for problem alcohol use and to carry out brief interventions. The aims of this study were to investigate the prevalence of documentation of problem alcohol use in patient records in Irish general practice, and to describe the documentation of its diagnosis and treatment.

Methods: General practitioners (GPs) affiliated with an Irish medical school were invited to participate in the study. One hundred patients were randomly selected from each participating practice using the practice software and the clinical records were reviewed for evidence of problem alcohol use. The following was recorded: patient demographics, whether problem alcohol use was documented, whether they had an intervention, a psychotropic medication or if a referral was made. Descriptive statistics and an estimate of the prevalence were calculated using SPSS and SAS software.

Results: Seventy one percent of the practices participated ($n = 40$), generating a sample of 3, 845 active patients. Only 57 patients (1.5%, 95% confidence interval 1 to 2%) were identified as having problem alcohol use in the previous two years. 29 (51%) of those with documented problem alcohol use were referred to other specialist services. 28 (49%) received a psychological intervention. 40 (70%) were prescribed psychotropic medications.

Conclusion: This is the first large scale study of patient records in general practice in Ireland looking at documentation of screening and treatment of problem alcohol use. It highlights the current lack of documentation of alcohol problems and the need to re-inforce positive attitudes among GPs in relation to preventive work.

Keywords: Alcoholism, Problem alcohol use, General practice, Primary care, Screening, Brief intervention

Background

A recent WHO report showed that almost half of Irish drinkers engage in heavy drinking on a regular basis, placing Ireland's binge drinking rates at the second highest of 174 countries studied [1]. According to the Central Statistics Office, Dublin, the current per capita alcohol consumption in Ireland is 10.9 l per person aged over fifteen years, a figure that has trebled over four decades, while in most other countries it has fallen [2]. The increase in per capita consumption is associated with an earlier age of commencing drinking [3] and a recent survey showed that half of Irish 15–16 year olds had consumed alcohol and 23% had been intoxicated at least once [4]. Furthermore, a study of third level students showed that two thirds were engaging in hazardous drinking [5]. These figures, particularly, are alarming as people with serious drug and alcohol problems commence drinking at a much earlier age than those without problems [6]. Ireland's unhealthy relationship with alcohol is therefore related to both the amount and pattern of alcohol consumption.

The socio-economic impact of alcohol in this country is enormous with a cost to the state of 3.7 billion yearly in terms of health, crime and work-place [7]. Alcohol misuse permeates all facets of Irish society and is a factor in: higher-risk sexual behaviour [8], almost half sexual assault cases [9]; in one quarter of marital disharmony and one third of domestic abuse incidents in this country [10]. There is a proven link to suicide [11], with alcohol detected in the blood of a half of suicide deaths in Ireland [12]. From a health perspective, alcohol is a

* Correspondence: Andrew.oregan@ul.ie
[1]Graduate Entry Medical School, Faculty of Education and Health Sciences, University of Limerick, Limerick, Ireland

causal factor in more than 60 medical conditions including hypertension, liver cirrhosis and depression [13] and is one of the most important causes of cancer in Ireland. It is a proven factor in the aetiology of cancers of the mouth, throat, stomach, liver and breast [14]. 28% of emergency department admissions to six of Ireland's main hospitals are due to alcohol with half of these being in the 18–30 year old age-group [15], mostly due to binge drinking.

Successive legislation has been largely ineffective in addressing the alcohol crisis but the seriousness of the problem has been recognised in recent legislation (Public Health [Alcohol] Bill, 2015) which includes evidence-based measures such as minimum unit pricing. Health strategy has emphasised the importance of resources and training for the preventative role of primary care. It is recognised that general practitioners (GPs) commonly see patients with a range of alcohol-related risks and problems (8–18% of patients presenting to primary care) and screening and brief interventions in this setting are proven to reduce misuse levels [16]. GPs have been identified as appropriate professionals to screen for those at risk of problem alcohol use and to conduct brief interventions to influence patients to think more actively about their alcohol consumption [17]. Despite the magnitude of the national alcohol problem and the detrimental effects on health and society, there is a surprising lack of data from general practice on the documentation of alcohol use and treatment.

The aims of this study, therefore, were to investigate the prevalence of documentation of problem alcohol use in patient records in Irish general practice, to describe the documented treatment of patients with problem alcohol use and their psychological comorbidities.

Methods

Participants

This study is part of a larger study on prevalence of psychological morbidity in adults attending general practice in Ireland, the methodology of which has been previously described [18]. All general practices affiliated with the University of Limerick Graduate Entry Medical School with a senior medical student on clinical placement in 2013 ($n = 56$ practices) were invited to participate in the study. As part of the medical school professional competencies curriculum, third year medical students are required to complete a clinical audit or research project and may do this while on any placement. A unique aspect of the curriculum is an 18-week general practice placement where faculty provide a standardised project for students with ethical approval, instructions on data retrieval and analysis, a coding sheet and supervision for the duration of the project. With this level of support and the suitability of electronic records to audit and research, the majority of students opt for the standardised project in general practice in conjunction with their GP tutors.

Practices affiliated with the School are broadly representative of practices nationally by size, urban/rural and patient eligibility for free care. Reporting functions of electronic practice management systems in all participating practices were used to generate a list of all patients aged 18 and over with a documented contact to the practice in the previous two years. A random sample of 100 adult patients was selected from this list in each practice using a random number function in Microsoft Excel. Inactive patients, e.g. temporary visitors or those known to have recently moved away or died were excluded from the sample.

Measures

Clinical records for a two year time period (2011–2013) were reviewed for the sample of patients by the senior medical student on placement in the practice and their supervising GP for any evidence of attending the practice with problem alcohol and/or substance use other than alcohol. Evidence included text in consultation notes; evidence of a pharmacological treatment or psychological intervention by the GP; evidence of a referral to another primary healthcare professional or specialist agencies and/or diagnostic coding.

Data was collected using an instrument validated for morbidity surveys in primary care in Ireland [19] which recorded the following information on all patients in the sample:

- Demographics: age, gender, eligibility for free care. The Republic of Ireland has the only health system in the European Union which does not offer universal coverage for primary care [20]. It has a mixed private-public system with 43% of the population eligible for a means-tested General Medical Services (GMS) card or doctor visit only card which is issued by the Health Service Executive. To qualify for a medical card the applicant must earn below a certain figure based on family size. GPs (who are self-employed) are paid a 'per capita' fee by the state for their care. These patients do not pay directly for GP consultations whereas patients without a card pay an average of €50 per consultation.
- Health service utilisation: total number of visits to the GP for any reason in the past year; any referral to or attendance at secondary care (including the emergency department) in the past year.

- Whether problem alcohol use or other substance use had been documented in the clinical records over the previous two years and if yes,
  - whether a referral to another agency was made;
  - whether psychotropic medication was received;
  - whether a psychological intervention was received and if yes, the type and delivery of the intervention.

Data was entered to an Excel file in each practice and anonymised datasets from all practices were merged together with practice characteristics (urban or rural, number of patients, number of staff). Ethical approval for the study was granted by the University Hospital Limerick Research Ethics Committee.

Statistical analysis

The proportion of patients with problem alcohol or substance use documented in the previous two years was estimated with a 95% confidence interval for the proportion, accounting for the structure of the dataset with patients clustered within practices. Demographic and healthcare utilisation variables were summarised using graphical and numeric descriptive statistics. For those patients with problem alcohol and/or substance use documented, information on treatment was summarised using graphical and numeric descriptive statistics. The association between categorical variables was tested using chi-square tests and median consultations rates were compared across groups using non-parametric tests. A 5% level of significance was used for all statistical tests. SPSS Statistics Version 21 for Windows and SAS software Version 9.2 for Windows (SAS Institute, Inc.) were used to carry out the analysis with the SAS procedure SURVEYFREQ used to account for clustering.

Results

Forty (71%) of the 56 practices affiliated with the Medical School agreed to participate. Practice characteristics of those who did not participate were similar to those who participated. Practice size ranged from less than one thousand to over three thousand registered patients. Twenty two (54%) practices indicated they were urban, 13 (33%) indicated they were rural and 5 (13%) indicated they were mixed urban/rural practices. Of the 4000 patient records sampled across 40 practices, 155 (4%) temporary visitors to the practice or those who were known to have died or moved away were excluded giving a sample of 3845 'active' patients.

Problem alcohol use

Fifty-seven (1.5%, 95% confidence interval 1 to 2%) were identified as having problem alcohol use documented in the previous two years. Of the 40 participating practices, 14 (35%) had no patients in their sample with documented problem alcohol use, 16 (40%) had up to 2% of their sample with documented problem alcohol use and 10 (25%) had between 2 and 8% of their sample with documented problem alcohol use. Patients with problem alcohol use were more likely to be male than those without any problem alcohol use documented (65% vs. 47%, $p = 0.007$). They were also more likely to be eligible for free GP care (72% vs 48%, $p < 0.001$), have been referred or attended secondary care in the past year (79% vs 50%, $p < 0.001$) and attend the GP more frequently (median of 5 vs 2 consultations a year, $p = 0.02$) (see Table 1).

The majority (72%) of those with problem alcohol use were identified from free text in consultation notes. Six patients (11%) had a diagnostic code entered for problem alcohol use. Four (7%) patients were identified from referral letters, four (7%) from both referral letters and consultation notes, one (2%) from a 'past history' page and one (2%) from a psychological assessment. Of the 57 patients with documented problem alcohol use, 22 (39%) also were documented as having depression, 21 (37%) stress and anxiety and 3 (5%) psychosis.

Twenty-three (0.6%, 95% confidence interval 0.4 to 0.9%) were identified as having substance use other than alcohol documented in the previous two years. The majority of practices ($n = 25$ practices, 63%) had no patients in their sample with documented problem substance use. Of the 23 patients with problem substance use, two (9%) were also identified as having problem alcohol use.

Twenty-nine (51%) of those with documented problem alcohol use were referred to other specialist services. 28 (49%) received a psychological intervention, mostly counselling or a brief intervention. The psychological intervention was given in a diverse range of settings including primary care teams (32%), rehabilitation or addiction services (21%), and Alcoholics Anonymous (4%). 40 (70%) were prescribed psychotropic medications during the two-year timeframe of the study, most commonly antidepressants (47%) and benzodiazepenes (37%). 16 (28%) had two or more drugs prescribed for psychological problems.

Discussion

Interpretation of findings

The high response rate to the study among general practices (70%; $n = 40$ practices) yielded a large study population ($n = 3845$ active patients) that is reflective of general practice nationally [21]. The proportion of patients with documented problem alcohol use was 1.5% (95% confidence interval 1 to 2%) and the proportion with documented substance use other than alcohol was 0.6%. Only two of the study population had documented co-existing drug and alcohol abuse. The percentage of patients that

Table 1 Demographics and healthcare utilisation by whether problem alcohol use was documented

	No problem alcohol use documented ($n = 3788$)	Documented problem alcohol use ($n = 57$)	*P*-value
Median Age (25th, 75th percentile)	46 (32, 61)	49 (36, 58)	0.45
Male	1777 (47%)	37 (65%)	0.007
Eligible for free GP care	1828 (48%)	41 (72%)	< 0.001
Any referral/attendance to secondary care in the past year	1910 (50%)	45 (79%)	< 0.001
Median GP consultations (25th, 75th percentile) in the past year	2 (1, 6)	5 (2, 7)	0.02

have documented problem alcohol use is very small with no patients with documented problem alcohol use in the samples from over a third of participating practices. Given how rare the documentation is, our study cannot explain the factors influencing documentation rates. Previous investigation of clinical documentation suggests that practices that have more user friendly software, as well as more clinician motivation and training, have superior documentation [22] but barriers and enablers to clinical documentation in this context requires further research.

Prevention in primary care in Canada, particularly preventive interventions that involve discussion, e.g. smoking cessation, are often not documented by the GP in the clinical notes [23]. In Ireland, coding is not routinely performed in general practice and notes are written in free text. A key motivator for good clinical note taking in Ireland is protection from litigation which is not relevant to the documentation of unstructured and un-resourced preventive screening. In this context, it is worth considering the outcome of a recent study that found no association between the quality of clinical documentation and the quality of care [24].

Factors that were found to be significant among those with documented problem alcohol use compared to those that did not were: male gender and eligibility for free GP care. The rates of co-morbid depression and anxiety were high in those with documented alcohol use (39 and 37% respectively). Approximately half of those with documented problem alcohol use were referred; half were given a psychological intervention and 70% were prescribed psychotropic medications.

Comparison with the literature

The documentation rate of problem alcohol use is very low considering that one fifth of patients that present routinely to general practice are likely to be excessive drinkers [25]. The figure is in fact consistent with international findings that, in the absence of interventions, problem alcohol use is underdiagnosed [26], with a large-scale American population study finding that only 5 .5% had been asked about their drinking by their GP [27]. Detection rates are similarly low in Irish hospitals with only 17% of attendees at a tertiary emergency department being asked about their alcohol consumption [28].

The high rate of psychiatric co-morbidities, especially depression and anxiety, and psychotropic prescribing among those identified with problem alcohol use is consistent with international findings, and most likely accounts for some of the higher health service utilisation by the this group. A large scale epidemiological study found that 40% of patients with alcohol abuse problems met the criteria for a psychiatric disorder, typically anxiety and depression [29]. Importantly, that study also highlighted that when problem alcohol use is identified and treated, this proportion falls considerably. The subgroup of patients with documented co-existing drug and alcohol use was very small and is most likely explained by lack of documentation rather than true prevalence.

The high intervention and referral rates in this study may be explained by the fact that those who are detected are more likely to be on the severe end of the spectrum and health related issues would have already surfaced. The hidden majority of problem alcohol users who are not documented could be the group that would benefit most from a brief intervention from their GP [30]. Most GPs, however, prefer not to do the counselling of non-dependent problem drinkers themselves, but to refer to a professional trained in behavioural interventions [31]. Anderson showed that the most important factors necessary for GPs to carry out interventions were: education, support and confidence [32].

Enablers and barriers to screening for problem alcohol use

The gap between actual practice and potential for preventive work has been previously reported, with busyness and lack of doctor confidence cited as the key barriers [33]. Time constraints, however, should no longer restrict a GPs ability to screen as physician-conducted screening can take 74 s and single question screening has been validated for use in primary care [34]. There may be deeper underlying deterrents for GPs in documenting problem alcohol use, including protection of their patients. GPs frequently answer questionnaires for health insurance companies relating to mortgage protection and employment suitability with their patients' permission. It may pose a dilemma for a GP on whether to include documented 'high-risk activities' such as binge drinking or alcohol addiction, so not documenting the finding may be an easier approach. Possibly, the high rates of alcohol abuse and dependence among physicians [35] may be a contributory factor in the reluctance to ask about alcohol problems in the general practice population. What is even more concerning is the societal psyche in relation to the alcohol problem which must also affect general practitioners, moving one commentator to write: *'We have moved from a cultural attitude to alcohol that was ambivalent, to a culture where public and private drunkenness are apparently acceptable'* [36].

Limitations

The study is dependent on the completeness of consultation notes and coding and previous research in general practice has emphasised the need to improve coding practices in primary care [37]. Given that GPs do not routinely document screening, the 1.5% of patients identified in the clinical notes with documented problem alcohol use cannot be taken as the true prevalence of those identified by their GP as having a problem with alcohol in practice. Furthermore, our results cannot give data on the epidemiology of problem alcohol use in the community, given that all subjects in this study were recruited from those that had attended their general practice within the previous two years. Practices involved in our study are similar to the national profile by demographic factors but may be more academically or research active than other practices because of their involvement with the medical school. It is possible, therefore that the figures reported in this study are higher than the national rate of documentation.

Suggestions for future research and policy

Highlighting the value of screening and intervention in general practice should be a public health priority because the GP, by simply asking about alcohol, can positively affect drinking behaviour [38]. Five to ten minutes of advice from a GP can lead to reductions of 25–35% in alcohol consumption that are maintained at six months and one year [17]. Training is perceived by GPs as the most useful enabler to perform alcohol screening, and the doctor-patient relationship is the most important feature for the patients, who believe that the GP has an important role to play [39]. The Irish College of General Practitioner guidelines state that GPs and practice nurses should screen routinely and opportunistically by asking about alcohol use and documenting the outcome [40]. Future research should focus on alternative methods for collecting data on alcohol use in general practice. There is an opportunity for qualitative studies with GPs to explore attitudes, barriers and potential enabling strategies to improve screening, intervention and the documentation of problem alcohol use in an Irish context.

Conclusion

This is the first large scale study of patient records in general practice in Ireland looking at documentation of screening and treatment of problem alcohol use. It highlights the current lack of documentation of alcohol problems in patient records and the need for training and discussion to improve confidence and re-inforce positive attitudes among GPs in relation to preventive work. GPs are ideally placed to detect and intervene due to frequent contact with problem alcohol use and the relationship they have with their patients. Ireland urgently needs a national conversation about its relationship with alcohol and on clinical and service organisation levels, GPs should be central to this.

Abbreviation

GP: General practitioner

Acknowledgements

The authors would like to acknowledge the contribution of the GPs affiliated to the Graduate Entry Medical School and senior medical students on placement in general practice who contributed to this project.

Funding

No external funding was received for this project.

Authors' contributions

AOR contributed to the study design, data collection, analysis and write-up. WC contributed to the study conception, design and write-up. LH contributed to the data collection, analysis and write-up. DM contributed to the study conception and design. AH contributed to the study conception, design, data collection, analysis and write-up. All authors read and approved the final manuscript.

Consent for publication

Not applicable.

Competing interests

The authors declare that they have no competing interests.

Author details

[1]Graduate Entry Medical School, Faculty of Education and Health Sciences, University of Limerick, Limerick, Ireland. [2]School of Medicine, University College Dublin, Health Sciences Centre, Belfield, Dublin, Ireland.

References

1. WHO: Global status report on alcohol and health, 2014. In.: World Health Organisation; 2014.
2. OECD: Health Statistics. In.: Organisation for Economic Co-operation and Development; 2014.
3. Smyth BP, Kelly A, Cox G. Decline in age of drinking onset in Ireland, gender and per capita alcohol consumption. Alcohol Alcohol. 2011;46(4):478–84.

4. Hibell B, Guttormsson U, Ahlström S, Balakireva O, Bjarnason T, Kokkevi A, Kraus L: The 2011 ESPAD Report. Substance Use among Students in 2012, 36:123–134.
5. Davoren MP, Shiely F, Byrne M, Perry IJ. Hazardous alcohol consumption among university students in Ireland: a cross-sectional study. BMJ Open. 2015;5(1):e006045.
6. DeWit DJ, Adlaf EM, Offord DR, Ogborne AC. Age at first alcohol use: a risk factor for the development of alcohol disorders. Am J Psychiatr. 2000;157(5):745–50.
7. Byrne S: Costs to society of problem alcohol use in Ireland. Dublin: Health Service Executive 2010.
8. Rundle K, Leigh C, McGee H, Layte R. Irish contraception and crisis pregnancy [ICCP] study. A survey of the general Population. 2004;
9. McGee H, Garavan R, de Barra M, Byrne J, Conroy R: The SAVI report: sexual abuse and violence in Ireland. 2002.
10. Health Do: Department of Health. Steering Group Report on a National Substance Abuse Strategy. In.: Department of Health; 2012.
11. Foster T, Gillespie K, McClelland R, Patterson C. Risk factors for suicide independent of DSM-III-R Axis I disorder. Case-control psychological autopsy study in Northern Ireland. Br J Psychiatry. 1999;175(2):175–9.
12. Bedford D, O'Farrell A, Howell F. Blood alcohol levels in persons who died from accidents and suicide. Ir Med J. 2006;99(3):80–3.
13. WHO: Global Status Report on Alcohol and Health. In. Geneva: World Health Organisation; 2011.
14. Martin J, Barry J, Goggin D, Morgan K, Ward M, O'Suilleabhain T. Alcohol-attributable mortality in Ireland. Alcohol Alcohol. 2010;45(4):379–86.
15. Mongan D: Health-related consequences of problem alcohol use. -3759 2007.
16. Whitlock EP, Polen MR, Green CA, Orleans T, Klein J. Behavioral counseling interventions in primary care to reduce risky/harmful alcohol use by adults: a summary of the evidence for the US preventive services task force. Ann Intern Med. 2004;140(7):557–68.
17. Anderson P. Effectiveness of general practice interventions for patients with harmful alcohol consumption. Br J Gen Pract. 1993;43(374):386–9.
18. Hickey L, Hannigan A, O'Regan A, Khalil S, Meagher D, Cullen W. Psychological morbidity among young adults attending primary care: a retrospective study. Early Interv Psychiatry. 2018;12(1):22–29. https://doi.org/10.1111/eip.12284.
19. Cullen W, O'Brien S, O'Carroll A, D O'Kelly F, Bury G. Chronic illness and multimorbidity among problem drug users: a comparative cross sectional pilot study in primary care. BMC Fam Pract. 2009;10(1):1.
20. Thomson S, Figueras J, Evetovits T, Jowett M, Mladovsky P, Maresso A, Cylus J, Karanikolos M, Kluge H: Economic crisis, health systems and health in Europe: impact and implications for policy: WHO regional Office for Europe; 2014.
21. Structure of General Practice in Ireland 1982–2015.
22. Hiddema-Van de Wal A, Smith R, van der Werf G, Meyboom-de Jong B. Towards improvement of the accuracy and completeness of medication registration with the use of an electronic medical record (EMR). Fam Pract. 2001;18(3):288–91.
23. Ngwakongnwi E, Hemmelgarn B, Quan H. Documentation of preventive screening interventions by general practitioners: a retrospective chart audit. BMC Fam Pract. 2010;11(1):21.
24. Edwards ST, Neri PM, Volk LA, Schiff GD, Bates DW. Association of note quality and quality of care: a cross-sectional study. BMJ quality & safety. 2014;23(5):406–13.
25. Kaner E, Heather N, Brodie J, Lock CA, McAvoy BR. Patient and practitioner characteristics predict brief alcohol intervention in primary care. Br J Gen Pract. 2001;51(471):822–7.
26. Fiellin DA, Reid MC, O'Connor PG. Screening for alcohol problems in primary care: a systematic review. Arch Intern Med. 2000;160(13):1977–89.
27. Hasin DS, Stinson FS, Ogburn E, Grant BF. Prevalence, correlates, disability, and comorbidity of DSM-IV alcohol abuse and dependence in the United States: results from the National Epidemiologic Survey on alcohol and related conditions. Arch Gen Psychiatry. 2007;64(7):830–42.
28. Nkire N, Udoh G, Elahi M, Cotter D, MacHale S. Screening and recording of patients' alcohol-use habit by clinicians in a tertiary accident and emergency unit in Ireland. Annals of medical and health sciences research. 2014;4(4):590–3.
29. Regier DA, Myers JK, Kramer M, Robins LN, Blazer DG, Hough RL, Eaton WW, Locke BZ. The NIMH epidemiologic catchment area program: historical context, major objectives, and study population characteristics. Arch Gen Psychiatry. 1984;41(10):934.
30. Kaner E, Bland M, Cassidy P, Coulton S, Dale V, Deluca P, Gilvarry E, Godfrey C, Heather N, Myles J. Effectiveness of screening and brief alcohol intervention in primary care (SIPS trial): pragmatic cluster randomised controlled trial. BMJ. 2013;346:e8501.
31. Spandorfer JM, Israel Y, Turner BJ: Primary care physicians' views on screening and management of alcohol abuse inconsistencies with national guidelines. J Fam Pract 1999, 48(11):899–899.
32. Anderson P, Kaner E, Wutzke S, Funk M, Heather N, Wensing M, Grol R, Gual A, Pas L. Attitudes and managing alcohol problems in general practice: an interaction analysis based on findings from a WHO collaborative study. Alcohol Alcohol. 2004;39(4):351–6.
33. Wilson GB, Lock CA, Heather N, Cassidy P, Christie MM, Kaner EF. Intervention against excessive alcohol consumption in primary health care: a survey of GPs' attitudes and practices in England 10 years on. Alcohol Alcohol. 2011;46(5):570–7.
34. Smith PC, Schmidt SM, Allensworth-Davies D, Saitz R. Primary care validation of a single-question alcohol screening test. J Gen Intern Med. 2009;24(7):783–8.
35. Oreskovich MR, Shanafelt T, Dyrbye LN, Tan L, Sotile W, Satele D, West CP, Sloan J, Boone S. The prevalence of substance use disorders in American physicians. Am J Addict. 2015;24(1):30–8.
36. Anderson R. Alcohol abuse and the Irish. Forum Clinical Focus. 2012;12(5):4–8.
37. Bhattarai N, Charlton J, Rudisill C, Gulliford MC. Coding, recording and incidence of different forms of coronary heart disease in primary care. PLoS One. 2012;7(1):e29776.
38. Kaner E, Beyer F, Dickinson H, Pienaar E, Campbell F, Schlesinger C, Heather N, Saunders J, Burnand B. Effectiveness of brief alcohol interventions in primary care populations. Cochrane Database Syst Rev. 2007;18;(2): CD004148. https://doi.org/10.1002/14651858.CD004148.pub3.
39. Field CA, Klimas J, Barry J, Bury G, Keenan E, Smyth BP, Cullen W. Problem alcohol use among problem drug users in primary care: a qualitative study of what patients think about screening and treatment. BMC Fam Pract. 2013;14(1):1.
40. Anderson RM, Joseph; Aherin, Adrian; Finegan, Pearse; Farren, Conor: Helping Patients with Alcohol Problems. In.: Irish College of General Practitioners; 2014.

20

Feasibility of an implementation strategy for the integration of health promotion in routine primary care

Alvaro Sanchez[1], Gonzalo Grandes[1*], Josep M. Cortada[2], Haizea Pombo[1], Catalina Martinez[1], Mary Helen Corrales[3], Enrique de la Peña[4], Justo Mugica[5], Esther Gorostiza[6] on behalf of the PVS group

Abstract

Background: Process evaluation is recommended to improve the understanding of underlying mechanisms related to clinicians, patients, context and intervention delivery that may impact on trial or program results, feasibility and transferability to practice. The aim of this study was to assess the feasibility of the Prescribe Healthy Life (PVS from the Spanish "*Prescribe Vida Saludable*") implementation strategy for enhancing the adoption and implementation of an evidence-based health promotion intervention in primary health care.

Methods: A descriptive study of 2-year implementation indicators for the PVS clinical intervention was conducted in four primary health care centers. A multifaceted collaborative modeling implementation strategy was developed to enhance the integration of a clinical intervention to promote healthy lifestyles into clinical practice. Process indicators were assessed for intervention reach, adoption, implementation, sustainability and their variability at center, practice, and patient levels.

Results: Mean rates of adoption by means of active collaboration among the three main professional categories (family physicians, nurses and administrative personnel) were 75% in all centers. Just over half of the patients that attended ($n = 11650$; 51.9%) were reached in terms of having their lifestyle habits assessed, while more than a third (33.7%; $n = 7433$) and almost 10% ($n = 2175$) received advice or a printed prescription for at least one lifestyle change, respectively. Only 3.7% of the target population received a repeat prescription. These process indicators significantly ($p < 0.001$) varied by center, lifestyle habit and patient characteristics. Sustainability of intervention components changed thorough the implementation period within centers.

Conclusions: The implementation strategy used showed moderate-to-good performance on process indicators related to adoption, reach, and implementation of the evidence-based healthy lifestyle promotion intervention in the context of routine primary care.

Sources of heterogeneity and instability in these indicators may improve our understanding of factors required to attain adequate program adoption and implementation through improved implementation strategies.

Keywords: Process evaluation, Implementation, Health promotion, Primary Health Care

* Correspondence: gonzalo.grandes@osakidetza.eus
[1]Primary Care Research Unit of Bizkaia, Basque Healthcare Service - Osakidetza, BioCruces Health Research Institute, Luis Power 18, 4ª planta, E48014 Bilbao, Spain
Full list of author information is available at the end of the article

Background

In the growing field of implementation research, the process of implementation of interventions is considered important in determining how to enhance their effectiveness, feasibility and sustainability [1, 2]. Further, the development, implementation and evaluation of complex health interventions all require careful consideration not only of outcomes obtained but also of the processes involved [3]. Process evaluations within trials explore the implementation, receipt and setting of an intervention, and help interpret the outcome results and ascertain the true implications of interventions in real practice [4, 5]. Further, this type of evaluation is particularly important in multisite trials, where the "same" intervention may be implemented and received in different ways, and consequently, may make it possible to assess fidelity and to monitor tolerable intervention doses and their variability. A better understanding of program implementation may also reveal opportunities for refining intervention content and delivery [6]. Lastly, process evaluation of intervention trials may inform future implementation and roll-out of the intervention in other contexts and settings, and indicate how interventions could move from research to practice [3, 5, 6].

The Prescribe Healthy Life (PVS from the Spanish "*Prescribe Vida Saludable*") strategy aims to optimize health promotion practice in primary and community care through implementation research [7]. Though no clinical intervention has a greater potential impact on public health than the promotion of healthy lifestyles, it remains far from being an integrated element of clinical practice, and hence, health promotion in primary care is an excellent example of the so-called "translational gap".

PVS follows a stepwise framework, appropriate for the design, evaluation and translation of complex interventions in clinical settings [3, 8]. In 2006, a preclinical phase was carried out to characterize the problem of health promotion integration, analyzing the causes of and barriers to change as well as the theoretical basis for developing solutions [7]. Then, in 2008, we conducted the phase I or modeling phase, in which four primary health care (PHC) centers, following an implementation strategy based on a collaborative and facilitated process [9], planned and designed intervention programs adapted to their specific contexts and resources, and identified strategies for change and mechanisms through which interventions should operate. This was done collaboratively among health care professionals, researchers, health service management, community workers and public health professionals. In the present paper, we describe the phase II pilot study conducted in the same four PHC centers with the goal of piloting and optimizing the previously designed intervention programs and their assessment procedures, and exploring the adoption, implementation, sustainability, acceptance and potential effectiveness and efficiency of the intervention programs.

The aim of the process evaluation reported in this paper was to assess the feasibility of the PVS implementation strategy for integrating healthy lifestyle promotion in PHC. Within the present study, feasibility concerns to the extent, likelihood, and manner in which an evidence-based health promotion intervention has been implemented as a direct result of performing an implementation strategy aimed at enhancing the adoption of the intervention [10]. Specifically, we describe PHC population-based indicators of the reach, adoption, implementation and sustainability of a healthy lifestyle promotion intervention in the context of routine primary care, and their variability at center, practice, and patient levels. We also identify socio-demographic and clinical characteristics associated with exposure to the intervention.

Methods

Study design and setting

A descriptive study of 2-year implementation indicators for the PVS clinical intervention was conducted in four PHC centers. The study protocol was approved by the Primary Care Research Committee of the Basque Health Service, Osakidetza, and by the Basque Country Clinical Research Ethics Committee (Ref: 6/2009). Our health service provides universal coverage that is free at the point of use, apart from co-payment for drugs, funded through regional general taxation. Each resident is included on the list of one practice under the care of a family physician or a pediatrician and a primary care nurse, who offer comprehensive primary care and access to hospital services. Primary care professionals work in full-time PHC teams at local centers providing health care for users in a defined geographical area.

Participants

The PVS implementation strategy has two main targets:

i) PHC centers and their staff, as the initiative seeks to improve health promotion practice through the mutual adaptation of evidence-based interventions and the center's organization; and
ii) primary care patients attending these health centers that fail to adhere to at least one of the following lifestyle recommendations: regular physical activity, healthy diet and abstinence from smoking.

PHC centers

Eligible centers were identified through the Medical Directors of the seven primary care organizations into which PHC is structured in the Basque Health System. Of the seven organizations, four agreed to collaborate and each selected one PHC center with the following eligibility criteria: (i) previous involvement in innovative health promotion programs or preventive practice optimization initiatives, (ii) the existence of community health promotion initiatives in their geographical area of influence, (iii) the presence of a positive attitude and cooperation among professionals, and (iv) the possibility of making changes in the organization of services. After explaining the study objectives and work plan in a meeting in each candidate center, we requested individual written commitment by a majority plus one of the staff in each of professional category (administrative personnel, nurses, family physicians, pediatricians, and others). The minimum required number of staff was obtained for all categories in all four centers. Health care professionals that committed to participate also gave written consent for the anonymous management and publication of data pertaining both to patients assigned to their practices and indicators related to their health care delivery activity.

PHC users

As public health programs, the PVS intervention programs aim to have an impact at the whole population level. Hence, their target population was all PHC users aged 10 to 65 years old registered with any of the collaborating PHC clinicians in any of the collaborating centers that attended the center during the program implementation period (from September 2011 to September 2013). We excluded patients who moved, those diagnosed with psychotic disorders, neurological degenerative diseases, or severe mental retardation, and those in residential care or with terminal illnesses.

Clinical intervention

The PVS clinical intervention targets three key aspects of a healthy lifestyle, namely, regular physical activity, a healthy diet and abstinence from smoking. The intervention is grounded in evidence-based theoretical models explaining behavior change: the Health Belief Model, the Theory of Planned Behaviour, the Transtheoretical model and Social-Cognitive Theory [7]. The multiple active intervention components and strategies are structured following the 5 A's (Ask, Advise, Agree, Assist, and Arrange follow-up) intervention framework [11], as it encompasses most of the evidence-based behavior modification techniques used to promote changes in the targeted lifestyles. It is considered that this strategy is useful in primary care for its simplicity, and low requirements for training and time, as well as for the scientific evidence supporting its effectiveness [7, 11–15].

Implementation strategy

The PVS implementation strategy worked at multiple levels: bottom-up primary care organizational change, top-down support from managers, community involvement, and the development of innovative e-health information and communication technologies [9]. Among the multiple specific implementation strategies used, three are directly related to the present study.

First, with the aim of adapting the clinical intervention to the context of each center where it was to be implemented and to redesign the health promotion delivery system, an action research-based collaborative modeling process was conducted in each of the centers with the active participation of PHC professionals and managers as well as researchers. Through a bottom-up decision making process based on discussion and consensus meetings among a multi-professional primary care team and community members guided by an external facilitator, staff in each center modeled and adapted the clinical intervention to their specific contexts and resources, and identified strategies for change, and mechanisms through which the interventions would operate. Between 10 and 13 working sessions were needed involving most of the primary care staff and at least one community-based organization. The process yielded multiple tailored healthy lifestyle intervention programs, varying between centers in the agents involved in each of the intervention actions as well as in the resources for their implementation and execution. Generally, within the collaborating PHC centers, administrative assistants, nurses and physicians were all involved in the PVS program but to different degrees. All professional categories were somewhat involved in the Assess step (A1), with considerable participation of administrative staff in order to perform the assessment before the medical consultation. Outside the center, individuals were themselves able to perform the assessment of healthy lifestyles through the PVS web questionnaire or a paper-based version of the same questionnaire delivered at community resources (e.g., company occupational health departments). The Advice and Agree steps (A2 and A3) were mainly delivered by family physicians, while the Assist step (A4) was mainly performed by nurses. All participants inside and outside the centers were involved in the Arrange follow-up (A5) process with particular involvement of administrative assistants and nurses. Based on reports by a sample of 32 professionals over 3 months of intervention piloting, the estimated mean time dedicated to each intervention component was 3, 7.84 and 13.67 min for assessing patient lifestyle (A1), and advising on (A2) and prescribing (A4) lifestyle change, respectively.

Second, an information and communication tool integrated in the electronic health record was developed in order to help and guide practitioners' clinical decision making related to diagnosis and therapeutic interventions in promoting healthy lifestyles. The functions of this software are the following: a) to identify people whose lifestyle habits have not been assessed and recorded; b) to assess patients' physical activity levels, diet, and smoking habits, complemented by paper-based questionnaires and a self-assessment website, c) to flag those not adhering to the recommendations; d) to identify high-priority populations for intervention based on data recorded in the electronic health records, e.g., age, motivation to change behavior, and chronic diseases; e) to guide health professionals in providing personalized and tailored advice based on effective communication of risks and benefits associated with lifestyle; f) to facilitate the prescription of plans for lifestyle modification, providing algorithms, evidence-based guidance and recommendations, warnings, timetables and information about community resources; f) to facilitate patient monitoring thorough the follow-up; and g) to integrate all the information and make it available to all staff of the center, thereby making it easier to track patients.

And lastly, there were audit and feedback strategies in the form of monthly tracking of process indicators related to patient reach and extent of implementation of intervention components. This auditing and feedback sought to maintain fidelity and intensity once initial implementation had been achieved.

Measurements

Process indicators pertaining to program execution and user socio-demographic (age, sex, socioeconomic status) and clinical (chronic health problems) characteristics were calculated from routine data extracted from the electronic health records of Osakidetza. The Primary Care Research Unit of Bizkaia (UIAPB) in conjunction with the Informatics Department of Osakidetza were responsible for the coordination and quality control of the process and execution of the study. This research unit is expressly authorized to retrieve and use data from the electronic health records for research by the owner thereof, namely, the Governing Board of Osakidetza. The data were kept confidential, anonymized, encrypted and managed centrally, in accordance with the Spanish laws on data protection and patient autonomy.

Specifically, within the program, healthy lifestyles were assessed with the 10-item PVS-Healthy Lifestyle Screening questionnaire. Briefly, content validity of this screening questionnaire was supported by an expert panel. Further, we conducted a pilot concurrent validity study in a sample of 126 patients. Firstly, we found that the physical activity screening items were acceptably correlated with total activity counts ($r = 0.46$; $p < 0.001$) and minutes of moderate-to-vigorous activity ($r = 0.34$; $p < 0.001$) measured with an ActiGraph GT3X accelerometer. Secondly, the two items used to screen fruit and vegetable consumption were well correlated with the total ($r = 0.50$; $p < 0.001$) score on a modified version of the Mediterranean Diet Adherence Screener used in the PREDIMED study [16] and with the specific items regarding fruit and vegetable consumption ($r = 0.54$; $p < 0.001$) on the PREDIMED Food Frequency Questionnaire [17]. Thirdly, the responses obtained in the tobacco use sub-scale showed a strong correlation with the level of carbon monoxide in exhaled air (CO in ppm) measured with a breath CO monitor ($r = 0.69$, $p < 0.001$) (data not published).

Using data extracted from health records for a 4-year period, we assessed whether each of the patients had any of nine groups of chronic diseases and also checked a list of 52 conditions and specific criteria defined for each condition to consider it active, based on the work of Orueta et al. [18]. For the purposes of this study, multimorbidity was defined as the coexistence of more than one health problem in the same patient considering these 52 conditions.

A Deprivation Index (DI), defined by census tract, developed and published in 2008 [19] was used as a socioeconomic status indicator. This index is an ordinal variable, categorized into five levels (DI quintiles), providing a measure of the socioeconomic characteristics of the population of census tracts. Its design allows the estimation of socioeconomic and environmental inequalities among inhabitants by census tract in Spain. The calculation takes into account the percentages of residents in a tract who are manual workers, unemployed, temporary employees, or have an poor level of educational attainment, overall and also specifically among young people, according to the most recent census data available (2001).

To assess the effectiveness of the PVS programs in terms of public health significance we used the RE-AIM (Reach, Efficacy, Adoption, Implementation, Maintenance) framework [20]. This framework underlines that to have a public health impact programs require more than efficacy. They must reach a diverse and representative sample of the at-risk population. Their adoption in specific practice/clinical settings must be realistic. Further, programs must be able to be implemented as intended. Lastly, they must also be maintained over time in a sustainable way by the individual and the practice/clinical setting. These dimensions together determine the overall impact of a program at the population level. Specifically, the process indicators assessed within the RE-AIM dimensions are:

Reach (Patient level)

Exposure of patients to the program at each center in terms of the percentage of the target population (patients 10 to 65 years old who attended the center at least once during the program implementation period) who had their lifestyle habits assessed, and consequently were exposed to the program.

Adoption (Practice/Center level)

Professional participation in the program: the percentage of professionals by professional category and percentage of practices (multidisciplinary health care professionals with an assigned list of patients, e.g., family physician plus nurse) in each center participating in the program who had performed at least one intervention component.

Implementation (Practice/Center level)

The percentage of practices that assessed at least 50% of their target population, gave advice to 25% and prescribed lifestyle change with a personalized plan to 10%.

Implementation (Patient level)

Reception of intervention components as intended in terms of the percentage of target patients whose lifestyle habits were assessed and included because they failed to adhere to at least one healthy lifestyle recommendation (I1: Included); the percentages of target patients (I2a: Advised-target) and included patients (I2b: Advised-included) who received advice; the percentages of target patients (I3a: Assisted-target), included patients (I3b: Assisted-included), and advised patients (I3c: Assisted-advised) who received a prescription for lifestyle change; and the percentages of target patients (I4a: Arranged-target), included patients (I4b: Arranged-included), and prescribed patients (I4c: Arranged-prescribed) who received a repeat prescription related to the same aspect of their lifestyle.

Maintenance

Sustainability of intervention program components over time in terms of the monthly rates of the aforementioned process indicators over 2 years.

Lastly, we also explored the association of patient sociodemographic and clinical characteristics with the likelihood of being assessed, advised or prescribed lifestyle changes.

Analysis

Data analysis was performed with SAS software. Frequencies and proportions were used to describe professional, practice and patient characteristics for continuous and categorical variables, respectively. Process indicators for each collaborating center and in total regarding adoption, reach and implementation were expressed as frequencies and percentages along with their corresponding 95% confidence intervals (CIs). Survival analysis was used to describe sustainability and compare the incidence of exposure to the intervention components (time until exposure to lifestyle assessment, advice, and prescription for lifestyle change) between the different centers. For univariate analysis of the association of time until exposure to the different intervention components with the comparison centers, cumulative survival probabilities over 24 months were estimated and compared using Kaplan-Meier curves along with the log-rank and Wilcoxon tests (SAS PROC LIFETEST, version 9.2, SAS Institute; 2008). Time to event or censoring was defined as the time between study entry (date of baseline interview) and date of exposure to the specific intervention component, or possible censoring at the end of the study (September 19, 2013), respectively.

Adjusted hazard ratios (AHRs) and 95% CIs describing relations between patient characteristics and the exposure to the intervention components were estimated using Cox proportional hazards models [21]. These models included health care center, sex, age, recorded chronic diseases, and the deprivation index as independent factors. The proportional hazard assumption was tested, introducing the interaction of each of the variables with time in the models. In the case of covariates for which the proportional hazard assumption was not satisfied, the Cox model was extended with time-dependent variables allowing hazard ratios to change over time.

Results

Practitioner team level (Center/professional level)

Adoption, Implementation & Maintenance

Table 1 describes the size and composition of the four collaborating PHC centers. Briefly, center size ranged from 14 to 36 staff mainly consisting of family physicians (range: 4 to 13), practice nurses (range: 5 to 13), pediatricians (range: 1 to 2) and administrative personnel (range: 4 to 6). Other professional categories included midwives, dentists and family planning physicians. Overall, 68 out of a total of 90 staff (75%) across professional categories (administrative personnel, nurses, family physicians, pediatricians, and others) initially committed in writing to participate in the study. This initial collaboration rate varied between centers ranging from 68 to 100% ($p < 0.01$). Within the centers, family physicians followed by nurses and administrative personnel were the most strongly represented categories, while pediatricians and especially midwives had the lowest rates of collaboration. As final unit of observation at center/professional level, we considered practices: the initial collaboration within centers ranged from 63 to 100% of practices with an overall participation of 84% from a total of 32.

Implementation of program components also varied between practices and centers. Specifically, rates of participation of practices in the execution of program components were not similar, except in one of the centers in which all teams collaborated and worked equally well. Overall, only 48% of practices assessed the lifestyles of 50% of all target patients that attended the center at least once during the program implementation period. Within centers, this rate of assessment was achieved by half or more than half of practices in three of the centers. However, only in two of the centers did half or more than half of collaborating practices reach levels of 25% or 10% of target patients being advised or prescribed lifestyle changes, respectively.

Table 1 Professional and practice level participation, and patient demographic and clinical characteristics, by center

	Center 1	Center 2	Center 3	Center 4	Total
Professional level					
Family physicians	11/13	5/6	3/4	4/4	23/27 (85%)
Nurses	9/13	6/8	4/5	6/6	25/32 (78%)
Administrative personnel	5/6	2/5	3/4	4/4	14/19 (74%)
Pediatricians	0/2	2/2	0/1	1/1	3/6 (50%)
Midwifes	0/2	0/1	–	1/1	1/4 (25%)
Others[a]	–	–	–	2/2	
Total	25/36 (69%)	15/22 (68%)	10/14 (71%)	18/18 (100%)	68/90 (75%)
Practice level					
Initial commitment	11/14	7/8	4/4	5/5	27/32 (84%)
Assessed (A1) 50% of target patients	2/11	4/7	2/4	5/5	13/27 (48%)
Advised (A2) 25% of target patients	4/11	5/7	1/4	5/5	15/27 (55%)
Assisted (A4) 10% of target patients	3/11	3/7	2/4	5/5	13/27 (48%)
Patient level					
Male sex	5126 (49.4%)	3215 (54.6%)	1266 (49.3%)	1760 (48.4%)	11367 (50.6%)
	(48.4%–50.4%)	(53.4%–55.9)	(47.4%–1.2%)	(46.8%–50.0%)	(49.9%–51.3%)
Age, years					
10–19	273 (2.6%)	551 (9.4%)	373 (14.5%)	367 (10.1%)	1564 (7%)
	(2.3%–2.9%)	(8.6%–10.1%)	(13.2%–5.9%)	(9.1%–11.15)	(6.6%–7.3%)
20–45	5713 (55.1%)	3585 (60.9%)	1214 (47.3%)	1881 (51.7%)	12393 (55.2%)
	(54.1%–56.0%)	(59.7%–62.2%)	(45.3%–9.2%)	(50.1%–3.4%)	(54.5%–55.8%)
46–65	4387 (42.3%)	1747 (29.7%)	981 (38.2%)	1387 (38.2%)	8502 (37.9%)
	(41.3%–43.2%)	(28.5%–30.8%)	(36.3%–40.1%)	(36.6%–9.7%)	(37.2%–38.5%)
Health problems					
Cancer[b]	215 (2.2%)	88 (1.6%)	41 (1.6%)	65 (1.8%)	409 (1.9%)
	(1.9%–2.4%)	(1.3%–2.0%)	(1.4%–2.3%)	(1.1%–2.2%)	(1.7%–2.1%)
Neurological disorder[a]	377 (3.8%)	206 (3.8%)	80 (3.2%)	165 (4.6%)	828 (3.9%)
	(3.4%–4.2%)	(3.4%/4.4%(	(2.5%–3.9%)	(3.9%–5.3%)	(3.6%–4.1%)
Cardiovascular disease[a]	1371 (13.8%)	610 (11.4%)	268 (10.8%)	481 (13.5%)	2730 (12.8%)
	(13.1%–14.5%)	(10.6%–12.3%)	(9.6%–12.1%)	(12.4%–14.6%)	(12.3%–13.2%)
Musculoskeletal disorder[a]	637 (6.4%)	311 (5.8%)	121 (4.9%)	268 (7.5%)	1337 (6.3%)
	(5.9%–6.9%)	(5.2%–6.4%)	(4.0%–5.7%)	(6.7%–8.4%)	(5.9%–6.6%)
Mental health problem[a]	1415 (14.2%)	1032 (19.3%)	357 (14.4%)	647 (18.2%)	3451 (16.2%)
	(13.5%–14.9%)	(18.2–20.4%)	(13.0%–15.8%)	(16.9%–19.5%)	(15.7%–16.7%)
Respiratory disease[a]	398 (4.0%)	342 (6.4%)	116 (4.7%)	211 (5.9%)	1067 (5.0%)
	(3.6%–4.4%)	(5.7%–7.0%)	(3.8%–5.5%)	(5.2%–6.7%)	(4.7%–5.3%)
Digestive disease[a]	415 (4.2%)	259 (4.8%)	84 (3.4%)	153 (4.3%)	911 (4.3%)
	(3.8%–4.6%)	(4.3%–5.4%)	(2.7%–4.1%)	(3.6%–5.0%)	(4.0%–4.5%)
Metabolism-related disease[a]	873 (8.7%)	383 (7.2%)	143 (5.8%)	257 (7.2%)	1656 (7.8%)
	(8.2%–9.3%)	(6.5%–7.8%)	(4.8%–6.7%)	(6.4%–8.1%)	(7.4%–8.1%)
Other[a]	621 (6.2%)	449 (8.4%)	157 (6.3%)	250 (7.0%)	1477 (6.9%)
	(5.8%–6.7%)	(7.6%–9.1%)	(5.4%–7.3%)	(6.2%–7.9%)	(6.6%–7.3%)
No chronic health problems	5885 (59.2%)	3098 (57.9%)	1560 (62.9%)	1954 (54.9%)	12497 (58.6%)
	(58.2%–60.2%)	(56.6%–59.3%)	(61.0%–64.8%)	(53.3%–56.6%)	(57.9%–59.3%)

Table 1 Professional and practice level participation, and patient demographic and clinical characteristics, by center *(Continued)*

Deprivation Index					
I	48 (0.5%)	230 (4.3%)	536 (21.4%)	87 (2.4%)	901 (4.2%)
	(0.3%–0.6%)	(3.7%–4.8%)	(19.8%–3.0%)	(1.9%–2.9%)	(3.9%–4.5%)
II	3456 (34.8%)	176 (3.3%)	1848 (73.8%)	2094 (58.8%)	7574 (35.4%)
	(33.8%–35.7%)	(2.8%–3.8%)	(72.1%–5.5%)	(57.2%–60.4%)	(34.8%–36.1%)
III	4867 (48.9%)	151 (2.8%)	43 (1.7%)	46 (1.3%)	5107 (23.9%)
	(48.0%–49.9%)	(2.4%–3.2%)	(1.2%–2.2%)	(0.9%–1.7%)	(23.3%–24.5%)
IV	907 (9.1%)	167 (3.1%)	35 (1.4%)	289 (8.1%)	1398 (6.6%)
	(8.5%–9.7%)	(2.6%–3.6%)	(0.9%–1.8%)	(7.2%–9.0%	(6.2%–6.95)
V	664 (6.7%)	4637 (86.5%)	43 (1.7%)	1043 (29.3%)	6387 (29.9%)
	(6.2%–7.2%)	(85.6%–87.4%)	(1.2%–2.2%)	(27.8%–30.8%)	(29.3%–30.5%)
Failure to adhere to ≥1 lifestyle recommendation	3206 (84.5%)	3070 (95.7%)	1536 (93.7%)	2693 (89.5%)	10505 (90.2%)
Insufficient physical activity	1979 (53.1%)	2250 (70.8%)	728 (61.9%)	1570 (58.3%)	6527 (60.6%)
Insufficient fruit and vegetable consumption	2507 (67.1%)	2766 (86.9%)	888 (76.6%)	1888 (70.1%)	8049 (74.7%)
Smoker	1009 (27.3%)	1146 (36.6%)	541 (33.8%)	978 (32.6%)	3674 (32.1%)

[a]Dentist and family planning physician
[b]$N = 21323$

Patient level

Reach, Implementation & Maintenance

A total sample of 22459 target patients aged 10 to 65 years old assigned to collaborating practices attended their PHC center at least once during program implementation period. As presented in Table 1, overall, half of the target patients were male (50.6%) and more than a half (55.2%) were young adults 20 to 45 years of age, with 37.9% and 7% of target patients being adults and adolescents, respectively. Approximately 40% of target patients had at least one chronic condition. The most prevalent diagnosed chronic health problems were mental health problems (16.2%) followed by cardiovascular (12.8%) and metabolism- related (7.8%) diseases.

Within centers, a higher percentage of women were present in the sample in center 2, and the age distribution of primary care users was slightly older in center 1. The most distinct characteristic of the populations was socioeconomic status (Table 1), with one of the centers having the vast majority of users in the lowest status (86.5%), while in two other centers users were mostly included in the three highest categories, and in the fourth center users were mostly in the second (59%) and lowest (29%) socioeconomic status categories.

Of the total sample of patients who attended the centers, 11650 (51.9%) had their lifestyle habits assessed (Table 2). The percentage of target patients reached ranged from 36.6 to 82.8% in collaborating centers. Among patients whose lifestyles were assessed, 10505 (90.2% of those assessed) did not adhere to at least one of the three healthy lifestyle recommendations considered and were therefore included in the intervention program (I1; see Table 1). Specifically, 32.1% of patients assessed and found to be eligible for the intervention were smokers, 74.7% did not consume five servings of fruits and vegetables a day, and 60.6% did not meet the recommended levels of aerobic physical activity (moderate intensity physical activity for ≥30 min 5 day/week or vigorous intensity activity for ≥20 min 3 day/week, or a combination of the two). The other 1145 (9.8%) adhered to recommendations on all three healthy lifestyles and were excluded from receiving the intervention. Among the collaborating centers, center 2 had the highest cumulative prevalence of unhealthy lifestyles.

Advice on change in at least one of the lifestyle habits was provided to a third (33.7%; $n = 7433$) of all target patients (I2a) and to 70.7% of included patients found not to adhere to at least one lifestyle recommendation when assessed (I2b) (Table 2). Regarding the areas in which advice was given, diet was the lifestyle on which the highest percentage of patients received advice (24.2% of target patients; 67.4% of those not eating five servings of fruits and vegetables a day). Advice for increasing physical activity was provided to 16.5% of target patients and 56.7% of those not reaching recommended physical activity levels, while advice on smoking cessation was given the least in terms of reaching target patients (10.6% of target patients; 65.1% of those identified as smokers at inclusion).

Regarding lifestyle prescription, 9.7% ($n = 2175$) of all target patients collaboratively designed and then received a printed prescription for at least one healthy lifestyle change (I3a), diet being the lifestyle most frequently addressed (6.4% of all target patients) followed by physical

Table 2 Implementation indicators at target and included patient population levels, by center and lifestyle habit

	Center 1	Center 2	Center 3	Center 4	Total
Target population	10373	5883	2568	3635	22459
A1 at least on 1 lifestyle	3792 (36.6%)	3209 (54.5%)	1640 (63.7%)	3009 (82.8%)	11650 (51.9%)
	(35.6–37.5%)	(53.3–55.8%)	(62.0–65.7%)	(81.5–84.0%)	(51.2–52.5%)
A2 at least on 1 lifestyle	2318 (22.3%)	2170 (36.9%)	809 (31.5%)	2136 (58.7%)	7433 (33.1%)
	(21.5–23.1%)	(35.6–38.1%)	(29.7–33.3%)	(57.2–60.4%)	(32.5–33.7%)
A4 at least on 1 lifestyle	840 (8.1%)	406 (6.9%)	377 (14.7%)	552 (15.2%)	2175 (9.7%)
	(7.6–8.6%)	(6.2–7.5%)	(13.3–16.1%)	(14.0–16.3%)	(9.3–10.1%)
A5 at least on 1 lifestyle	231 (2.2%)	198 (3.4%)	177 (6.9%)	218 (6.0%)	824 (3.7%)
	(1.9–2.5%)	(2.95–3.8%)	(5.9–7.9%)	(5.2–6.7%)	(3.4–3.9%)
Physical Activity (PA)					
A1_PA	3727 (35.9%)	3176 (54%)	1176 (45.8%)	2692 (74.1%)	10771 (48.0%)
	(35.0–36.8%)	(52.7–55.3%)	(43.9–47.7%)	(72.6–75.5%)	(47.3–48.6%)
A2_PA	1097 (10.6%)	1148 (19.5%)	386 (15%)	1071 (29.5%)	3702 (16.5%)
	(10.0–11.2%)	(18.5–20.5%)	(13.6–16.4%)	(28.0–30.9%)	(16.0–17.0%)
A4_PA	315 (3%)	123 (2.1%)	161 (6.3%)	194 (5.3%)	793 (3.5%)
	(2.7–3.4%)	(1.7–2.4%)	(5.3–7.2%)	(4.6–6.1%)	(3.3–3.8%)
A5_PA	50 (0.5%)	38 (0.6%)	68 (2.6%)	43 (1.2%)	199 (0.9%)
	(0.3–0.6%)	(0.4–0.8%)	(2.0–3.2%)	(0.8–1.5%)	(0.8–1.0%)
Diet (DT)					
A1_DT	3737 (36%)	3182 (54.1%)	1159 (45.1%)	2693 (74.1%)	10771 (48.0%)
	(35.1–36.9%)	(52.8–55.4%)	(43.2–47.0%)	(72.7–75.5%)	(47.3–48.6%)
A2_DT	1688 (16.3%)	1848 (31.4%)	486 (18.9%)	1407 (38.7%)	5429 (24.2%)
	(15.6–17.0%)	(30.2–32.6%)	(17.4–20.4%)	(37.1–40.3%)	(23.6–24.7%)
A4_DT	549 (5.3%)	319 (5.4%)	217 (8.5%)	353 (9.7%)	1438 (6.4%)
	(4.9–5.7%)	(4.8–6.0%)	(7.4–9.5%)	(8.7–10.7%)	(6.1–6.7%)
A5_DT	154 (1.5%)	176 (3%)	110 (4.3%)	144 (3.9%)	584 (2.6%)
	(1.2–1.7%)	(2.5–3.4%)	(3.5–5.1%)	(3.3–4.6%)	(2.4–2.8%)
Tobacco (TB)					
A1_TB	3698 (35.6%)	3133 (53.3%)	1599 (62.3%)	2997 (82.4%)	11427 (50.9%)
	(34.7–36.6%)	(52.0–54.5%)	(60.4–64.1%)	(81.2–83.7%)	(50.2–51.5%)
A2_TB	652 (6.3%)	836 (14.2%)	227 (8.8%)	676 (18.6%)	2391 (10.6%)
	(5.8–6.7%)	(13.3–15.1%)	(7.7–9.9%)	(17.3–19.7%)	(10.2–11.0%)
A4_TB	99 (1%)	60 (1%)	40 (1.6%)	67 (1.7%)	266 (1.2%)
	(0.8–1.1%)	(0.8–1.3%)	(1.1–2.0%)	(1.4–2.3%)	(1.0–1.3%)
A5_TB	42 (0.4%)	17 (0.3%)	4 (0.2%)	34 (0.9%)	97 (0.4%)
	(0.3–0.5%)	(0.1–0.4%)	(0.0–0.3%)	(0.6–1.2%)	(0.3–0.5%)

Note: A1 refers to Assess; A2 refers to Advise; A4 refers to Assist with a prescription for change; and A5 refers to arrange follow-up with a repeat prescription

activity and smoking cessation (3.5% and 1.25% of all target patients, respectively). From those included in the program with unhealthy lifestyles, 20.7% received a prescription for at least one lifestyle change (I3b), while 29.3% of those who received advice regarding lifestyle changes finally ended up designing and receiving a personalized lifestyle change plan (I3c). Further, of those who received dietary advice, 26.5% were also prescribed dietary changes, while prescriptions regarding increasing physical activity and smoking cessation were provided to 21.4% and 11.1% of those advised, respectively.

Only 3.7% of the target population received repeat prescriptions and consequently the full 5 A's intervention over the course of the program (I4a), again with diet being the lifestyle addressed in most cases (2.6% for diet; 1% for physical activity and 0.4% for smoking cessation). The percentage of patients with a repeat prescriptions rose to 7.8% and 37.9% in included patients' (I4b) and in those with a previous prescription (I4c), respectively. Multiple-lifestyle intervention indicators were as follows: 4.7% of the target population ($n = 1057$) received advice on all three lifestyles considered and 12.7% ($n = 2861$) received it on two. This corresponded to only 35 patients who attended the centers (0.15%) receiving a prescription to change physical activity, diet and smoking habits, while in 609 (2.7%) modifications in two aspects of patient lifestyles were planned and prescribed.

Figure 1 illustrates the cumulative exposure of patients to the main intervention components in the four collaborating centers over the 2-year program implementation period. There was a significant between-center difference in the monthly rate for assessment (A1), advice (A2) and prescription of a healthy lifestyle change (A4) (Log-rank test of equality for survival distributions < 0.001). Furthermore, 'center' did not satisfy the proportionality assumption ($P <$ 0.001 for the interaction between center and time) and hence was included in an extended Cox model as a time-dependent variable (Table 3). As an example, during the first 3 months, compared to the reference center (center 1), exposure to assessment was 3.42, 8 and 6 times more likely in centers 2, 3 and 4, respectively. Patients of these three centers were more than 4 times more likely than those in center 1 to be exposed to advice, and 2 to 4.22 times more likely to receive a prescription for lifestyle change.

With respect to the other variables included in the model, most patient personal and clinical characteristics where also associated with the implementation of the different intervention components (Table 3). Specifically, the hazard ratio for exposure to components of the healthy lifestyle promotion intervention was higher in women than in men (AHR of being assessed in men: 0.83; 95% CI: 0.80–0.86) and increased with patient age, 1.05-fold for every 5 years of age. Some of the chronic conditions were also related to exposure to intervention components. The hazard ratio for exposure to assessment, advice and prescription for lifestyle change was significantly higher in those with cardiovascular, musculoskeletal, respiratory, digestive, and metabolism-related diseases, among other conditions, than in patients without these conditions. Among these chronic health problems, cardiovascular diseases had the strongest association with being assessed (AHR: 1.41; 95% CI: 1.33 to 1.49), advised (HR: 1.51; 95% CI: 1.42 to 1.62), and receiving a prescription for lifestyle change (AHR: 1.87; 95% CI: 1.67 to 2.09).

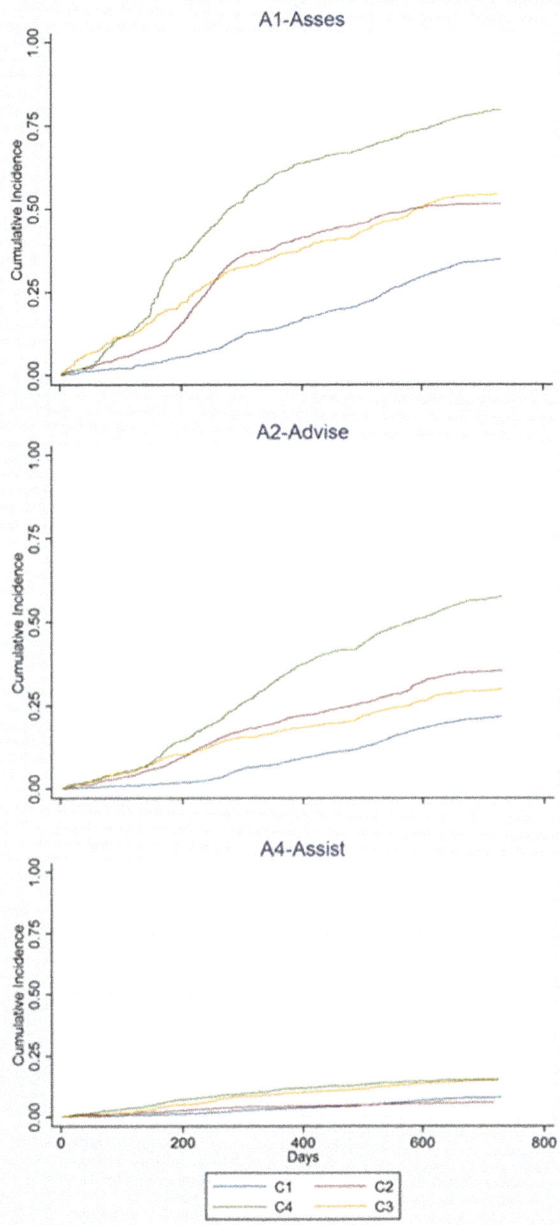

Fig. 1 Cumulative exposure of patients to the main intervention components in the four collaborating centers over the 2-year program implementation period

Discussion

Results of this pilot study showed that the PVS implementation strategy was feasible and achieved modest-to-good improvement in clinical practice regarding adoption, reach, and implementation of an evidence-based healthy lifestyle promotion intervention in the context of routine primary care. The main contribution of this study is the description of the significant heterogeneity observed in the assessed process indicators associated with lifestyle habits, patient characteristics, settings and implementation timeframe.

Overall, rates of adoption within centers were high in the three main professional categories considered, family physicians, nurses and administrative personnel. During the 2-year period of program implementation, more than the half of all the primary care users aged 10 to 65 years

Table 3 Characteristics of target population associated with exposure to the main intervention components: Assessment of lifestyles (A1), Advice on lifestyle change (A2), and Prescription of lifestyle change (A4)

Variables			Adjusted Hazard Ratio (95% CI)		
			Assessed (A1)	Advised (A2)	Prescribed (A4)
Age (unit = 5 years)			1.05 (1.04–1.06)	1.04 (1.03–1.05)	1.04 (1.02–1.06)
Sex		Female	1.00	1.00	1.00
		Male	0.83 (0.80–0.86)	0.84 (0.80–0.88)	0.68 (0.63–0.74)
Cardiovascular disease		No	1.00	1.00	1.00
		Yes	1.41 (1.33–1.49)	1.51 (1.42–1.62)	1.87 (1.67–2.09)
Musculoskeletal disorder		No	1.00	1.00	1.00
		Yes	1.19 (1.11–1.28)	1.15 (1.05–1.25)	1.20 (1.04–1.39)
Mental health problem		No	1.00	1.00	1.00
		Yes	1.09 (1.04–1.14)	1.18 (1.11–1.25)	1.15 (1.03–1.28)
Respiratory disease		No	1.00	1.00	1.00
		Yes	1.25 (1.15–1.35)	1.36 (1.24–1.49)	1.51 (1.29–1.77)
Digestive disease		No	1.00	1.00	1.00
		Yes	1.12 (1.03–1.23)	1.12 (1.01–1.24)	1.25 (1.06–1.49)
Metabolism-related disease		No	1.00	1.00	1.00
		Yes	1.25 (1.17–1.34)	1.26 (1.16–1.36)	1.32 (1.16–1.51)
Other chronic health problem		No	1.00	1.00	–
		Yes	1.13 (1.05–1.21)	1.14 (1.05–1.24)	–
Deprivation Index		High	1.00	1.00	1.00
		Medium	1.18 (1.10–1.27)	1.17 (1.10–1.25)	1.14 (0.98–1.33)
		Low	1.16 (1.10–1.22)	1.19 (1.11–1.27)	1.25 (1.11–1.42)
Center		Center 1	1.00	1.00	1.00
	0–3 months	Center 2	3.42 (3.00–3.90)	4.23 (3.47–5.16)	3.24 (2.47–4.25)
		Center 3	8.54 (7.54–9.66)	5.04 (4.07–6.25)	2.06 (1.46–2.89)
		Center 4	6.19 (5.48–7.00)	4.54 (3.70–5.56)	4.22 (3.25–5.47)
	3–6 months	Center 2	2.97 (2.52–3.48)	7.43 (5.77–9.56)	2.62 (1.78–3.88)
		Center 3	3.55 (2.93–4.30)	6.91 (5.22–9.15)	6.55 (4.57–9.38)
		Center 4	8.96 (7.78–10.32)	10.59 (8.27–13.57)	6.38 (4.54–8.97)
	6–12 months	Center 2	4.42 (4.02–4.85)	2.81 (2.49–3.18)	0.95 (0.73–1.23)
		Center 3	2.37 (2.08–2.70)	1.43 (1.20–1.69)	2.16 (1.71–2.73)
		Center 4	5.69 (5.17–6.27)	4.45 (3.97–4.99)	2.03 (1.64–2.52)
	12–24 months	Center 2	1.01 (0.92–1.12)	1.52 (1.37–1.68)	0.41 (0.32–0.53)
		Center 3	1.26 (1.12–1.42)	1.01 (0.89–1.15)	1.24 (1.01–1.52)
		Center 4	2.50 (2.27–2.75)	2.91 (2.65–3.19)	0.91 (0.75–1.11)

old were reached in the four centers in terms of having their lifestyles assessed. This level of reach should be considered notably high, given that the program has been implemented in "real world" conditions in primary care, among those attending routine appointments, and thus represents general and unselected sample of the primary care population for the groups covered. Other studies evaluating the feasibility of lifestyle screening in routine context have attained reach rates ranging from 49.6 to 86.7%, though these figures have been attained in shorter exposure periods or/and with limited sample sizes [22–24].

Research on healthy lifestyle promotion in clinical settings has established that intensive counseling in the form of advice and the use of behavioral change techniques are some of the active components that help individuals initiate and maintain health-related behavior change [7]. The PVS implementation strategy aimed to enhance the integration and feasibility of the execution of these effective intervention components

[9]. PVS centers have been able to provide advice on change in at least one of the lifestyles considered to a third of patients who attended the centers and almost 10% of these patients have collaboratively designed and then received a printed prescription for at least one lifestyle change. Other implementation trials aiming to improve the promotion of healthy lifestyles have also shown positive results in terms of increasing screening and intervention rates [25–29]. However, as observed in other studies [30, 31], a full 5 A's intervention is rarely performed, only 4% of patients receiving all components in relation to at least one aspect of their lifestyle.

These process and performance indicators regarding adoption, reach and implementation varied between lifestyle habits, patient characteristics and centers. First, regarding lifestyle habits, higher percentages of patients received advice and a prescription for change in the case of physical activity and diet once these had been assessed, while smoking habits has been the lifestyle most commonly assessed but with the lowest rates of advice and prescription. This variability in the priority given to the healthy lifestyles was a result of the implementation strategy used, which sought to help collaborating centers adapt the intervention program to their actual context and resources in order to enhance its integration in routine service delivery in PHC. In this adaptation process, they were instructed to prioritize both the lifestyles to be addressed and strategies to re-organize the delivery of preventive actions within centers. Considering that 90% of patients assessed in this study failed to adhere to at least one of the lifestyle recommendations considered, it seems reasonable to apply some sort of prioritization strategy to deal with work overload and maximize feasibility of a population-level healthy lifestyle promotion program in the context of routine primary care. Further research is warranted as to identify what are the best cut-off points for attaining the optimal balance between feasibility and workload when identifying individuals in need of a healthy lifestyle promotion intervention.

Second, the delivery of health promotion actions has been found to be associated with various personal and clinical characteristics of the targeted population. Regarding patients' intra-personal characteristics, the likelihood of being assessed, receiving advice and being prescribed lifestyle changes increased with age and was higher in women than men. Those with chronic health conditions (e.g., cardiovascular disease) were also more likely to receive each of the intervention components. A possible explanation for these associations is that health care providers have targeted and prioritized their healthy lifestyle promotion actions to those more likely to face fewer obstacles to changing their lifestyle, such as, older patients who may have more free time (as they are working less or retired completely and have fewer obligations); or to those that would potentially benefit the most, such as those with a chronic health problem. Indeed, selective and targeted counseling of patients prioritizing among other factors patient with known health risks or readiness for change has been documented [32] and is currently recommended in order to maximize their impact [33, 34].

Moreover, factors beyond personal characteristics, such as socioeconomic status also influenced the implementation of intervention components. Specifically, each of the main intervention components were more likely to be received by those with higher socioeconomic status. Therefore, it seems that intra- and extra-personal characteristics of target populations may also explain variability in the integration and implementation of healthy lifestyle promotion and the feasibility of this type of intervention [32, 35].

Third, PHC center has been observed to be a great source of variability in program adoption, reach and implementation indicators. Overall, relatively high rates of adoption by staff have been attained in all the centers. This is not surprising given that written commitment from the majority of staff within the different categories was a requirement for study participation. However, actual rates of involvement and contribution differed: while in one of the centers all staff committed to participate and did so, in other centers complete participation was not attained. These rates of adoption may have a direct impact on both the actual reach of the program and the implementation of intervention components as could be observed in the present study. On the one hand, in the center in which all staff participated, more than 80% of the target population was reached in terms of the identification of at least one healthy lifestyle, and almost 60% received advice on lifestyle changes, as well as the highest percentage of target users (comparing with other centers) received a prescription of a lifestyle change plan. Additionally, within collaborating professionals, all of them actually showed good performance in terms of indicators of implementation. On the other hand, the center with the lowest rates of adoption obtained the poorest rates of implementation of intervention components at practices and patient levels (e.g., 37% of target patients assessed and only 2 out of 11 collaborating practices assessed at least 50% of target users seen during the program implementation period).

Furthermore, rates of adoption by staff and reach at the patient level may have contributed substantially to the observed variability in implementation rates at the center level. Specifically, the likelihood of being exposed to intervention components of advice and prescription for lifestyle change was 4 times more likely in the center with the highest rates of adoption and reach than the center with the lowest rates of adoption and reach. The likelihood of exposure to the intervention program in the other two centers with intermediate rates of adoption and reach was also significantly higher than in the center with the lowest rates. In this sense, based on the actual adoption and implementation of intervention components across collaborating health centers, we may distinguish three levels of implementation performance: high, medium and low.

Variability in program adoption by professionals, program reach and implementation indicators between different sites has also been reported in other implementation trials [24, 36]. Centers each have different contexts and thus implementation strategies must be targeted and adapted to those specific contexts. Even after a hypothetical adaptation, results and products would be context specific. That is, context is crucial, meaning that interventions may be implemented in different ways in different settings and thus outcomes may also vary [37–39].

And finally, another important finding of the present study is that the sustainability or the extent of exposure to intervention components over time differed between centers and varied thorough the implementation period within centers, probably reflecting intermittent efforts and continuous adaptation to the multiple unstable contextual and organizational factors in the centers, to the innovation itself, the providers, the processes involved and the interaction of all of these factors [40–42]. We should recognize that in the present implementation study competition with other initiatives, in particular those imposed by health system management, structural changes and staff movements, lack of ongoing training of staff, and technical problems with the information and communication tool may all have hindered ideal implementation of intervention components throughout the implementation period [see accompanying paper by Martinez et al.].

The present study has several limitations. First, the process evaluation refers to a prospective cohort study performed in four selected centers and the observational nature of the study together with the absence of a comparison group mean that it is not possible to attribute the results obtained to the implementation strategy alone. Although collaborating centers are apparently diverse, they may not be representative of all PHC centers in our health service. In addition, though we have described some characteristics regarding representativeness (in terms of PHC size and composition, socioeconomic status of catchment populations, and so on), missed information regarding other specific characteristics of the context may hinder interpretation of results. Though the external validity of the study may be questioned, implementation trials aim to conduct a broad evaluation of the translation of proven-efficacy interventions into routine care, assessing results in heterogeneous, unselected populations and real-life clinical settings [43, 44]. Another limitation relates to difficulties interpreting the results obtained, especially those concerning variability between centers/settings and the nature of changes or reasons for intermittent sustainability. Consequently, a qualitative inquiry study has also been performed to explore staff perceptions of the program implementation and its results [see accompanying paper by Martinez et al.].

The main strengths of the study are that it has been conducted at the population level and the quality of data assessed, as these were recorded in and subsequently retrieved from an established electronic health record.

Conclusions

Implementation research must be the priority in order to first transform our health systems into continuously learning organizations and consequently enact the final step of translating scientific knowledge to real-life clinical settings in an effort to close the translational gap. In doing so, engagement of all stakeholders is crucial, especially of those who interact with patients and are the actual providers of health care. However, contexts are heterogeneous and unstable and an adequate program adoption and implementation may not always be achieved. Identifying the factors behind implementation heterogeneity may help us to tailor implementation strategies, but comparative effectiveness research is needed to determine the best theoretically grounded and operationalized implementation strategies to improve clinical practice.

Abbreviations

5 A's: Ask, Advise, Agree, Assist, and Arrange follow-up; A1: Assessment of healthy lifestyles; A2: Advice on healthy lifestyle change; A4: Prescription of a healthy lifestyle change; AHR: Adjusted hazard ratio; CI: 95% confidence interval; DI: Deprivation Index; I1: Included: percentage of target patients whose lifestyle habits were assessed and included because they failed to adhere to at least one healthy lifestyle recommendation; I2a: The percentage of target patients who received advice; I2b: The percentage of included patients who received advice; I3a: The percentage of target patients who received a prescription for lifestyle change; I3b: The percentage of included patients who received a prescription for lifestyle change; I3c: The percentage of advised patients who received a prescription for lifestyle change; I4a: The percentage of target patients who received a repeat prescription related to the same aspect of their lifestyle; I4b: The percentage of included patients who received a repeat prescription related to the same aspect of their lifestyle.; I4c: The percentage of prescribed patients who received a repeat prescription related to the same aspect of their lifestyle.; PHC: Primary Health Care; PREDIMED: *Prevención con Dieta Mediterranea* study; PVS: *Prescribe Vida Saludable* study; RE-AIM: Reach, Efficacy, Adoption, Implementation, Maintenance framework; UIAPB: The Primary Care Research Unit of Bizkaia

Acknowledgements

We gratefully acknowledge all the PVS participants who contributed to the focus groups and the representatives of the public health department who accompanied the facilitator in the interviews (see Additional file 1: Members of the PVS group).

Funding
The PVS project was supported by the Carlos III Health Institute of the Spanish Ministry of Economy and Competitiveness, co-financed by the European Regional Development Fund (research grant PS09/01461), the Health Department of the Basque Government (research grants 2007111009, 2009111072, and 2011111145), the Basque Foundation for Social and Health Care Innovation (grant CA-2012-086), the Basque Research Center in Chronicity-Kronikgune (grant 11/056), and the Spanish Primary Care Research Network for Prevention and Health Promotion (redIAPP RD06/0018/0018 and RD12/0005/0010). The funding body had no role in the design of the study and collection, analysis, and interpretation of data and in writing the manuscript.

Authors' contributions
GG and AS conceived the idea and are the study guarantors. They are primarily responsible for the study design and planning, coordination and supervision, analysis and interpretation of results. AS and GG were responsible for the analysis of results and drafted the manuscript. JMC and HP collaborated in the study design, obtained funding, and were responsible for study coordination. MHC, EP, JM, and EG were local leaders at the primary care centers and contributed to implementation and interpretation of the process. All contributors have critically reviewed the manuscript and approved this version submitted for publication to Implementation Science.

Competing interests
The authors declare that they have no competing interests.

Author details
[1]Primary Care Research Unit of Bizkaia, Basque Healthcare Service - Osakidetza, BioCruces Health Research Institute, Luis Power 18, 4ª planta, E48014 Bilbao, Spain. [2]Deusto Primary Health Care Center, Bilbao-Basurto Integrated Care Organization– Osakidetza, BioCruces Health Research Institute, Luis Power 18, E48014 Bilbao, Spain. [3]La Merced Primary Health Care Center, Bilbao-Basurto Integrated Care Organization – Osakidetza, Luis Iraurrizaga 1, 48003 Bilbao, Spain. [4]Sondika Primary Health Care Center, Uribe Integrated Care Organization – Osakidetza, Lehendakari Agirre 41, 48160 Sondika, Spain. [5]Beasain Primary Health Care Center, Goieri-Alto Urola Integrated Care Organization – Osakidetza, Bernedo s/n, 20200 Beasain, Spain. [6]Matiena Primary Health Care Center, Barrualde-Galdakao Integrated Care Organization – Osakidetza, BioCruces Health Research Institute, Trañabarren 13-Bajo, 48220 Abadiño, Spain.

References
1. Peters DH, Adam T, Alonge O, Agyepong IA, Tran N. Implementation research: what it is and how to do it. BMJ. 2013;347:f6753.
2. Neta G, Glasgow RE, Carpenter CR, Grimshaw JM, Rabin BA, Fernandez ME, Brownson RC. A Framework for Enhancing the Value of Research for Dissemination and Implementation. Am J Public Health. 2015;105(1):49–57.
3. Medical Research Council. Developing and evaluating complex interventions: new guidance. London: Medical Research Council; 2008.
4. Saunders RP, Evans MH, Joshi P. Developing a process-evaluation plan for assessing health promotion program implementation: a how-to guide. Health Promot Pract. 2005;6(2):134–47.
5. Grant A, Treweek S, Dreischulte T, Foy R, Guthrie B. Process evaluations for cluster-randomised trials of complex interventions: a proposed framework for design and reporting. Trials. 2013;14:15.
6. Steckler A, Linnan L. Process Evaluation for Public Health Interventions and Research. San Francisco: Jossey-Bass; 2002.
7. Grandes G, Sánchez A, Cortada JM, Balague L, Calderon C, Arrazola A, Vergara I, Millan E. For the "Prescribe Vida Saludable" group, Is integration of healthy lifestyle promotion into primary care feasible? Discussion and consensus sessions between clinicians and researchers. BMC Health Serv Res. 2008;8:213.
8. Medical Research Council. A framework for development and evaluation of complex interventions to improve health. London: Medical Research Council; 2000.
9. Sanchez A, Grandes G, Cortada JM, Pombo H, Balague L, Calderon C. Modelling innovative interventions for optimising healthy lifestyle promotion in primary health care: 'Prescribe Vida Saludable' phase I research protocol. BMC Health Serv Res. 2009;9:103.
10. Bowen DJ, Kreuter M, Spring B, Cofta-Woerpel L, Linnan L, Weiner D, Bakken S, Kaplan CP, Squiers L, Fabrizio C, Fernandez M. How we design feasibility studies. Am J Prev Med. 2009;36(5):452–7.
11. Goldstein MG, Whitlock EP, DePue J. Planning Committee of the Addressing Multiple Behavioral Risk Factors in Primary Care Project. Multiple behavioral risk factor interventions in primary care. Summary of research evidence. Am J Prev Med. 2004;27:61–79.
12. Sanchez A, Bully P, Martinez C, Grandes G. Effectiveness of physical activity promotion interventions in primary care: A review of reviews. Prev Med. 2015;76(Suppl):S56–67.
13. Richards J, Hillsdon M, Thorogood M, Foster C. Face-to-face interventions for promoting physical activity. Cochrane Database Syst Rev. 2013;9, CD010392.
14. Bhattarai N, Prevost AT, Wright AJ, Charlton J, Rudisill C, Gulliford MC. Effectiveness of interventions to promote healthy diet inprimary care: systematic review and meta-analysis of randomised controlled trials. BMC Public Health. 2013;13:1203.
15. Stead LF, Buitrago D, Preciado N, Sanchez G, Hartmann-Boyce J, Lancaster T. Physician advice for smoking cessation. Cochrane Database Syst Rev. 2013;5, CD000165.
16. Schröder H, Fitó M, Estruch R, Martínez-González MA, et al. A short screener is valid for assessing Mediterranean diet adherence among older Spanish men and women. J Nutr. 2011;141(6):1140–5.
17. de la Fuente-Arrillaga C, Vázquez-Ruiz Z, Bes-Rastrollo M, et al. Reproducibility of a food frequency questionnaire (FFQ) validated in Spain. Public Health Nutr. 2010;13:1364–72.
18. Orueta JF, García-Álvarez A, García-Goñi M, Paolucci F, Nuño-Solinís R. Prevalence and costs of multimorbidity by deprivation levels in the Basque country: a population based study using health administrative databases. PLoS ONE. 2014;9(2):e89787.
19. Domínguez-Berjón MF, Borrell C, Cano-Serral G, Esnaola S, Nolasco A, et al. Constructing a deprivation index based on census data in large Spanish cities (the MEDEA project). Gac Sanit. 2008;22:179–87.
20. Glasgow RE, Vogt TM, Boles SM. Evaluating the public health impact of health promotion interventions: the RE-AIM framework. Am J Public Health. 1999;89(9):1322–7.
21. Cox DR. 1972) Regression models and life tables (with discussion. J R Stat Soc. 1972;34:187–220.
22. Krist AH, Phillips SM, Sabo RT, Balasubramanian BA, Heurtin-Roberts S, Ory MG, Johnson SB, Sheinfeld-Gorin SN, Estabrooks PA, Ritzwoller DP, Glasgow RE, MOHR Study Group. Adoption, reach, implementation, and maintenance of a behavioral and mental health assessment in primary care. Ann Fam Med. 2014;12(6):525–33.
23. Krist AH, Woolf SH, Frazier CO, Johnson RE, Rothemich SF, Wilson DB, Devers KJ, Kerns JW. An electronic linkage system for health behavior counseling effect on delivery of the 5A's. Am J Prev Med. 2008;35(5):S350–8.
24. Rodriguez HP, Glenn BA, Olmos TT, Krist AH, Shimada SL, Kessler R, Heurtin-Roberts S, Bastani R. Real-world implementation and outcomes of health behavior and mental health assessment. J Am Board Fam Med. 2014;27(3):356–66.
25. Aspy CB, Mold JW, Thompson DM, Blondell RD, Landers PS, Reilly KE, Wright-Eakers L. Integrating screening and interventions for unhealthy behaviors into primary care practices. Am J Prev Med. 2008;35(5 Suppl): S373–80.
26. Goodwin MA, Zyzanski SJ, Zronek S, Ruhe M, Weyer SM, Konrad N, Esola D, Stange KC. A clinical trial of tailored office systems for preventive service delivery. The Study to Enhance Prevention by Understanding Practice (STEP-UP). Am J Prev Med. 2001;21(1):20–8.
27. Hogg W, Lemelin J, Moroz I, Soto E, Russell G. Improving prevention in primary care: Evaluating the sustainability of outreach facilitation. Can Fam Physician. 2008;54(5):712–20.
28. Grunfeld E, Manca D, Moineddin R, Thorpe KE, Hoch JS, Campbell-Scherer D, Meaney C, Rogers J, Beca J, Krueger P, Mamdani M, BETTER Trial Investigators. Improving chronic disease prevention and screening in primary care: results of the BETTER pragmatic cluster randomized controlled trial. BMC Fam Pract. 2013;14:175.

29. Harris MF, Chan BC, Laws RA, Williams AM, Davies GP, Jayasinghe UW, Fanaian M, Orr N, Milat A, CN SNAP Project Team. The impact of a brief lifestyle intervention delivered by generalist community nurses (CN SNAP trial). BMC Public Health. 2013;13:375.
30. Carroll JK, Antognoli E, Flocke SA. Evaluation of physical activity counselling in primary care using direct observation of the 5As. Ann Fam Med. 2011; 9(5):416–22.
31. Sherson EA, Yakes Jimenez E, Katalanos N. A review of the use of the 5 A's model for weight loss counselling: differences between physician practice and patient demand. Fam Pract. 2014;31(4):389–98.
32. Bock C, Diehl K, Schneider S, Diehm C, Litaker D. Behavioral counseling for cardiovascular disease prevention in primary care settings: a systematic review of practice and associated factors. Med Care Res Rev. 2012;69(5):495–518.
33. Lin JS, O'Connor E, Whitlock EP, Beil TL. Behavioral counseling to promote physical activity and a healthful diet to prevent cardiovascular disease in adults: a systematic review for the U.S. Preventive Services Task Force. Ann Intern Med. 2010;153:736–50.
34. Grandes G, Sánchez A, Torcal J, Sánchez-Pinilla RO, Lizarraga K, Serra J, PEPAF Group. Targeting physical activity promotion in general practice: characteristics of inactive patients and willingness to change. BMC Public Health. 2008;8:172.
35. Damschroder LJ, Aron DC, Keith RE, Kirsh SR, Alexander JA, Lowery JC. Fostering implementation of health services research findings into practice: a consolidated framework for advancing implementation science. Implement Sci. 2009;4:50.
36. Wilcox S, Parra-Medina D, Felton GM, Poston MB, McClain A. Adoption and implementation of physical activity and dietary counseling by community health center providers and nurses. J Phys Act Health. 2010;7(5):602–12.
37. Dickinson LM, Dickinson WP, Nutting PA, Fisher L, Harbrecht M, Crabtree BF, Glasgow RE, West DR. Practice context affects efforts to improve diabetes care for primary care patients: a pragmatic cluster randomized trial. J Gen Intern Med. 2015;30(4):476–82.
38. Hawe P, Shiell A, Riley T. Complex interventions: how "out of control" can a randomised controlled trial be? BMJ. 2004;328(7455):1561–3.
39. Datta J, Petticrew M. Challenges to evaluating complex interventions: a content analysis of published papers. BMC Public Health. 2013;13:568.
40. Wiltsey Stirman S, Kimberly J, Cook N, Calloway A, Castro F, Charns M. The sustainability of new programs and innovations: a review of the empirical literature and recommendations for future research. Implement Sci. 2012;7:17.
41. Durlak JA, DuPre EP. Implementation matters: a review of research on the influence of implementation on program outcomes and the factors affecting implementation. Am J Community Psychol. 2008;41(3–4):327–50.
42. Greenhalgh T, Macfarlane F, Barton-Sweeney C, Woodard F. "If we build it, will it stay?" A case study of the sustainability of whole-system change in London. Milbank Q. 2012;90(3):516–47.
43. Glasgow RE, Lichtenstein E, Marcus AC. Why don't we see more translation of health promotion research to practice? Rethinking the efficacy-to-effectiveness transition. Am J Public Health. 2003;93:1261–7.
44. Pinnock H, Epiphaniou E, Taylor SJ. Phase IV implementation studies. The forgotten finale to the complex intervention methodology framework. Ann Am Thorac Soc. 2014;11(2):S118–22.

21

Strengthening general practice/family medicine in Europe—advice from professionals from 30 European countries

Natalia Zarbailov[1], Stefan Wilm[2], Howard Tandeter[3], Francesco Carelli[4] and Mette Brekke[5*]

Abstract

Background: Substantial variations are still to be found in the strength of general practice/family medicine (GP/FM) across Europe regarding governance, workforce competence and performance, as well as academic development and position. Governments are encouraged by the WHO to secure high quality primary health care to their population, a necessity for reaching the goal "Health for all". The present study aimed at investigating the opinions of council members of the European Academy of Teachers in General Practice (EURACT) on necessary actions to strengthen the position of GP/FM in their country.

Methods: The study used a mixed methods exploratory sequential design. EURACT representatives from 32 European countries first participated in brain-storming on how to strengthen GP/FM in Europe. Later, representatives from 37 countries were asked to individually score the relevance of the proposed actions for their country on a 9-point Likert scale. They were also asked to evaluate the status of GP/FM in their country on four dimensions.

Results: Respondents from 30 European countries returned complete questionnaires. To build and secure GP/FM as an academic discipline comprising teaching and research was seen as essential, regardless the present status of GP/FM in the respective country. To build GP/FM as a specialty on the same level as other specialties was seen as important in countries where GP/FM held a strong or medium strong position. The importance of common learning objectives and a defined bibliography were stated by respondents from countries where GP/FM presently has a weak position.

Conclusions: In order to strengthen GP/FM throughout Europe, EURACT and other professional organizations must establish common goals and share expertise between countries. To influence decision makers through information on cost-effectiveness of a GP/FM-based health care system is also important.

Keywords: General practice, Family medicine, Europe, EURACT, Quality improvement, Mixed methods

Background

Primary Health Care was identified as central to achieve the goal "Health for all" launched by WHO at the Alma Ata conference in 1978 [1]. Thirty years later WHO encouraged all countries to orient their health care systems towards a strengthened primary health care [2], with general practice/family medicine (GP/FM) as core of primary medical care. There is increasing evidence that a strong primary health care system is more likely to provide better population health, more equity in health throughout the population, and better use of economic resources, compared to systems oriented towards specialty care [3–5].

In the "WHO global strategy on integrated people-centered health services 2016–2026" [6] building strong primary care-based systems is highlighted as a necessity. The document states that strong primary care services are essential for reaching the entire population and guaranteeing universal access to services. This includes ensuring adequate funding, appropriate training, and connections to other services and sectors [6]. The strength of GP/FM in a country can be assessed by outcome measures covering several dimensions: governance, economic conditions, workforce development, accessibility, comprehensiveness,

* Correspondence: mette.brekke@medisin.uio.no
[5]Department of General Practice, Institute of Health and Society, University of Oslo, P.O. Box 1132 018, Blindern, Norway

continuity, and coordination of care [7]. How GP/FM is defined as a clinical specialty, if and how it is taught on undergraduate level in medical schools, as well as its position in research, are also important markers of its strength and position [8, 9].

Substantial variations are still to be found in the strength of GP/FM across Europe – regarding governance, workforce development and performance [7], as well as academic development and position [10]. It is still possible to graduate from a European medical school without having learned the principles of GP/FM and without any clinical teaching in a GP's office [10].

Each country is responsible for improving development of primary care and securing and sustaining its position. European professional organizations should facilitate such an improvement, like the European Academy of Teachers in General Practice/Family Medicine (EURACT) [11] did by its statement to encourage all medical faculties and departments across Europe to implement teaching and training programs of GP/FM into their curriculum [9] and to develop a minimal core curriculum [12]. EURACT was launched in March, 1992 as the European educational wing and network organization of World Organization of Family Doctors (WONCA) [13]. EURACT has over 800 members in nearly 40 countries. Its overall aim is to foster and maintain high standards of care in European GP/FM by promoting GP/FM as a discipline by learning and teaching. Council members are elected among the EURACT members in each country. The present study aimed at investigating these council members' opinions on necessary actions to strengthen the position of GP/FM in their country – in order to get a European overview.

Methods

Study design

The study used a mixed methods exploratory sequential design [14]. This design begins with a qualitative data collection and analysis phase, which builds to the subsequent quantitative phase. Participants first launched possible actions needed to strengthen GP/FM in Europe through brain-storming. Later, they individually scored the relevance of the proposed actions for their country on a questionnaire.

Participants

The participants were GPs from 32 (brain-storming process) or 30 (questionnaire study) European countries plus Israel, who at the time of the study were elected council members of EURACT [11]. EURACT council members are elected by and out of all EURACT members in their respective country. As EURACT is an organization dedicated to teaching in GP/FM, their members are mainly experienced academic GPs involved in undergraduate teaching, vocational training and/or continuous medical education. Most – but not all – also work part time in clinical practice and most have research experience. To be elected as a EURACT council member requires that the person stands a trusted and respected position among academic GPs in his/her country.

The election period is 3 years, but may be extended. At present, EURACT has all together 38 council members from 37 European countries plus Israel. Out of these, 15 are men and 23 are women, and most are between 40 and 65 years of age. These council members represent countries with a great variety of GP/FM's academic development and position as well as in the profession's strength in the health care system.

Data collection

Data collection consisted of a brain-storming process and a subsequent questionnaire study and took place from October 2013 until December 2014. The EURACT council meets twice a year on different locations. During a meeting in October 2013 in Tirana, Albania [15], the council members were asked to brain-storm in two consecutive sessions around the question: "Which activities to strengthen general practice/family medicine are relevant for European countries?" Representatives from 32 countries out of the 37 member countries (by Oct 2013) were present at the meeting and participated in the brain-storming. The research question, the design of the study and the sessions were planned in advance by the authors, whereas the other council members were not informed about the content of the study beforehand. The sessions took place in plenary and were conducted by two of the authors (HT, NZ).

All council members were active in the process. The facilitating question was "Which activities to strengthen general practice/ family medicine are relevant for *your* country?" The answers of the participants were protocoled verbatim and generated a list of more than 60 possible actions.

The two facilitators revised the list and agreed upon doublets, which were deleted. Otherwise, the items were kept in the original version proposed during the session. This resulted in a list of 50 items.

This list of 50 possible actions to strengthen GP/FM in Europe was subsequently sent to the 37 EURACT representatives by e-mail. They were asked to score the importance of the individual items for their country by means of a 9-poins Likert scale from 1 (strongly disagree that this action is important to strengthen GP/FM in my country) to 9 (strongly agree), with 5 being neutral. Main outcome was the panelists' evaluation of each statement as scored on the Likert scale. Respondents were also asked to evaluate the status of GP/FM in their country on four dimensions: At policy/governance level, at academic/university level, at population acceptance level and the importance for health care system progress – by means of the scores low, medium and high. Based on these scores, the countries were grouped in "high level", "medium level" and "low level" countries.

Statistics

The scores from the questionnaire study were plotted into SPSS version 22. For each criterion, mean scores with standard deviation (SD) was calculated. Agreement on importance for a statement was obtained if the mean score minus one SD exceeded 5 (called "final score"). Subgroup analyses were carried out for "high level", "medium level" and "low level" countries.

Results

Out of the 37 EURACT representatives asked to score the importance of the 50 possible actions needed to strengthen GP/FM, 30 returned complete questionnaires.

The 50 items with mean score (min – max) on a 9-point Likert scale and SD, as well as the "final score" are shown in Table 1 in decreasing order of importance.

For 26 out of the 50 items, mean score minus one SD ("final score") exceeded 5. These 26 items were grouped by the authors into the following five categories: Actions to strengthen GP/FM as an academic discipline, Actions to develop GP/FM as a specialty, Actions to influence decision makers, Organizational work, and Personal work. The five categories are shown in Table 2 with the item with the highest "final score" on top.

The respondents' ratings of GP/FM development in their country on policy/governance level, on academic/ university level, on population acceptance level and regarding importance for health care system progress are shown in Table 3. Thirteen out of the 30 countries obtained a total high development score, 11 a medium score, whereas six countries scored low.

Based upon subgroup analyses on the 50 items for the countries labelled as high, medium and low level countries (data not shown in Table), the ten items with highest score in each group were identified (Table 4).

To establish and strengthen GP/FM as an academic discipline was seen as essential in all the three groups, as several of the top score items addressed this theme. To build GP/FM as a specialty on the same level as other specialties was seen as important in high- and medium score countries. The low-score countries did not prioritize this statement, whereas the importance of common learning objectives and a defined bibliography were stated – both important issues in the building of a specialty. Low score countries valued "To use experts' help and invite experienced colleagues from other countries to establish a GP/ FM university department", while high score countries agreed on the importance of "To look at what specific help individual countries need". Actions to inform and influence policy makers about the importance of GP/FM were listed by all three groups, as were "To keep working and proving yourself" and "To work on good examples".

Discussion

There was substantial agreement on actions needed to strengthen GP/FM among EURACT council members from 30 European countries. The proposed actions were oriented towards two main themes: First, to improve the quality of GP/FM as a profession, and second, to optimize the circumstances under which the GP's work is carried out. Actions to improve quality focused on two main tasks: to build and secure GP/FM as an academic discipline comprising teaching and research and to develop GP/ FM as a clinical specialty.

General practice is probably the only health care setting where patients can freely address their worries and present several, unrelated and often complex problems [16]. Ageing and increasingly multi-morbid populations demand that multiple problems have to be dealt with in consultations [17]. To deal repeatedly with such complaints within brief encounters and to translate them into medically sound actions is said to be the most challenging intellectual exercise in clinical medicine [18]. Thus, to work as a GP demands a specific type of competence, more comprehensive and different from traditional knowledge regarding diseases and their treatment [5, 19]. This has implications for medical education, both undergraduate, and in particular for GPs' vocational training.

The quality level of GP/FM services still varies between European countries [20]. An example is Norway, where until now there has been no mandatory postgraduate training for GPs at all. In our study, respondents saw actions to develop GP as a specialty as highly important – and "to build the same level of specialty as other disciplines" got top score (Table 2).

Actions to strengthen undergraduate GP/FM teaching were also agreed upon as important, like "to list competencies for undergraduate level", and "to introduce a special course on GP/FM for first year students and early clinical exposure". It is still possible to graduate from a European medical school without having been exposed to a GP/FM curriculum [10]. EURACT will continue to launch efforts so that all medical students will complete a GP/FM curriculum [12], as well as a GP/FM clerkship [9].

High quality GP/FM undergraduate and postgraduate teaching requires a correspondingly high academic level of the profession, as seen as essential by our study participants. This also comprises "investment in research and common research projects" (Table 2). It is widely accepted that knowledge borrowed or adapted from other specialties is insufficient to create an evidence base for

Table 1 Possible actions to strengthen general practice/family medicine (GP/FM) in Europe – scores on a 9-point Likert scale (1 = strongly disagree on importance, 9 = strongly agree, n = 30 respondents)

Possible action to strengthen GP/FM in Europe	Mean score	Min - max	SD	Final score
To keep family doctors as leaders of GP/FM university departments	8.36	5–9	0.99	7.37
To build the same level of specialty as other disciplines	8.29	3–9	1.54	6.75
To train academic teaching staff, to run "Training of Trainers"	7.96	5–9	1.35	6.61
To create a network of GP/FM university departments	7.89	5–9	1.29	6.60
To develop staff and invest in academic development, motivate young staff to build an academic career	7.66	5–9	1.08	6.58
To have strong leaders	7.89	4–9	1.32	6.57
To remind that to prepare doctors for primary care is a priority for Ministry of Health and universities	7.82	4–9	1.36	6.46
To look at what specific help individual countries need	7.54	5–9	1.31	6.24
To keep working and proving yourself	7.68	4–9	1.43	6.18
To invest in research and common research projects	7.60	3–9	1.45	6.15
To know existing statement papers and create a common list of documents, bibliography and selected readings	7.57	4–9	1.45	6.12
To build a strong scientific society	7.83	1–9	1.74	6.09
To introduce a mentor system with one to one teaching and create a list of tutors for teaching	7.39	3–9	1.52	5.87
To empower EURACT, make transparency and visibility	7.32	4–9	1.49	5.83
To list the competencies for undergraduate level	7.39	4–9	1.69	5.70
To establish common learning objectives	7.25	1–9	1.65	5.60
To create a link between academics and policy makers	7.23	4–9	1.63	5.60
To collaborate with other organizations	7.10	3–9	1.61	5.49
To find a "right person" to get in touch with Minister of Health, rector, etc.	7.11	3–9	1.71	5.40
To use public opinion for political pressure	7.10	4–9	1.71	5.39
To find what are the patient's needs and make patients our partners	6.96	3–9	1.44	5.32
To stress the cost- effectiveness	7.07	1–9	1.84	5.23
To involve media to show leaders and/or popular persons	6.75	4–9	1.53	5.22
To make GP/FM attractive - "sexy"	6.89	4–9	1.69	5.20
To introduce a special course on GP/FM for first year students and early clinical exposure	7.00	3–9	1.87	5.13
To work on good examples	7.36	1–9	2.20	5.16
To introduce certification for GP/FM educators	6.79	1–9	1.83	4.96
To use experts' help and invite experienced colleagues from other countries to establish a GP/FM university department	7.04	1–9	2.12	4.92
To provide databases and web resources	6.75	3–9	1.88	4.87
To learn from those who succeed to establish a GP/FM University Department	6.96	1–9	2.15	4.81
To present goals at national conferences	6.83	1–9	2.02	4.81
To use modern technology	6.71	1–9	1.94	4.77
To use help of whole Europe	6.71	1–9	1.97	4.69
To show documents to the governments and media	6.25	4–9	1.58	4.67
To prepare a position paper to define university curriculum and include GP/FM in university curriculum	7.10	1–9	2.52	4.58
To look at the common GP/FM curriculum in the country	6.54	3–9	2.01	4.53
To write an open letter, describe who you are, what are your goals and objectives, what is done already, what are your future aspirations, offer yourself as an expert, volunteer to help	6.32	2–9	1.83	4.49
To organize educational research on "the best curriculum"	6.68	1–9	2.21	4.47
To know what others do, find common points with specialists and look for specialists' allies and help, share and collaborate with them	6.11	4–9	1.69	4.42
To exchange teachers	6.43	1–9	2.19	4.11
To post an English version of the curriculum on the university website	6.29	1–9	2.39	3.90
To implement a GP/FM approach in other subjects/disciplines	6.21	1–9	2.42	3.88

Table 1 Possible actions to strengthen general practice/family medicine (GP/FM) in Europe – scores on a 9-point Likert scale (1 = strongly disagree on importance, 9 = strongly agree, *n* = 30 respondents) *(Continued)*

To improve European legislation	5.80	1–9	2.20	3.60
"Touch the hearts"/ show movies	5.86	1–9	2.42	3.44
To define what is GP/FM	5.43	1–9	2.69	2.74
To organize GP/FM training for other specialists	4.04	1–9	2.69	1.35
To push deans to specialize in GP/FM	3.54	1–8	2.50	1.04
To organize workshops on cardiology, hematology, neurology etc. for GPs	3.46	1–9	2.29	.67
To stop fighting	3.54	1–9	3.01	.53
To start fighting	3.43	1–9	3.02	.41

Final score = mean score − 1 SD

Table 2 Important actions to strengthen general practice/family medicine (GP/FM) in Europe (Final score = mean score minus 1 SD on a 9-point Likert scale, 1 = strongly disagree on importance, 9 = strongly agree, *n* = 30 respondents)

	Mean score	SD	Final score
Actions to strengthen GP/FM as an academic discipline			
To keep family doctors as leaders of GP/FM departments – the teaching process and decision making	8.36	0.99	7.37
To train academic staff, to run "Training of Trainers"	7.96	1.35	6.61
To create a network of GP/FM university departments	7.89	1.29	6.60
To develop staff and invest in academic development, motivate young staff to build an academic career	7.66	1.08	6.58
To invest in research and common research projects	7.60	1.45	6.15
To build a strong scientific society	7.83	1.74	6.09
Actions to develop GP/FM as a specialty			
To build the same level of specialty as other disciplines	8.29	1.54	6.75
To know existing statement papers and create a common list of documents, bibliography and selected readings	7.57	1.45	6.12
To introduce a mentor system with one to one teaching and create a list of tutors for teaching	7.39	1.52	5.87
To list competencies for undergraduate level	7.39	1.69	5.70
To establish common learning objectives	7.25	1.65	5.60
To make GP/FM attractive - "sexy"	6.89	1.69	5.20
To introduce a special course on GP/FM for first year students and early clinical exposure	7.00	1.87	5.13
Actions to influence decision makers			
To have strong leaders	7.89	1.32	6.57
To remind that to prepare doctors for primary care is a priority for Ministry of Health and universities	7.82	1.36	6.46
To create a link between academics and policy makers	7.23	1.63	5.60
To find a "right person" to get in touch with Minister of Health, rector, etc. – direct your efforts to decision makers	7.11	1.71	5.40
To use public opinion for political pressure	7.10	1.71	5.39
To find what are the patient's needs and make patients our partners	6.96	1.44	5.32
To stress the cost- effectiveness	7.07	1.84	5.23
To involve media to show leaders and/or popular persons	6.75	1.53	5.22
Organizational work			
To look at what specific help individual countries need	7.54	1.31	6.24
To empower EURACT, make transparency and visibility	7.32	1.49	5.83
To collaborate with other organizations	7.10	1.61	5.49
Personal work			
To keep working and proving yourself	7.68	1.43	6.18
To work on good examples	7.36	2.20	5.16

Importance = Final score > 5.0

Table 3 Respondents' rating of general practice/family medicine development in their country (n = 30)

Country	Policy/Governance Low = 1 Medium = 2 High = 3	Academic/University Low = 1 Medium = 2 High = 3	Population acceptance Low = 1 Medium = 2 High = 3	Health care system progress Low = 1 Medium = 2 High = 3	General Score Low = 4–6 Medium = 7–9 High = 10–12
High(n = 13)					
Netherlands	3	3	3	3	12
Israel	3	3	3	3	12
United Kingdom	3	3	3	3	12
Denmark	3	3	3	2	11
Estonia	2	3	3	3	11
Turkey	2	3	3	3	11
Bosnia-Herzegovina	2	2	3	3	10
Germany	3	2	3	2	10
Lithuania	1	3	3	3	10
Malta	2	3	3	2	10
Norway	2	3	3	2	10
Portugal	2	3	2	3	10
Romania	2	2	3	3	10
Medium (n = 11)					
Croatia	2	3	2	2	9
Czeck Rep.	2	3	2	2	9
Finland	2	3	2	2	9
Slovenia	2	3	2	2	9
Sweden	3	2	2	2	9
Italy	1	1	3	3	8
Montenegro	2	2	2	2	8
Poland	1	2	3	2	8
Slovakia	2	2	2	2	8
Spain	2	1	3	2	8
Bulgaria	2	2	1	2	7
Low (n = 6)					
Austria	1	1	2	2	6
Georgia	1	2	1	2	6
Macedonia	1	2	1	2	6
Moldova	2	1	1	2	6
Russia	1	2	2	1	6
Serbia	1	1	2	2	6

the comprehensive medical care that takes place in general practice [8, 21, 22]. Investment in and level of GP/FM research, however, varies among European countries [23, 24], and generally still has potential for improvement [25].

The second main theme proposed by our respondents as essential was to optimize the structural conditions for GP/FM. Strong primary care does not emerge spontaneously, but requires facilitating political and economic circumstances. In a recent paper Schäfer et al. investigated changes in the breadth of services provided by GPs in 28 European countries from 1993 to 2012 and possible explanations for these changes [20]. They found that conditions on the national level were associated with changes in the service profile of GPs. In countries with stronger growth of health care expenditures the service profiles had expanded. This reality seems clear to our informants, as they propose several actions to

Table 4 Top ten items for countries with high, medium and low rating of general practice/family medicine (GP/FM) status. Scores on a 9-point Likert scale (mean score minus 1SD)

Rank	Item	Score
Countries with high rating (*n* = 13)		
Rank	Item	Score
1	To develop staff and invest in academic development, motivate young staff to build an academic career	7.22
2	To build the same level of specialty as other disciplines	7.15
3	To have strong leaders	7.13
4	To keep family doctors as leaders of GP/FM departments	7.06
5	To create a link between academics and policy makers	6.76
6	To look at what specific help individual countries need	6.51
7	To collaborate with other organizations	6.30
8	To create a network of GP/FM university departments	6.27
9	To keep working and proving yourself	6.09
10	To train academic staff, to run "Training of Trainers"	6.06
Countries with medium rating (*n* = 11)		
Rank	Item	Score
1	To build a strong scientific society	7.62
2	To keep family doctors as leaders of GP/FM departments	7.56
3	To build the same level of specialty as other disciplines	7.43
4	To train academic staff, to run "Training of Trainers"	6.97
5	To have strong leaders	6.75
6	To introduce a mentor system with one to one teaching and create a list of tutors for teaching	6.75
7	To remind that to prepare doctors for primary care is a priority for Ministry of Health and universities	6.61
8	To keep working and proving yourself	6.61
9	To develop staff and invest in academic development, motivate young staff to build an academic career	6.57
10	To establish common learning objectives	6.56
Countries with low rating (*n* = 6)		
Rank	Item	Score
1	To create a network of GP/FM university departments	8.25
2	To keep family doctors as leaders of GP/FM departments	7.50
3	To establish common learning objectives	7.36
4	To post an English version of the curriculum on the university website	7.35
5	To train academic staff, to run "Training of Trainers"	7.29
6	To remind that to prepare doctors for primary care is a priority for Ministry of Health and universities	7.29
7	To use experts' help and invite experienced colleagues from other countries to establish a GP/FM university department	7.00
8	To know existing statement papers and create a common list of documents, bibliography and selected readings	6.96
9	To introduce a mentor system with one to one teaching and create a list of tutors for teaching	6.96
10	To work on good examples	6.90

influence national health policy: through strong leaders and academia, through media and public opinion, as well as with the help of patients (Table 2). "To stress the cost- effectiveness" is another action proposed by our respondents to help influence health policy in their country. The favourable cost-effectiveness of a GP/FM oriented health care system versus one based upon specialists and hospitals has been clearly stated [2–4].

While stronger primary care could be seen as a common solution when facing limited resources, European countries have responded differently to these challenges. WHO defines health policy as "decisions, plans and actions that are undertaken to achieve specific health goals within a society" [26]. Mackenbach et al. investigated variations in health policy regarding ten areas of preventive tasks in 43 European countries and found striking variations between countries in process and outcome indicators of health policy [27]. They concluded that substantial health gains can be achieved if all countries would follow best practice, but that this depends on both the "will" and the "means" of governments to implement such a health policy.

Our study participants were asked to rank the position of GP/FM in their country on several dimensions, leading to a label of "high", "medium" or "low" (Table 3). Several studies have investigated the performance of primary care systems in Europe in terms of quality, equity and costs [7, 28–32]. We could have used data from these studies for our subgroup analyses – although some were not published at the time the present study was planned. However, their labeling only showed minor deviations compared to the ranking done by the EURACT representatives [7, 30] which we therefore view as reliable for the purpose of this study. There were only minor variations between the three groups in what was considered important, as shown in Table 4 (even if the study is too small to allow for reliable statistical analysis on this matter). Countries where GP/FM has a high position were open to "look at what specific help individual countries need", whereas the "low position" countries expressed the wish to "use experts' help and invite experienced colleagues from other countries to establish a GP/FM university department". As Seifert et al. point out regarding Central- and Eastern European countries: There is a need for continuous exchange of expertise between countries – e.g. to promote and secure academic infrastructure and CME [23].

The strength of our study was that representatives from 32 countries participated in creating the list of the 50 possible actions, securing that a multitude of opinions were exposed, and that 30 representatives subsequently carried out the scoring. One limitation of the study was that we were not able to obtain questionnaire data from some countries: Albania, Belgium, Greece, Hungary, Ireland, Latvia and Switzerland, due to non-response. A further limitation was the subjective character of the responses, coming from just one person representing one country, even if the participants stand a trusted position in their respective countries.

Conclusion

EURACT and other professional organizations have a responsibility to promote a strong and high quality GP/FM throughout Europe. This implies to establish common goals and to share expertise between countries. The aims are that every European medical school should have an undergraduate GP/FM curriculum and a residency. Vocational training should be accessible and mandatory. The academic position of GP/FM should be strengthened, and research should be facilitated. Working conditions must be improved – so decision makers must be influenced, by information on cost-effectiveness and potential health gains through a health care system based on strong GP/FM.

Abbreviations

EURACT: European Academy of Teachers in General Practice/Family Medicine; GP/FM: General practice/family medicine; SD: Standard deviation; WHO: World Health Organization; WONCA: World Organization of Family Doctors

Acknowledgments

We want to express our gratitude to the EURACT council members who participated in the data collection.

Authors' contributions

NZ, SW, HT, FC, and MB participated in the planning of the study, NZ, SW, FC, and HT collected the data, MB plotted the data and carried out the data analyses, NZ drafted the first version of the paper, MB revised the paper, with the help of SW, FC and HT. All authors read and approved the final manuscript.

Funding

Not applicable.

Competing interests

The authors declare that they have no competing interests.

Author details

[1]Family Medicine Department, State University of Medicine and Pharmacy "Nicolae Testemitanu", Bd. Stefan cel Mare 165, MD-2004 Chisinau, Republic of Moldova. [2]Institute of General Practice, Heinrich-Heine-University, Werdener Str. 4, D-40227 Düsseldorf, Germany. [3]Department of Family Medicine and Siaal research center for family medicine and primary care, Ben-Gurion University of the Negev, Beer-Sheva, Israel. [4]University of Milan, Francesco Sforza 35, Milan, Italy. [5]Department of General Practice, Institute of Health and Society, University of Oslo, P.O. Box 1132 018, Blindern, Norway.

References

1. UNICEF, World Health Organization. International Conference on Primary Health Care. Geneva: USSR Alma Ata; 1978.
2. World Health Organization 2008: The World Health Report 2008 – primary health care (now more than ever). http://www.who.int/whr/2008/whr08_en.pdf. Accessed 22 Jan 2017.
3. Starfield B. Primary care: an increasingly important contributor to effectiveness, equity, and efficiency of health services. Gac Sanit. 2012; 26:20–6. http://www.ncbi.nlm.nih.gov/pubmed/22265645. Accessed 22 Jan 2017
4. Macinko J, Starfield B, Erinosho T. The impact of primary healthcare on population health in low- and middle-income countries. J Ambul Care Manage. 2009;32:150–71. https://depts.washington.edu/sphnet/wp-content/uploads/2013/01/Macinko.pdf Accessed 22 Jan 2017
5. Kringos DS, Boerma WGW, Hutchinson A, van der Zee J, Groenewegen PP. The breadth of primary care: a systematic literature review of its core dimensions. BMC Health Serv Res. 2010;10:65. http://www.biomedcentral.com/1472-6963/10/65 Accessed 22 Jan 2017
6. WHO global strategy on people-centered and integrated health services, World Health Organization (2015). http://www.who.int/servicedeliverysafety/areas/people-centred-care/global-strategy/en/ Accessed 22 Jan 2017.
7. Kringos DS, Boerma WGW, Bourgueil Y, et al. The strength of primary care in Europe: an international comparative study. Br J Gen Pract. 2013;63(616): e742–50. doi:https://doi.org/10.3399/bjgp13X674422.
8. Pavličević I, Švab I. Family medicine defines its academic niche: the split initiative. Acta Med Acad. 2012;41:1–3.
9. Carelli F. EURACT Statement on Family Medicine Undergraduate Teaching. European J Gen Pract 2014; doi:https://doi.org/10.3109/13814788.2014.946009.
10. Brekke M, Carelli F, Zarbailov N, et al. Undergraduate medical education in general practice/family medicine throughout Europe – a descriptive study. BMC Med Edu. 2013;13:157. http://www.biomedcentral.com/1472-6920/13/157 Accessed 22 Jan 2017
11. http://euract.woncaeurope.org/ Accessed 22 Jan 2017.
12. Tandeter H, Carelli F, Timonen M, et al. A 'minimal core curriculum' for family medicine in undergraduate medical education: a European Delphi survey among EURACT representatives. Eur J Gen Pract. 2011;17:217–20.
13. http:///globalfamilydoctor.com Accessed 22 Jan 2017.
14. Creswell JW. A concise introduction to mixed methods research. Thousand Oaks: Sage; 2015.
15. Report of EURACT council meeting, Tirana, 3–5 October 2013. http://euract.woncaeurope.org/sites/euractdev/files/pages/council-meetings-and-reports/2013_october_3-5_tirana_albania_-_euract_autumn_council_meeting.pdf. Accessed 3 Apr 2017.
16. Bjørland E, Brekke M. What do patients bring up in consultations? Scand J Prim Health Care 2015; doi: https://doi.org/10.3109/02813432.2015.1067518.
17. Salisbury C, Johnson L, Purdy S, Valderas JM, Montgomery AA. Epidemiology and impact of multimorbidity in primary care: a retrospective cohort study. Br J Gen Pract. 2011;61(582):e12–21. doi:https://doi.org/10.3399/bjgp11X548929.
18. Loxtercamp D. What a doctor is good for. BMJ. 2014;349:g6894.
19. Kirkengen AL, Ekeland TJ, Getz L, Hetlevik I, Ulvestad E, Vetlesen AJ. What constitutes competence? That depends on the task. Scand J Prim Health Care. 2013;31:65–6.
20. Schäfer W, Boerma W, Spreeuwenberg P, Schellevis F, Groenewegen P. Two decades of change in European general practice profiles: conditions associated with the developments in 28 countries between 1993 and 2012. Scand J Prim Health Care 2016; doi:https://doi.org/10.3109/02813432.2015.1132887.
21. Stange KC, Miller WL, McWhinney I. Developing the knowledge base of family practice. Fam Med. 2001;33:286–97.
22. Graffy J. Engaging family practitioners in research: are we getting it right? Fam Pract. 2008;25:69–70.
23. Seifert B, Svab I, Madis T, Kersnik J, Windak A, Steflova A, Byma S. Perspectives of family medicine in central and Eastern Europe. Fam Pract. 2008;25:113–8.
24. Hummers-Pradier E, Scheidt-Nave C, Martin H, Heinemann S, Kochen MM, Himmel W. Simply no time? Barriers to GPs' participation in primary care research. Fam Pract. 2008;25:105–12.
25. Sullivan F, Butler C, Cupples M, Kinmonth AL. Primary care networks in the United Kingdom. BMJ. 2007;334:1093–4.

"I can't bend it and it hurts like mad": direct observation of gout consultations in routine primary health care

Anthony Dowell, Caroline Morris*, Lindsay Macdonald and Maria Stubbe

Abstract

Background: Gout is the most common form of inflammatory arthritis and is associated with considerable co-morbidity. It is usually managed in the primary care setting with a combination of lifestyle modification and pharmacological therapy. This study describes patterns of communication about gout observed in interactions between patients and primary care practitioners during routine consultations.

Methods: Secondary analysis of video-recordings of individual healthcare consultations between patients and a range of primary care practitioners (including general practitioners, practice nurses, podiatrists and dietitians) from an archived database. Consultations that included any discussion about gout were eligible for inclusion (n = 31) and were not restricted to those where gout was the main presenting complaint. The consultation transcripts were analysed using a qualitative inductive approach from clinical and linguistic perspectives and supplemented with visual observation of the interactions.

Results: Two main themes emerged from the data; the importance of gout and 'telling' versus 'listening' in consultations. The first theme had two distinct strands; gout as an incidental part of the consultation and the impact of gout on patients. A trend towards more didactic practitioner communication encompassed by the second theme occurred at many different consultation points including diagnosis, in more general post-diagnosis discussion, and when discussing biochemical test results and lifestyle advice. In contrast, when discussion about treatment with medicines occurred a tendency towards a greater degree of listening to patients was observed.

Conclusion: Our observation of the communication patterns in these consultations illustrates an inherent complexity of gout consultations in primary care. Gout may be more important to patients than is often apparent to practitioners in routine consultations. Consultation management needs to take into account the impact of the condition and the balance of information provided around lifestyle advice versus long-term management with medicines.

Keywords: Communication, Consultation, General practice, Gout, Primary health care, Qualitative research

Background

Gout is recognised as the most common form of inflammatory arthritis and occurs as a response to the deposition of monosodium urate crystals in the joints [1]. It is associated with a range of co-morbidities including diabetes, hypertension and obesity; it is a chronic condition manifested by acute flares and chronic monosodium urate crystal deposition with differing management options; [1] it is usually managed in primary care. Effective management is by advocating a combination of lifestyle modification and pharmacological therapy [1, 2]. In contrast to some other chronic conditions (e.g. asthma), a clearly defined target value for a biochemical test result (serum urate level $\leq$ 0.36 mmol/L) is associated with better outcomes for patients whose symptoms recur [1, 2].

Challenges to effective primary care management include doctors' and patients' perceptions of the condition and the need to address gout and its co-morbidities within short consultation time-frames [3]. In line with primary care consultations for other conditions, gout may be the patient's main presenting complaint or surface incidentally

* Correspondence: caroline.morris@otago.ac.nz
Department Primary Health Care & General Practice, University of Otago, 23a Mein Street, Wellington, New Zealand

during the consultation, and be raised by either the patient or their doctor [4, 5].

A number of primary care based qualitative [6–14] and quantitative [15–17] studies have investigated patient and/or practitioner experiences and perceptions of gout. Evidence shows that the condition adversely affects sufferers' lives in a substantive way. Gout is the cause of considerable pain and has a negative impact on patients' home, work and social lives [6–8, 10–13]. Furthermore, the diagnosis can be a source of stigma for patients resulting from the stereotypes that exist around the condition's perceived link to lifestyle and alcohol use [10–13].

Although doctors are aware that a gout diagnosis is a potential source of stigma for patients, [12] feelings of being stigmatised may contribute to sub-optimal management, [18] alongside a lack of patient [6–8, 12, 13, 19] or practitioner [12, 14, 18] knowledge about the appropriate management of the condition.

Patients and practitioners often have differing views about gout and the ease with which it can be managed, [9] with management perceived by doctors as being further complicated by the presence of patient co-morbidities. [12, 14] Although treatment guidelines exist, [20–22] they are not always applied by clinicians in practice [18, 19].

Some patients are aware of specific food or drinks precipitating a personal acute gout attack, [12] while others show a lack of awareness that lifestyle modification may be one way of managing the condition, [19] and poor awareness of common food triggers [16, 23]. Although modifying lifestyle and diet is a recognised part of gout management [1, 2] and recommendations encompassing these areas form part of national guidelines for gout management, [20, 21] the evidence supporting their inclusion is low in the evidence hierarchy. More recently the question of the balance of information provision to patients about lifestyle measures versus management with medicines has been raised as an important issue to address [11, 14].

There is a significant body of research dating back to the 1970s involving the direct observation of patient-health professional communication [24]. In the past two decades interactional sociolinguistics and conversation analysis methodologies have been used to unpack the "background orientations, individual experiences, sensibilities, understandings, and objectives that inhabit the medical visit" [25]. Previous work demonstrates the ways in which doctors and patients often pursue quite different agendas in the history-taking phase of the consultation. While pursuing their biomedical agenda, doctors may suppress patients' expressions of their "lifeworld" concerns and circumstances even though these often had a real bearing on their medical problems and outcomes [26].

Previous qualitative research with gout patients and the primary care practitioners involved in their care has taken place outside of the consultation setting thus relying on participant recall of the events that took place. To date, no previous study has explored directly observed interactions between patients with gout and the practitioners who care for them during routine consultations. This study aims to provide an initial description of the language and patterns of communication relating to gout observed in interactions between these parties within the day to day context of primary care consultations. A clearer understanding of the consultation process has the potential to help identify ways of improving patient care.

Methods

Data source

Consultation data are sourced from the Applied Research on Communication in Health (ARCH) Corpus at the University of Otago, Wellington, New Zealand (see Table 1). The collection of all Corpus data and guidelines for subsequent use have been approved by the national New Zealand Health and Disability Ethics Committee [27].

Table 1 Background information about the ARCH Corpus database [27]

This Corpus houses a digitally stored collection of patient / practitioner consultation data that includes video-recorded consultations and verbatim transcripts.

Included data has been collected since 2003 as part of funded studies.

These studies include the:

- Interaction Study (IS) exploring clinical decision-making when rationing is explicit;
- Tracking Study (TS) exploring communication processes throughout a single complete episode of care of patients referred from primary to secondary care;
- Diabetes Study (DS) tracking the contact of newly diagnosed patients with Type 2 diabetes with healthcare professionals over a six-month period.

The combined dataset for the IS and TS comprised an unselected sample of 183 routine consultations involving 15 general practitioners recorded in 21 participating general practices in the Wellington region of New Zealand between 2004 and 2007. The data for the DS was purposively collected in Wellington and Auckland; for this study, 36 patients newly diagnosed with type 2 diabetes were recruited prospectively via 21 general practices (6 of which had participated in the previous studies) and tracked for a period of 6 months between 2008 and 2011. Their consultations with general practitioners and nurses at the general practice and related consultations with allied health professional staff were video-recorded.

All consultations were made in the course of 'practice as usual' and are therefore typical of routine interactions occurring in New Zealand healthcare.

Written consent was sought from participants in these original studies to use their data for secondary analysis.

At the time of sampling the ARCH Corpus included 418 video-recorded consultations recorded between 2003 and 2011, 337 of which were eligible for inclusion. These comprised 247 individual patients, 30 general practitioners, 31 nurses and 15 other practitioners.

Identification of gout consultations

The ARCH Corpus includes a Microsoft Access database populated with full demographic information about every participant, research site information and free text content logs of each consultation. The logs are prepared by a research nurse according to a standard template and include information about the main topics discussed, outcomes of the consultation (including prescriptions and referrals), and a minute by minute summary of key events and content. The logs thus capture any complaint or topic mentioned incidentally in a consultation, in addition to the main presenting complaint(s). The database and logs link electronically to full verbatim transcripts and the original audio and video-recordings to facilitate subsequent more detailed analysis, but the latter cannot be queried directly via the database.

A query was run on the Microsoft Access database using the keyword "gout". It is theoretically possible that not all potentially relevant consultations in the Corpus were identified, but this is unlikely as gout is a readily identifiable topic of discussion. A subsequent cross-check using the names of common gout medicines as search terms did not yield any additional consultations. The purpose was the construction of a relevant dataset adequate for the purpose of undertaking a descriptive qualitative analysis, not to investigate frequency of occurrence.

The term gout was present in the logs of 31 individual patient consultations with primary care practitioners. The aim was not specifically to identify consultations where gout is the main presenting complaint, but rather to observe how gout is addressed in the context of routine consultations. Twenty of the consultations analysed originated from the DS (see Table 1), and the majority of those contained elements of a more structured consultation format based on a national protocol for diabetes care. The remaining 11 general practitioner (GP) consultations were derived from the IS study (n = 5) and the TS study (n = 6) respectively. Brief demographic characteristics of the patients and practitioners included in these consultations are shown in Table 2.

Table 2 Demographic characteristics of patients and practitioners involved in the gout consultations (n = 31)

Patient characteristics

- 18 individual patients
  - Male n = 13; female n = 5
  - Age: mean 54 years; median 52 years
  - Age range: 36 to 67 years

Health practitioner characteristics

- 17 individual practitioners
  - General practitioners n = 10
  - Nurses n = 4
  - Podiatrists n = 2,
  - Dietitian n = 1

Data analysis

This study was based on the verbatim transcripts and video-recordings of interactions between patients and practitioners. Themes were derived iteratively using a qualitative inductive approach, [28–30] following the process shown in Table 3; our overarching aim being to report on the emerging range of issues and communication styles without pre-conceived assumptions.

Table 3 Data analysis process

1. CM identified and coded conversation sequences related to gout in the transcripts. CM then reviewed the video-recordings to confirm and enrich the analysis. A note was made of any important contextual non-verbal communication from either party e.g. nodding of the head, smiling, sighing, listening attentively, examining the patient, turning away from the patient.
2. Initial coding included:
   - how gout was introduced into a consultation and by whom
   - the location within the consultation
   - the importance of the condition from the patient perspective
   - diagnosis and treatment of the condition
   - emphasis placed on biochemical test results and dietary and lifestyle advice
3. Themes and sub-themes were identified from the data. Initial interpretations of the clinical relevance and importance of the themes derived were debated and discussed between CM, a pharmacist and experienced qualitative researcher, and AD, the general practitioner member of the project team.
4. LM and MS, researchers with experience in linguistics, contributed to a second round of discussion and interpretation. Examples of refinements at this point include:
   - "Gout as an incidental part of the consultation" and "Impact of gout for patients" being combined as sub-themes of the overarching theme "The importance of gout"
   - A linguistic interpretative viewpoint to the differences observed around lifestyle and medicines
   - Acknowledgement of the importance and possible ambiguity of 'semi-verbal' communication (e.g. the use of "mm" by participants)
5. Disagreements were resolved by consensus.
6. All authors reviewed and agreed the final themes and interpretation

Results

Two key and important themes that emerged from our data relating to the importance of gout and telling versus listening in consultations are the focus of this paper and described in more detail below. These, together with other themes identified from the dataset are shown Table 4.

The importance of gout

To aid interpretation of the results contextual background information about the 31 gout consultations is shown in Table 5.

Table 4 Themes derived from the data

Themes that are the focus of this paper
• The importance of gout
- Gout as an 'incidental' part of the consultation
- The impact of gout on patients
• 'Telling' versus 'listening' in consultations
Medicine-related themes[a]
• Level of patient knowledge
• Patient attitudes to medicines
• Attributes of practitioner communication
- Delivery and content of information provided
- Taking the opportunities presented
Other themes
• Patient interpretation of symptoms
• Patient understanding of gout management
• Patient understanding of uric acid levels

[a]Described in detail elsewhere [40]

The data show that gout is perceived as an important issue by patients and practitioners in two distinct ways. Firstly, gout can 'intrude' into the consultation, even when it is not the prime reason for consulting; it is the presenting complaint in only two consultations. Secondly, when patients introduce the condition by name or describe symptoms of gout it becomes clear that it has a significant impact on their well-being. The abbreviations used in the quotations below are as follows: GP = general practitioner; NS = nurse; PT = patient; POD = podiatrist; DIET = dietitian.

Gout as an 'incidental' part of the consultation

In many consultations conversations about gout stem from the practitioner's general review of the patient or during a consultation about a different, but related, morbidity e.g. diabetes:

> *NS: "If we can check everything [blood tests] ... it's part of the annual review that's very important ... we also check your uric acid, that's for, you know, your gout" (DS-NS27–02)*

Three patients intentionally and explicitly re-focus their diabetes review visits to gout by raising the issue at the beginning of the consultation. Following a very short discussion about their weight this patient abruptly changes the subject to gout symptoms:

> *PT: "Right now ... look, [patient shows GP their foot], I can't touch it, I can't bend it and it hurts like mad ... [I've had it] for a week and a half ... it hurts" (DS-GP29–01)*

Re-focusing a consultation to gout is not always patient-driven. This GP makes gout a focus right at the start of the consultation despite the patient's primary reason for visiting being influenza-like symptoms:

> *GP: "You saw [Doctor's name] since I last saw ... and he thought you had resistant gout" (IS-GP02–03)*

A lengthy dialogue then ensues around gout and its treatment before the patient sighs heavily and clearly and deliberately re-focuses the consultation to the presenting complaint.

On other occasions gout is merely alluded to in passing; most commonly relating to a previously prescribed medicine:

> *"... and I also gave you some [medicine name] for your gout back then as well" (TS-GP03–12)*

The impact of gout on patients

Gout is an important topic of patient concern that may be raised within a consultation with any member of the primary care team (including GPs, nurses, dietitians, podiatrists) in this dataset. The personal impact of the condition and more general aspects of management are all discussed, irrespective of whether the patient is currently experiencing an acute disease flare. Furthermore, counter to an often anecdotally perceived clinical picture of easily managed gout flares restricted to a single anatomical area, patients highlight both the severity and the duration of attacks:

> GP consultation:
>
> *PT: "at night it is really swollen and I've had to put my foot out of the bed ... night-time it is worse ... and I've been wearing [sandals] because I can't have anything touch it ..." (DS-GP29–01)*
> Podiatrist consultation:
> *PT: "I had a big wave of gout for a little while [that] lasted for about a good three weeks, it took a while to wear off"*
> *POD: oh you poor thing, ... whereabouts did it affect you the most?*
> *PT: ... "it started from my toes, round to my ankle and then it just stayed there for a while and it just slowly headed up this way [points up the leg]." (DS-HP07-01b)*

Patients also comment on the impact of the lifestyle changes they make to help manage their condition. Most patients with diagnosed disease are aware of some of their potential dietary triggers:

> *PT: "I used to eat mussels but it gives me a lot of trouble with my gout ... I keep away from foods that make me sick ... " (DS-NS14-02a)*

Table 5 Contextual information about 18 individual patient's gout consultations (n = 31)

Consultation Identifier*	Patient age (years)	Practitioner	Incidental or presenting complaint (PC)	Initiator of gout conversation	Point of consultation gout first mentioned	Discussion length; context	Gout medicines mentioned	Lifestyle advice/ diet mentioned	Uric acid levels mentioned
DS-GP01-04	41–50	GP	Incidental	Patient	Early	Short; no current symptoms	Yes	Yes	Yes
DS-NS10-01	41–50	Nurse	Incidental	Practitioner	Late	In passing[#]	No	Yes	Yes
DS-NS14-02a	51–60	Nurse	Incidental	Practitioner	Late	In passing[#]	No	Yes	No
DS-GP19-02b	51–60	GP	Incidental	Patient	Start	Substantive; no current symptoms	Yes	Yes	Yes
DS-NS14-02b	51–60	Nurse	Incidental	Patient	Start	Short; No current symptoms	Yes	Yes	No
DS-GP29-01	41–50	GP	Incidental	Patient	Start	Substantive; acute flare, new diagnosis	Yes	Yes	Yes
DS-NS13-01a	31–40	Nurse	Incidental	Patient	Middle	Short; patient thought they had gout	No	Yes	Yes
DS-NS13-01b	31–40	Nurse	Incidental	Practitioner	Early	Short; following up discussion of previous visit where patient thought they had gout	Yes	No	No
DS-GP18-01	31–40	GP	Incidental	Practitioner	Middle	Substantive; discussion of preventive therapy	Yes	No	No
DS-HP06-01a	31–40	Dietitian	Incidental	Patient	Start	Short; struggling with gout	Yes	Yes	No
DS-HP07-01a	31–40	Podiatrist	Incidental	Patient	Start	Substantive; no current symptoms	Yes	Yes	No
DS-NS13-01c_GP18	31–40	Nurse & GP	Incidental	Patient	Start	Substantive; acute flare	Yes	No	No
DS-HP06-01b	31–40	Dietitian	Incidental	Practitioner	Start	Substantive; acute flare	Yes	Yes	No
DS-HP07-01b	31–40	Podiatrist	Incidental	Practitioner	Start	Substantive; no current symptoms	Yes	No	No
DS-NS13-01d_GP18	31–40	Nurse & GP	Incidental	Patient	Early	Substantive; acute flare subsiding	Yes	No	Yes
DS-NS13-04d_GP21	61–70	Nurse & GP	Incidental	Patient	Start	Short; mention of recent flare	No	No	Yes
DS-NS25-01	51–60	Nurse	Incidental	Practitioner	Early	In passing[#]	Yes	No	No
DS-NS27-02	41–50	Nurse	Incidental	Practitioner	Close	In passing[#]	Yes	No	Yes
DS-HP10-02a	41–50	Podiatrist	Incidental	Patient	Middle	Short; making conversation	Yes	No	No
DS-HP10-02b	41–50	Podiatrist	Incidental	Patient	Middle	Short; making conversation	Yes	Yes	Yes
IS-GP02-03	41–50	GP	Incidental	Practitioner	Start	Substantive; no current symptoms	Yes	No	No

Table 5 Contextual information about 18 individual patient's gout consultations (n = 31) *(Continued)*

Consultation Identifier*	Patient age (years)	Practitioner	Incidental or presenting complaint (PC)	Initiator of gout conversation	Point of consultation gout first mentioned	Discussion length; context	Gout medicines mentioned	Lifestyle advice/ diet mentioned	Uric acid levels mentioned
IS-GP02–14	41–50	GP	PC	Patient	Start	Substantive; acute flare, pre-existing diagnosis	Yes	No	Yes
IS-GP03–06	61–70	GP	Incidental	Practitioner	Late	In passing[#]	Yes	No	Yes
IS-GP07–05	61–70	GP	Incidental	Practitioner	Start	In passing[#]	Yes	No	No
IS-GP07–06	41–50	GP	Incidental	Practitioner	Middle	In passing[#]	Yes	No	No
TS-GP03–08	51–60	GP	Incidental	Practitioner	Middle	In passing[#]	Yes	No	No
TS-GP03–12	61–70	GP	Incidental	Practitioner	Start	In passing[#]	Yes	No	No
TS-GP03–17	61–70	GP	Incidental	Practitioner	Middle	Short; gout considered before being eliminated	Yes	No	No
TS-GP08–10	51–60	GP	Incidental	Practitioner	Early	In passing[#]	Yes	No	Yes
TS-GP09–05	41–50	GP	PC	Patient	Start	Substantive; acute flare, pre-existing diagnosis	Yes	Yes	No
TS-GP14–04	61–70	GP	Incidental	Practitioner	Middle	Substantive; no current symptoms	Yes	No	No

GP General practitioner
*Consultations prefixed by DS were part of the Diabetes Study, IS the Interaction Study and TS the Tracking Study; a brief description of each study is shown in Table 1
[#]In the context of general patient review / medicines and/or blood test review

Despite this knowledge, there is, however, a sub-theme of continuing to eat foods which patents knew they should avoid.

> *PT: "... I ate all these wrong kind of foods and I gave myself gout which is a real drag cos I haven't had an attack for ages, but it's totally self-inflicted ... I ate all kinds of shell fish and [expletive] chocolate and all the things that triggered it" (TSGP09–05)*

The ways in which patients in our data typically conceptualised gout and their experience of its symptoms and management are clearly displayed in the language used in these excerpts to describe symptoms and the degree to which discomfort is beyond what is considered normal. As shown in the podiatrist consultation this usually elicits a sympathetic response which serves to validate the severity of the patient's reported symptoms and potentially demonstrates the justification for medical attention.

'Telling' versus 'listening' in consultations

Despite demonstrating high levels of professional expertise in patient management, practitioners often appeared to find patient-centred approaches to gout communication challenging. In this dataset practitioners tended to employ a more didactic style of communication by 'telling' rather than listening, often framing information in a biomedical way that is likely to be out of step with the patient's 'lived' experience.

The 'telling' consultation style can be observed at the beginning of a patient's gout 'career' as shown in the following consultation where gout is discussed for the first time. The GP comprehensively examines the foot while eliciting information about symptoms and the limits they place on the patient's ability to function. The patient maintains eye contact and listens attentively as the GP explains the aetiology of the condition in a biomedical way, identifying uric acid as the cause, but linking back to the symptoms the patient is experiencing:

> *GP: "We call it gout ... there is one acid called uric acid ... if the level in the blood is high it forms crystals and they deposit in the joint and make the joint painful - it is painful and swells up at times " (DS-GP29–01)*

Although the patient immediately responds by articulating their difficulty in managing the pain, particularly at night, the GP moves straight into providing information on treatment options and lifestyle changes. The didactic approach means there is little attempt to identify the patient's understanding of gout or the psychological or social impact of the condition.

This communication style persists in more general gout discussions following diagnosis. Here, the patient volunteers that they take medicines for gout. The podiatrist immediately provides information while looking down at the patient's feet, without first ascertaining the patient's knowledge of their condition:

POD: "The gout tablet allopurinol is to prevent you having a gout attack"

PT: The colchicine
POD: "That's for when you get the attack ... Gout's very painful as well, it's a type of arthritis, it causes intense pain and inflammation in a joint usually in these ones [points to the toes] but I have seen it round the ankles and down the sides of the feet ... if they leave it untreated you can get damage to the joints which is permanent damage ..." (DS-HP10-02b)

As uric acid levels are a defined biochemical marker for the diagnosis of gout, GPs often discuss this condition with patients from a biochemical perspective:

GP: "OK, it looks to me like you're doing well with the diabetes and the gout. The uric acid level in that last blood test was normal and we probably should get you to have another blood test at some stage so I might just print you [off a blood test form]." (DS-NS13-01d_GP18)

The GP gave information about uric acid levels without any discussion about how the patient currently felt about their gout or its impact on them.

In this cohort patients often appeared to have little understanding of the importance and meaning of uric acid levels, although one did raise the issue in a routine diabetes check when the nurse is discussing their diet:

PT: "... [I'm] cutting down [on certain foods], because of my cholesterol and my uric acid ..."

This immediately precipitates a short conversation that focuses on information provision:

NS: "Do you suffer from gout? Yeah, and you've had good information about things that trigger your gout? Do you go on the internet at all?"

PT: now and then
NS: "OK, so I'm just going to write up your care plan and we're really nearly there" (DS-NS10-01)

Conversations around dietary triggers for gout are a feature of many consultations spanning all practitioner groups. In the following example the GP appears to assume that the patient already has dietary information, rather than taking the opportunity to elicit the patient's understanding of triggers for gout and what it means to them personally. The patient's reply precipitates an information giving approach from the GP:

GP: "... you've got information about the foods to avoid with regard to your gout"

PT: I don't have any information about that, but I just think in my mind that I don't really eat too much red meat, maybe fish, but I haven't had any information about that
GP: "OK well I'll give you something to read about that, about the sorts of food to avoid [and] what tends to precipitate it; but the things you said are all the things that tend to bring it on and so just try to eat those in moderation or avoid them if they do cause flare-ups. Some of the other main things are shell fish, also alcohol, beer and carbonated drinks as well like fizzy drinks" (DS-GP19-02b)

At this point the patient volunteers information about their diet which the GP assesses and then reframes biomedically in the context of uric acid levels:

PT: "I avoid them all except sea food, I ate mussels, is that OK"?
GP: Did it cause any symptoms after you had the mussels?
PT: No
GP: "if you're having small amounts and you don't get symptoms that should be OK although your uric acid level in your blood ... it is still high" (DS-GP19-02b)

The patient maintains eye contact throughout the conversation and nods his head indicating an unspoken acknowledgment of what has been said.

Similar conversations with other practitioners are also framed in a biomedical way, with a focus remaining on 'telling' the patient rather than attempting to gain an understanding of their perspective. In this podiatrist consultation the patient mentions a pamphlet about diet precipitating this response:

POD: "I think it's about the only type of arthritis that it's been proven that certain food will have an effect on it and you're supposed to avoid foods that are high in uric acid I think like shell fish ... and alcohol." (DS-HP10-02b)

Medicines play a key role in the optimal management of gout. In this topic area the style of consultation was observed to move away from a didactic one towards a greater degree of listening to the patient. In the following example the GP negotiates options and checks that the patient is happy with a decision before it is finalised:

GP: "we should be probably giving you something to prevent the gout"

PT: oh OK, cos I do get it quite regularly especially in my ankle and my toe and it just throbs and I know that runs in my family
GP: we'd start you with a low [dose] - you can choose to start the tablet now or we can put it off for a while, it's up to you really ...
PT: just do it, just get it over and done with
GP: "[so], we start with a low dose and sometimes it can flare it up a little bit so it's probably good to do it now if you haven't got any gout ... it's probably better to just get this a little bit sorted out for you if we can" (DS-GP18-01)

Many patients were willing to consider long-term preventive treatment and others were very positive about it. Although there were no examples of patients refusing allopurinol specifically, some patients are less than comfortable with medicines per se:

PT: "... I don't like tablets ... I don't want to take any more tablets ..." (DS-GP19-02b)

In this case the GP acknowledges the patient's view and carefully introduces the possibility that allopurinol may be the best option if the clinical situation alters. The patient non-verbally indicates their acceptance by a nod of their head:

GP: "... so I think if you do start having regular flare-ups then we should look again at putting you back on allopurinol." (DS-GP19-02b)

Discussion

To our knowledge, this study is the first to directly observe conversations about gout in routine primary care consultations. It provides insights into how the importance of gout is framed by both patients and practitioners in primary care, and the way in which gout stories are elicited and placed in the context of management.

In line with other studies, our results show that gout has a significant impact on patients' functionality and well-being [6–8, 10–13]. It can be the cause of significant pain as shown by the demeanour of patients as they described their symptoms in the consultation, and can have a substantial impact on their lives. A notable feature is the use of "extreme case formulations" [31] (e.g. *"a big wave of gout", "I can't have anything touch it", "all the things that triggered it"*). Phrases such as these, along with the body language at the time of their utterance clearly convey the impact on the patient and also serve to strengthen the legitimacy of their description in the face of possible doubt [31]. Patients also clearly articulated the discomfort they were experiencing and how it persists or varies over time, reinforcing their justification for seeking medical attention [32].

Whether the issue of gout arose as a presenting complaint or as an incidental part of the consultation practitioners clearly listened to patients' concerns and were sympathetic but in the cases studied moved quickly to a biomedical framing of the condition. Understandably the patient focus is on the pain they are experiencing, while the practitioners' focus remains on disease management. Irrespective of circumstances, in common with other studies investigating chronic disease, often only limited time was spent attempting to understand the patient's perspective and the wider impact of the disease. The use of a biomedical model, language and framing heightens the challenge of exploring the psychosocial implications of gout in the consultation [33].

Although patients voiced agendas usually focus on symptoms, [34] doctors may also have an agenda [5]. A similar gap in the conceptualisation of illness has been previously identified in a study of a diverse range of general practice consultations [5] and specifically in diabetes, [33] with patients focusing on physical symptoms while doctors focused on prevention, medicines and tests. In this dataset gout was more often raised as an incidental part of the consultation rather than a presenting complaint, a feature that has also been described in relation to osteoarthritis [4].

GP consultations are known to be complex with many involving several patient problems covering multiple disease areas [5]. It is well known that there is time pressure to adequately consider issues raised incidentally, or beyond the presenting reason for encounter. GPs have previously described areas of differential prioritisation. [4] Influencing factors include patient safety, prioritising problems where they considered they could be most helpful and prioritising areas where financial incentives exist. Issues that were introduced at a later point in the consultation were sometimes perceived as unproblematic for the patient [4]. In the present study gout was rarely the presenting complaint, and the GP conversations illustrate the challenges faced when a condition of concern to the patient is not presented as a high priority within the consultation agenda.

A key finding from this study, clearly identified by the verbal interaction and additional insight gained from viewing the body language, is the different priority given to 'listening' and 'telling' in gout consultations when discussing lifestyle versus medicines. In this sample there was a more didactic focus on 'telling' patients what to do when lifestyle issues such as diet are discussed irrespective of the current status of the patient's condition. The didactic 'telling' style of lifestyle advice has parallels with other studies of directly observed consultations where rather than adjusting information to the specific situation of a patient only generic information about lifestyle behaviour is provided [35]. We have previously noted a similar tendency in diabetes-related lifestyle discussions in the larger set of consultations analysed for the DS, from which the dataset for the current study was drawn [36]. The impact on patients' lives of recommended lifestyle changes for chronic conditions such as gout can be significant, and a patient's life circumstances may in turn influence their willingness and ability to accept and follow the advice proffered where this conflicts with the patient's non-medical priorities [37–39].

Consultation conversations became more measured with a greater focus on listening when the topic is treatment with medicines. With medicines practitioners often asked open questions and took a more patient-centred approach. This feature of our dataset has been described in more detail elsewhere [40]. This difference may arise because treatment with medicines is perceived as potentially more problematic clinically, resulting in the "tentative hedging" we observed.

A gout diagnosis is a recognised source of stigma for patients due to its association with negative lifestyle choices. [8, 10, 11, 13]. A focus on lifestyle by practitioners may amplify this, leading patients to feel that they are being judged [11] and that their condition will not be taken seriously, [18] thereby making them less likely to seek help [14]. Indeed, some primary care practitioners have expressed frustration that patients' gout symptoms persist because they do not adhere to dietary advice [14]. In addition, other work has identified that some practitioners lack confidence in the treatment of gout, [12] are unfamiliar with treatment guidelines, [12, 18, 19] place a higher priority on lifestyle advice [14] and focus on treating acute attacks underestimating the long-term complications of the disease [18, 19]. A key challenge for practitioners is likely to be finding the optimal balance between the delivery of lifestyle advice and advice around the more effective, but potentially more challenging conversation of treatment with medicines [11].

In this study patients were willing to talk about gout to any available practitioner. It is thus important that primary care practitioners make use of opportunities for a more pro-active approach to gout management, especially as part of a multidisciplinary team. Gout management strategy 'packages' (information / education; tight monitoring; reassurance) with more clearly defined practitioner roles have been shown to be effective in specialist hospital clinic practice, and it is possible that elements of this approach might be of use in primary care [41].

A strength of the study is the direct observation of gout discussions in routine consultations. This provides an opportunity to see how gout is made relevant in consultations where it has not been the prime reason for the encounter. We were also able to view interactions between patients and a range of primary care practitioners. This provides information about interactions within the context of the primary care team, aligning with the desired trend towards better integration of the wider team in chronic disease management [42]. A potential limitation of the study is that differences may exist between patients who did not consent to being videoed and therefore not included in the database used for the study and those who were happy to be recorded and therefore included. A further limitation includes the possibility that the presence of the video-recorder may have led participants to behave differently from 'normal'. However, while all appear aware that the consultation is being recorded at the beginning, this diminishes as the core business of the consultation proceeds [43]. Although this study was conducted within the New Zealand healthcare system, the commonalities of long-term condition management in many high-income countries give the findings international relevance.

Conclusions

This study illustrates an inherent complexity of gout consultations in primary care. Gout may be more important to patients than is often apparent to practitioners in routine consultations. Consultation management needs to take into account the impact of the condition and the balance of information provided around lifestyle advice versus long-term management with medicines.

Abbreviations

ARCH: Applied research on communication in health; DIET: Dietitian; DS: Diabetes study; GP: General practitioner; IS: Interaction study; NS: Nurse; POD: Podiatrist; PT: Patient; TS: Tracking study

Acknowledgments

The data archived in the ARCH Corpus of Health Interactions were originally collected as part of research projects funded by the New Zealand Health Research Council, the Royal Society of New Zealand Marsden Fund, the New Zealand Lotteries Health Research Fund and the University of Otago Research Committee. The authors thank all participants for generously allowing their consultations to be recorded and archived, and acknowledge the input of Lesley Gray, Rachel Tester and other colleagues and research assistants from the ARCH Group, Kevin Dew, another member of the ARCH group, from the School of Social and Cultural Studies, Victoria University of Wellington, New Zealand and Barbara Docherty, Devi-Ann Hall, Timothy Kenealy, Debbie Raphael and Nicolette Sheridan from the Faculty of Medical and Health Sciences, The University of Auckland, New Zealand.

Funding

The funders of the studies from which these data are drawn (see "Acknowledgements") had no part in the design of the original studies that provided the data for secondary analysis that was used for this article. In addition, they had no involvement in the collection, analysis and interpretation of data for this article or the decision to submit it for publication. No external funding source was secured for this work; all authors completed it in within their paid University employment time.

Authors' contributions

AD, LM and MS designed the studies from which these data are drawn. LM undertook fieldwork and data collection. CM viewed and reviewed recorded data and with AD was responsible for the initial data analysis and interpretation. All authors contributed to the final interpretation. CM drafted the manuscript and all authors read and approved the final manuscript.

Authors' information

AD is a practising GP and Professor of Primary Health Care and General Practice. CM is a practising pharmacist with a pharmacy practice PhD. LM is a registered nurse with a postgraduate qualification in nursing and linguistics. MS is an experienced health communication researcher with a PhD in applied sociolinguistics.

Ethics approval and consent to participate

The collection of all Corpus data and guidelines for subsequent use have been approved by the national New Zealand Health and Disability Ethics Committee. [27] All participants whose data is held in the ARCH Corpus provided written informed consent to participation in the original studies, for the archiving of the data for future unspecified use in research and education, and for the publication of de-identified excerpts in future publications. Each of the original studies on which this manuscript is based have been approved by the following New Zealand National Health and Disability Ethics Committee (Study reference numbers: IS - Wellington Ethics Committee 03/09/090; TS - Central Region Ethics Committee CEN/05/12/096; DS - Lower South Regional Ethics committee LRS/08/09/041). Permission to access the data for the purposes of this study was granted by the ARCH Governance Group [27].

Consent for publication

Written informed consent was obtained from all participants for the use of de-identified data and transcript excerpts in academic publications (as is the case here).

Competing interests

The authors declare that they have no competing interests.

References

1. Roddy E, Mallen CD, Doherty M. Gout. Br Med J. 2013;347:f5648. https://doi.org/10.1136/bmj.f5648.
2. Ting K, Graf SW, Whittle L. Update on the diagnosis and management of gout. Med J Aust. 2015;203:86–8.
3. Dalbeth N. Management of gout in primary care: challenges and potential solutions. Rheumatology. 2013;52:1549–50.
4. Paskins Z, Sanders T, Croft PR, Hassell AB. The identity crisis of osteoarthritis in general practice: a qualitative study using video-stimulated recall. Ann Fam Med. 2015;13:537–44.
5. Salisbury C, Procter S, Stewart K, Bowen L, Purdy S, Ridd M, et al. The content of general practice consultations: cross-sectional study based on video recordings. Br J Gen Pract. 2013; https://doi.org/10.3399/bjgp13X674431.
6. Te Karu L, Bryant L, Elley CR. Maori experiences and perceptions of gout and its treatment: a kaupapa Maori qualitative study. J Prim Health Care. 2013;5:214–22.
7. Martini N, Bryant L, Karu LT, Aho L, Chan R, Miao J, et al. Living with gout in New Zealand: an exploratory study into People's knowledge about the disease and its treatment. J Clin Rheumatol. 2012;18:125–9.
8. Lindsay K, Gow P, Vanderpyl J, Logo P, Dalbeth N. The experience and impact of living with gout: a study of men with chronic gout using a qualitative grounded theory approach. J Clin Rheumatol. 2011;17:1–6.
9. Harrold LR, Mazor KM, Velten S, Ockene IS, Yood RA. Patients and providers view gout differently: a qualitative study. Chronic Ill. 2010;6:263–71.
10. Richardson JC, Liddle J, Mallen CD, Roddy E, Prinjha S, Ziebland S, et al. "Why me? I don't fit the mould… I am a freak of nature": a qualitative study of women's experience of gout. BMC Womens Health. 2015; https://doi.org/10.1186/s12905-015-0277-z.
11. Liddle J, Roddy E, Mallen CD, Hider SL, Prinjha S, Ziebland S, et al. Mapping patients' experiences from initial symptoms to gout diagnosis: a qualitative exploration. BMJ Open. 2015; https://doi.org/10.1136/bmjopen-2015-008323.
12. Vaccher S, Kannangara DRW, Baysari MT, Reath J, Zwar N, Williams KM, et al. Barriers to Care in Gout: from prescriber to patient. J Rheumatol. 2016;43:144–9.
13. Chandratre P, Mallen CD, Roddy E, Liddle J, Richardson J. "You want to get on with the rest of your life": a qualitative study of health-related quality of life in gout. Clin Rheumatol. 2016;35:1197–205.
14. Humphrey C, Hulme R, Dalbeth N, Gow P, Arroll B, Lindsay K. A qualitative study to explore health professionals' experience of treating gout: understanding perceived barriers to effective gout management. J Prim Health Care. 2016;8:149–56.
15. Dalbeth N, Petrie KJ, House M, Chong J, Leung W, Chegudi R, et al. Illness perceptions in patients with gout and the relationship with progression of musculoskeletal disability. Arthritis Care Res. 2011;63:1605–12.
16. Harrold L, Mazor K, Peterson D, Naz N, Firneno C, Yood R. Patients' knowledge and beliefs concerning gout and its treatment: a population based study. BMC Musculoskelet Disord. 2012;13:180. https://doi.org/10.1186/1471-2474-13-180.
17. Harrold LR, Mazor KM, Negron A, Ogarek J, Firneno C, Yood RA. Primary care providers' knowledge, beliefs and treatment practices for gout: results of a physician questionnaire. Rheumatology. 2013;52:1623–9.
18. Doherty M, Jansen TL, Nuki G, Pascual E, Perez-Ruiz F, Punzi L, et al. Gout: why is this curable disease so seldom cured? Ann Rheum Dis. 2012;71:1765–70.
19. Spencer K, Carr A, Doherty M. Patient and provider barriers to effective management of gout in general practice: a qualitative study. Ann Rheum Dis. 2012;71:1490–5.
20. Jordan KM, Cameron JS, Snaith M, Zhang W, Doherty M, Seckl J, et al. British Society for Rheumatology and British health professionals in rheumatology guideline for the management of gout. Rheumatology. 2007;46:1372–4.
21. Khanna D, Fitzgerald JD, Khanna PP, Bae S, Singh MK, Neogi T, et al. 2012 American College of Rheumatology guidelines for management of gout. Part 1: systematic nonpharmacologic and pharmacologic therapeutic approaches to hyperuricemia. Arthritis Care Res. 2012;64:1431–46.
22. Zhang W, Doherty M, Bardin T, Pascual E, Barskova V, Conaghan P, et al. EULAR evidence based recommendations for gout. Part II: management. Report of a task force of the EULAR standing committee for international clinical studies including therapeutics (ESCISIT). Ann Rheum Dis. 2006;65:1312–24.
23. Shulten P, Thomas J, Miller M, Smith M, Ahern M. The role of diet in the management of gout: a comparison of knowledge and attitudes to current evidence. J Hum Nutr Diet. 2009;22:3–11.
24. Byrne PS, Long BE. Doctors talking to patients: a study of the verbal behaviours of doctors in the consultation. London: Her Majesty's Stationary Office; 1976.
25. Heritage J, Maynard DW. Introduction: analyzing interaction between doctors and patients in primary care encounters. In: Heritage J, Maynard DW, editors. Communication in medical care: interaction between primary care physicians and patients. Cambridge: Cambridge University Press; 2006. p. 1–21.
26. Mishler EG. The discourse of medicine: dialects of medical interviews. Norwood, NJ: Ablex; 1984.
27. ARCH. Corpus of health interactions. Wellington: University of Otago. http://www.otago.ac.nz/wellington/research/arch/corpus/. Accessed 7 Sept 2017.
28. Boyatzis R. Thematic analysis and code development: transforming qualitative information. London: Sage Publications; 1998.
29. Braun V, Clarke V. Using thematic analysis in psychology. Qual Res Psychol. 2006;3:77–101.
30. Fereday J, Muir-Cochrane E. Demonstrating rigor using thematic analysis: a hybrid approach of inductive and deductive coding and theme development. Int J Qual Methods. 2006;5:80–92.
31. Pomerantz A. Extreme case formulations: a way of legitimizing claims. Hum Stud. 1986;9:219–29.
32. Maynard DW, Heritage J. Conversation analysis, doctor–patient interaction and medical communication. Med Educ. 2005;39:428–35.
33. Freeman J, Loewe R. Barriers to communication about diabetes mellitus. Patients' and physicians' different view of the disease. J Fam Pract. 2000;49:507–12.
34. Barry CA, Bradley CP, Britten N, Stevenson FA, Barber N. Patients' unvoiced agendas in general practice consultations: qualitative study. Br Med J. 2000;320:1246–50.
35. Noordman J, Koopmans B, Korevaar JC, van der Weijden T, van Dulmen S. Exploring lifestyle counselling in routine primary care consultations: the professionals' role. Fam Pract. 2013;30:332–40.
36. Barton J, Dew K, Dowell A, Sheridan N, Kenealy T, Macdonald L, et al. Patient resistance as a resource: candidate obstacles in diabetes consultations. Sociol Health Ill. 2016; https://doi.org/10.1111/1467-9566.12447.
37. Balfe M. Diets and discipline: the narratives of practice of university students with type 1 diabetes. Sociol Health Ill. 2007;29:136–53.

38. Schoenberg NE, Amey CH, Coward RT. Stories of meaning: lay perspectives on the origin and management of noninsulin dependent diabetes mellitus among older women in the United States. Soc Sci Med. 1998;47:2113–25.
39. Sheridan NF, Kenealy TW, Kidd JD, Schmidt-Busby JI, Hand JE, Raphael DL, et al. Patients' engagement in primary care: powerlessness and compounding jeopardy. A qualitative study. Health Expect. 2015;18:32–43.
40. Morris C, Macdonald L, Stubbe M, Dowell A. "It's complicated" - talking about gout medicines in primary care consultations: a qualitative study. BMC Fam Pract. 2016;17:114. https://doi.org/10.1186/s12875-016-0515-y.
41. Rees F, Jenkins W, Doherty M. Patients with gout adhere to curative treatment if informed appropriately: proof-of-concept observational study. Ann Rheum Dis. 2013;72:826–30.
42. World Health Organization. Primary health care: now more than ever. Geneva: World Health Organization; 2008.
43. Dowell A, Macdonald L, Stubbe M, Plumridge E, Dew K. Clinicians at work: what can we learn from interactions in the consultation? N Z Fam Physician. 2007;34:345–50.

23

A qualitative evidence synthesis to explore healthcare professionals' experience of prescribing opioids to adults with chronic non-malignant pain

Fran Toye[1*], Kate Seers[2], Stephanie Tierney[2] and Karen Louise Barker[3]

Abstract

Background: Despite recent guidelines suggesting that patients with chronic non-malignant pain might not benefit, there has been a significant rise in opioid prescription for chronic non-malignant pain. This topic is important because an increasing number of HCPs are prescribing opioids despite very limited evidence for long-term opioid therapy for chronic non-malignant pain outside of end-of-life care. To better understand the challenges of providing effective treatment, we conducted the first qualitative evidence synthesis to explore healthcare professionals' experience of treating people with chronic non-malignant pain. We report findings that explore healthcare professionals' experience of prescribing opioids to this group of patients.

Methods: We searched five electronic bibliographic databases (Medline, Embase, CINAHL, PsychINFO, AMED) from inception to November 2015 and screened titles, abstracts and full texts of potential studies. We included studies in English that explored healthcare professionals' experience of treating adults with chronic non-malignant pain. Two reviewers quality appraised each paper. We used the methods of meta-ethnography developed and refined for large reviews, and the GRADE-CERQual framework to rate confidence in review findings.

Results: We screened 954 abstracts and 184 full texts, and included 77 studies in the full review. 17 of these 77 studies included concepts that explored the experience of prescribing opioids. We abstracted these concepts into 6 overarching themes: (1) Should I, shouldn't I? (2) Pain is Pain; (3) Walking a fine line; (4) Social guardianship; (5) Moral boundary work; (6) Regulations and guidelines. We used the GRADE-CERQual framework to evaluate confidence in findings. A new overarching concept of 'ambiguity' explains the balancing required around the factors taken into account when prescribing opioids. Managing this ambiguity is challenging and these findings can inform healthcare professionals dealing with these decisions.

Conclusions: This conceptual model demonstrates the complexity of making a decision to prescribe opioids to someone with chronic non-malignant pain. Although opioid prescription is underpinned by the therapeutic aim of alleviating pain, this aim may be misplaced. This has implications for education in light of the new regulations for opioid prescription. Findings also demonstrate that the decision is influenced by intra- and interpersonal factors and broader external concerns.

Keywords: Chronic pain, Analgesic, opioid, Qualitative research, Qualitative evidence synthesis, Meta-ethnography

* Correspondence: Francine.toye@ouh.nhs.uk
[1]Nuffield Orthopaedic Centre, Oxford University Hospitals NHS Foundation Trust, Windmill Road, Oxford OX3 7HE, UK
Full list of author information is available at the end of the article

Background

Population estimates suggest that around 25% of adults around the world suffer with moderate or severe pain [1–5] and for between 6 and 14% of these adults pain can be severe and disabling [5, 6]. Each year over five million people in the UK develop chronic non-malignant pain [7], and healthcare professionals (HCPs) can find it a challenge to effectively treat this pain. For example, they can find it difficult if they are unable to offer the patient a solution [8], or if they have to refuse patients' requests for a particular test or treatment [9, 10]. Despite recent USA [11] and UK guidelines [12] suggesting that patients with chronic non-malignant pain might not gain benefits, opioids are commonly prescribed for uncontrolled persistent pain, and there has been a significant rise in opioid prescription [13–18]. Survey data suggest that around 12% of UK patients with chronic non-malignant pain are prescribed strong opioids, mainly by GPs [1]. As many as 20% of patients with non-malignant pain symptoms receive an opioid prescription [19].

In order to better understand the challenges of providing effective treatment, we aimed to explore healthcare professionals' experience of treating patients with chronic non-malignant pain by conducting a qualitative evidence synthesis in this area. A full report of HCPs experience of treating patients with chronic non-malignant pain is being published by the NIHR Journals library [20]. We aimed to focus on the experience of treating chronic pain conditions with no clear attributable biomedical cause. Qualitative evidence synthesis aims to systematically search for and integrate findings in order to increase our understanding of complex processes of care, and thus improve the experience and quality of that care. As part of this review, we found a body of evidence that specifically explored healthcare professionals' (HCPs) experience of prescribing opioid medication to patients with chronic non-malignant pain. This topic is important because an increasing number of HCPs are prescribing opioids despite very limited evidence for long-term opioid therapy for chronic non-malignant pain outside of end-of-life care [18].

Methods

We used the methods of meta-ethnography developed, refined and reported in a previous qualitative evidence synthesis of patients' experience of chronic non-malignant musculoskeletal pain [21]. There are seven stages to meta-ethnography: getting started, deciding what is relevant, reading the studies, determining how studies are related, translating studies into each other, synthesising translations and expressing the synthesis [22].

Search strategy

We searched five electronic bibliographic databases (Medline, Embase, CINAHL, PsychINFO, AMED) from inception to end of November 2015 using terms adapted from the InterTASC Information Specialists' Sub-Group (ISSG) Search Filter Resources [23–26]. We combined thesaurus terms from each database with free text terms for qualitative research as a subject, and for pain as a subject (Table 1). Previous research suggests that citation checks, hand searching, grey literature or PhD searches do not necessarily add value to large meta-ethnographies. For example, Toye and colleagues found that 95% of studies were identified in the first three databases searched [21, 27]. FT and KLB screened the titles, abstracts and full text of potential studies for relevance. Any disagreement was discussed and resolved with a third reviewer.

Inclusion/exclusion criteria

We included studies written in English that explored HCPS' experience of treating adults with chronic non-malignant pain. We used a broad search strategy that included 'PAIN' as both a thesaurus and free text term in order to encompass all chronic non-malignant pain conditions. We excluded acute pain, head pain, arthritis (including osteoarthritis and rheumatoid arthritis), patient experience and studies where HCP experience could not be disentangled from the experience of others. Our focus was on non-specific chronic non-malignant pain. We did not include HCPs experience of treating patients with arthritis as, after consultation with our advisory group of clinicians and patients, we felt it likely that treating conditions with bio-medically attributable causes would be qualitatively different. At the outset of this study, we had intended to only include HCPs experience of treating chronic non-malignant *musculoskeletal* pain in order to mirror a previous QES of patients' experience of chronic non-malignant musculoskeletal pain [21]. However our preliminary reading indicated that HCPs experience of treating chronic non-malignant pain was not boundaried to a particular body system, but was a summative experience that cuts across conditions.

Quality appraisal

Although there are many suggested frameworks, there is no consensus on what makes a qualitative study good [28, 29]. We used three methods of quality appraisal to frame our discussions regarding inclusion: (a) The Critical Appraisal Skills Programme (CASP) questions for appraising qualitative research [30]; (b) constructs from a qualitative study embedded in a previous large meta-ethnography [31]; (c) a global appraisal of whether the study was: a 'key paper' ('conceptually rich and could potentially make an important contribution to the synthesis'); a satisfactory paper; a paper that is irrelevant to the synthesis; a methodologically fatally flawed paper [29]. Two reviewers appraised each paper, and if they were unable to reach an

Table 1 Example search terms – Medline: (a) qualitative subject headings); (b) qualitative free text terms; (c) pain subject headings; (d) pain free text terms

(I) QUALITATIVE SUBJECT HEADINGS	exp QUALITATIVE RESEARCH exp. INTERVIEWS AS TOPIC exp. FOCUS GROUPS NURSING METHODOLOGY RESEARCH ATTITUDE TO HEALTH
(II) QUALITATIVE FREE TEXT TERMS	Qualitative ADJ5 (theor* OR study OR studies OR research OR analysis) ethno.ti,ab emic OR etic. ti,ab phenomenolog*.ti,ab hermeneutic*.ti,ab heidegger* OR husserl* OR colaizzi* OR giorgi* OR glaser OR strauss OR (van AND kaam*) OR (van AND manen) OR ricoeur OR spiegelberg* OR merleau).ti,ab constant ADJ3 compar*.ti,ab focus ADJ3 group*.ti,ab grounded ADJ3 (theor* OR study OR studies OR research OR analysis).ti,ab narrative ADJ3 analysis.ti,ab discourse ADJ3 analysis.ti,ab (lived OR life) ADJ3 experience*.ti,ab (theoretical OR purposive) ADJ3 sampl*.ti,ab (field ADJ note*) OR (field ADJ record*) OR fieldnote*.ti,ab participant* ADJ3 observ*.ti,ab action ADJ research.ti,ab (digital ADJ record) OR audiorecord* OR taperecord* OR videorecord* OR videotap*).ti,ab (cooperative AND inquir*) OR (co AND operative AND inquir*) OR (co-operative AND inquir*) .ti,ab (semi-structured OR semistructured OR unstructured OR structured) ADJ3 interview*.ti,ab (informal OR in-depth OR indepth OR "in depth") ADJ3 interview*.ti,ab ("face-to-face" OR "face to face") ADJ3 interview*.ti,ab "IPA" OR "interpretative phenomenological analysis".ti,ab "appreciative inquiry".ti,ab (social AND construct*) OR (postmodern* OR post-structural*) OR (post structural* OR poststructural*) OR (post modern*) OR post-modern* OR feminis*).ti,ab humanistic OR existential OR experiential.ti,ab
(III) PAIN SUBJECT HEADINGS	exp BACK PAIN/OR exp. CHRONIC PAIN/OR exp. LOW BACK PAIN/OR exp. MUSCULOSKELETAL PAIN/OR exp. PAIN/OR exp. PAIN CLINICS/. exp. FIBROMYALGIA/ exp. PAIN MANAGEMENT/
(IV) PAIN FREE TEXT TERMS	(chronic* OR persistent* OR long-stand* OR longstand* OR unexplain* OR un-explain*) fibromyalgia "back ache" OR back-ache OR backache "pain clinic" OR pain-clinic* pain adj5 syndrome*

agreement, the study was sent to another reviewer for the final decision. We utilised the GRADE-CERQual framework [32] which aims to help reviewers to assess and describe how much confidence readers can place in review findings. GRADE-CERQual suggest four domains of interest: (1) 'Methodological limitations' concern the conduct of the primary study; (2) 'Relevance' is the extent to which the primary studies are applicable to the review; (3) 'Adequacy of data' is an 'overall determination of the degree of richness and quantity of data supporting a review finding'; (4) Coherence considers how well the findings are grounded in the primary studies [32].

Data extraction and synthesis

Two reviewers read each paper to develop a list of the concepts from the primary papers. If they agreed that there was no clear concept then it was not included in the analysis. Translating studies into each other involves comparing concepts in order to sort them into conceptual categories [22]. All reviewers sorted the concepts into categories with shared meaning. Through constantly comparing and discussing these categories they started to see similarities and differences that allowed further abstraction into the final conceptual categories. The final analytic stage, 'synthesising translations' involved integrating the conceptual categories into a conceptual framework. We planned to develop a line of argument synthesis, which involves 'making a whole into something more than the parts alone imply' [22] (page 28). This is achieved by comparing concepts and developing 'a grounded theory that puts the similarities and differences between studies into interpretive order' [22] (page 64).

Results

We report findings that explored HCPs' experience of prescribing opioids to patients with chronic non-malignant pain. A full report of HCPs experience of treating patients with chronic non-malignant pain is being published by the NIHR Journals library [20]. The results of the systematic search are shown in Fig. 1. We screened 954 potentially relevant studies and excluded 770 after screening the abstracts. We retrieved 184 full text articles and excluded 101. We excluded 16 studies that were not qualitative or that included limited qualitative data, and 85 studies that we agreed were out of scope (for example, they did not present the HCP voice, or they did not explore the experience of chronic non-malignant pain). Full details of study exclusions are being published elsewhere [20]. Of the 83 studies remaining, we unanimously excluded a further six on the grounds of methodological report. After reading and extracting concepts from the remaining 77 studies, the reviewers identified 17 studies that included concepts specific to the experience of prescribing opioids to patients with chronic non-malignant pain [33–49]. Table 2 gives the author, year, country, participants, data collection, analytic method and aim of the 17 studies included. Findings are drawn from 486 HCPs from different geographic locations; USA (n = 10), UK (n = 4), Canada (n = 2), Spain (n = 1) (Table 2).

All reviewers discussed and organised the concepts into 18 conceptual categories. Only a single concept did not fit into a conceptual categories (Barry 2010: Patient Factors - Cost of Specialty Pain Management [34]). This described how some HCPs felt their patients were concerned about the costs and coverage of specialty pain management and therefore might only be relevant to healthcare systems that are not free at point of delivery. All four reviewers further abstracted the 18 conceptual categories into 6 themes that underpin HCPs' experience of prescribing opioids to patients with chronic non-malignant pain. A core concept overarching all six themes was a sense of ambiguity surrounding opioid prescribing.

Confidence in review findings (GRADE -CERQual assessment)

Indicators of confidence in our review findings as recommended in the GRADE -CERQual framework [32] are shown in Table 3. Both reviewers rated all studies as satisfactory. Twelve studies were directly relevant and aimed to explore the experience of opioid prescription [33–35, 37–39, 41, 43, 44, 46, 48, 49]. The remaining

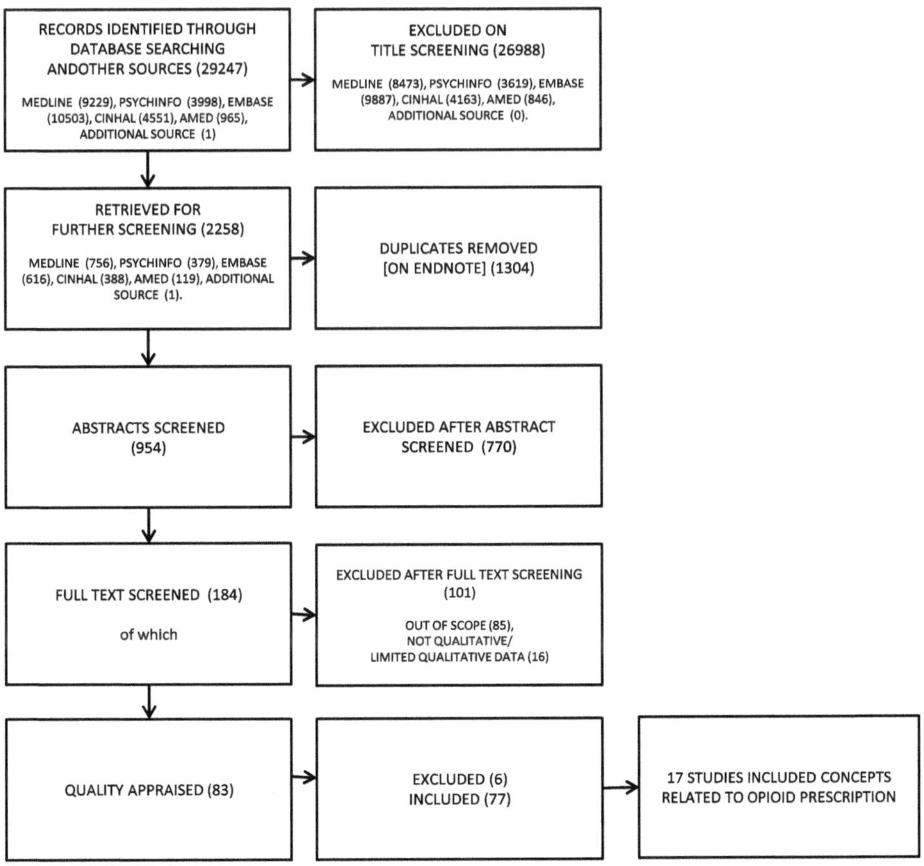

Fig. 1 Flow Chart showing results of systematic search: this figure give the records identified, screened, retrieved, appraised and included in the review

Table 2 Characteristics of 17 studies that included concepts exploring the experience of prescribing opioids to patients with chronic non-malignant pain

AUTHOR YEAR	COUNTRY	PARTICIPANTS	DATA COLLECTION	ANALYSIS	AIM OF STUDY
BALDACCHINO 2010 [33]	SCOTLAND, UK	29 physicians	2 focus groups/19 interviews	Framework analysis	To describe physicians' attitudes and experience of prescribing opioids for chronic non-cancer pain with a history of substance abuse.
BARRY 2010 [34]	USA	23 physicians	Semi-structured interview	Grounded theory	To identify barriers and facilitators to opioid treatment of chronic non-cancer pain patients
BERG 2009 [35]	USA	16 physicians and 'assistants'	Semi-structured interview	Thematic analysis	To explore providers' perceptions of ambiguity, and then to examine their strategies for making diagnostic and treatment decisions to manage chronic pain among patients on methadone maintenance therapy.
BRIONES-VOZMEDIANO 2013 [36]	SPAIN	9 mixed HCPs: (GPs, physicians, physiotherapists, rheumatologists, psychologists, psychiatrist)	Semi-structured interview	Discourse Analysis	To explore experiences of fibromyalgia management, namely diagnostic approach, therapeutic management and the health professional-patient relationship.
ESQUIBEL 2014 [37]	USA	21 family practitioners	In-depth interviews	Immersion-crystallization	To explore the experiences of adults receiving opioid therapy for relief of chronic non-cancer pain and that of their physicians
FONTANA 2008 [38]	USA	9 advanced practice nurses	Semi-structured interview	No specific method identified	To critically examine subjective factors that influence prescribing practices of registered nurses for patients with chronic non-malignant pain.
GOOBERMAN-HILL 2011 [39]	UK	27 general practitioners	Semi-structured interview	Thematic analysis	To explore GPs' opinions about opioids and decision-making processes when prescribing 'strong' opioids for chronic joint pain.
KAASALAINEN 2007 [40]	CANADA	66 mixed HCPs: (Physicians ($n = 9$), registered practical nurses)	Semi-structured interviews/ focus groups	Grounded theory	To explore the decision-making process of pain management of physicians and nurses and how their attitudes affect decisions about prescribing and administering pain medications among older adults in long-term care.
KAASALAINEN 2010B [42]	CANADA	53 Mixed HCPs: (15 Registered nurses, 6 registered practical nurses, 4 physicians, 20 unlicensed care practitioners, 2 pharmacists, 2 physiotherapists, 4 administrators)	6 focus groups/interviews	Case-study analysis	To: (1) explore barriers to pain management and those associated with implementing a pain management program in long-term care (LTC); (2) to develop an inter-professional approach to improve pain management in LTC.
KILARU 2014 [41]	USA	61 emergency physicians	Semi-structured interview	Grounded theory	To identify key themes regarding emergency physicians' definition, awareness, use, and opinions of opioid prescribing guidelines.
KREBS 2014 [43]	USA	14 primary care physicians	Semi-structured interview	Immersion-crystallisation	To understand physicians' and patients' perspectives on recommended opioid management practices and to identify potential barriers to and facilitators of guideline-concordant opioid management in primary care.

Table 2 Characteristics of 17 studies that included concepts exploring the experience of prescribing opioids to patients with chronic non-malignant pain *(Continued)*

AUTHOR YEAR	COUNTRY	PARTICIPANTS	DATA COLLECTION	ANALYSIS	AIM OF STUDY
MCCRORIE 2015 [44]	UK	15 general practitioners	2 focus groups	Grounded theory	To understand the processes which bring about and perpetuate long-term prescribing of opioids for chronic, non-cancer pain.
RUIZ 2010 [45]	USA	19 mixed HCPs: (14 primary care physicians, 5 nurse practitioners)	3 focus groups 9 semi-structured interviews	Grounded theory	To explore the attitudes of primary care clinicians (PCPs) toward chronic non-malignant pain management in older people.
SEAMARK 2013 [46]	UK	22 general practitioners	Interviews/focus groups	Thematic analysis	To describe the factors influencing GPs' prescribing of strong opioid drugs for chronic non cancer pain.
SIEDLECKI 2014 [47]	USA	48 nurses	Interviews	Grounded theory	To explore and understand nurses' assessment and decision-making behaviours related to the care of patients with chronic pain in the acute care setting.
SPITZ 2011 [48]	USA	26 Mixed HCPs: (23 physicians, 3 nurse practitioners)	Focus groups	Thematic analysis	To describe primary care providers' experiences and attitudes towards, as well as perceived barriers and facilitators to prescribing opioids as a treatment for chronic pain among older adults.
STARRELS 2014 [49]	USA	28 physicians	Open ended telephone interview	Grounded theory	To understand primary care providers' experiences, beliefs and attitudes about using opioid treatment agreements for patients with chronic pain.

Table 3 Confidence in review findings – GRADE -CERQual assessment

REVIEW FINDING	METHODOLOGICAL LIMITATIONS (NUMBER OF SATISFACTORY STUDIES)	RELEVANCE (PARTIAL OR DIRECT)	ADEQUACY (NUMBER OF CONCEPTS)	COHERENCE* (NUMBER OF STUDIES OUT OF 17)	OVERALL ASSESSMENT OF CONFIDENCE
SHOULD I, SHOULDN'T I?	ALL	9 DIRECT	19	9 [34–39, 43, 44, 48]	HIGH CONFIDENCE
PAIN IS PAIN	ALL	5 DIRECT, 1 PARTIAL	8	6 [33, 39, 40, 42, 46, 48]	MODERATE CONFIDENCE
WALKING A FINE LINE	ALL	9 DIRECT, 1 PARTIAL	16	8 *[33, 35, 39–41, 45, 46, 48]*	MODERATE CONFIDENCE
SOCIAL GUARDIANSHIP	ALL	10 DIRECT, 1 PARTIAL	17	11 [33–35, 37–39, 41, 43, 45, 46, 48]	HIGH CONFIDENCE
MORAL BOUNDARY WORK	ALL	12 DIRECT, 2 PARTIAL	27	14 [33–35, 37–39, 41, 43–49]	HIGH CONFIDENCE
REGULATIONS AND GUIDELINES	ALL	8 DIRECT	18	8 [34, 35, 38, 39, 41, 43, 48, 49]	MODERATE CONFIDENCE

five studies were partially relevant and included themes related to opioid prescription. Table 3 shows the number of concepts and the number of studies out of 17 supporting each review finding. We rated our confidence in the review finding as high when it was supported by more than half of the studies. However, there is currently no agreed way of making an assessment of confidence for qualitative synthesis.

Thematic analysis

Our synthesis supports six themes that can help to understand HCPs experience of prescribing opioids to patients with chronic non-malignant pain: (1) Should I, shouldn't I? (2) Pain is Pain; (3) Walking a fine line; (4) Social guardianship; (5) Moral boundary work; (6) Regulations and guidelines. We have illustrated each theme with examples of narrative from the primary studies.

Should I, shouldn't I?

The theme 'should I, shouldn't I?' describes the sense of uncertainty about when to prescribe opioids, and a feeling of ambiguity about the effects of medication. This feeling was heightened by an observation that, in similar circumstances, other HCPs seemed to make different clinical decisions:

> When we're practicing alongside other people who have come to completely different conclusions, it really makes you think ... have I been making the wrong decisions; did we get different information and come to different conclusions? Do we have different values that underlie our decision-making? [35] (physician, USA)

HPCs found it harder to approach analgesic prescribing where the disease aetiology was unknown, for example, in fibromyalgia.

> Because you don't really know what's happening there. The aetiology of the disease is not really known and you have few means of knowing what you're doing. You're treating the pain and you don't know why there is no response [36] (rheumatologist, Spain)

> They are in pain, you give them something for the pain and: 'it doesn't do me any good ... it relieved the pain a little but the pain has come back' ... . No matter what you give them, the pain doesn't go away [36] (GP, Spain)

There was a sense that clinical education did not prepare HCPs adequately for these decisions.

> We took an advanced pharm[acology] class, and we discussed it in one lecture, but that was it. Isn't that ridiculous considering how many people we see in pain? [38] (practise nurse, USA)

Uncertainty was also compounded by the sense that specialist referrals were either restricted or unproductive. Some HCPs felt unsupported in managing the most difficult cases and explored the possibility of more specialist services: for example, for patients with chronic pain and substance abuse:

> Often I find that they are not accomplishing any more than I was and [patients] are often sent back to me with them [pain specialists] essentially saying, 'we did our best.' It's very frustrating, because if they were easy patients they wouldn't have been seeing them ... they wouldn't have been referred ... I would love for there to be a separate clinic where I could refer patients for management of their chronic pain and substance abuse simultaneously. Kind of take me out of the picture [34] (physician, USA)

Pain is pain

The theme 'pain is pain' is underpinned by the ideal that if a person is in pain then the primary aim of the HCP should be to relieve pain. Some felt that even addiction should not be a barrier to opioid prescription and described the stigma against patients with addiction:

> I had a guy last week who'd been stabbed and he'd been in ITU ... and he had to discharge himself because they wouldn't give him any pain control ... he wasn't even getting his prescribed dose of methadone he was getting under dosed for his addiction and his pain control ... there's a protocol ... but they choose not to know about it and it's just pure stigma. [33] (physician, UK)

> At the end of the day, if someone's got chronic pain it doesn't matter if they're addicted to painkillers if it sorts out their quality of life [39] (GP, UK)

However, although in *theory* 'pain is pain', HCPs described factors that would make them less likely to prescribe opioids in practice for chronic non-malignant pain. For example, whereas for malignant pain the aim might be to achieve complete pain relief, in non-malignant pain the HPC would need to consider the balance of risks and benefits of long term opioid prescription over time:

> I don't regard them [malignant and non-malignant pain] the same ... with [malignant pain] ... your aim always is to get complete relief of pain ... over a finite period of time. For chronic pain ... you've got to weigh up ... the potential side effects... I think there has to be an acceptance that you are not necessarily going to get them pain free because they've got the rest of their lives to live as well ... so your two end points are different [46] (GP, UK)

Some HCPs queried whether enough attention was given to chronic non-malignant pain when the focus was mainly on pain control in palliative patients.

> The only people in my practice that I prescribe [opioids] to would be people who are palliative ... . [on the other hand] we tend to focus too much on pain control for palliation as opposed to just everyday clients. Certainly nobody wants to die in pain, but nobody wants to live in pain either [40] (physician, Canada)

Walking a fine line

The theme 'walking a fine line' describes the need for HCPs to carefully balance the benefits and adverse effects of opioids. On the one hand, emphasising adverse effects might lead to unnecessary pain; on the other hand, emphasis on pain control might lead to harm or abuse. Some HCPs felt that treating pain should take priority over the risk of opioid misuse when making prescribing decisions.

> I mean there are two mistakes you make. You can make the mistake of under treating or of giving medicines that end up being sold or used for unintended purposes. You're going to make errors both ways, and I think it's generally better to risk opiates being misused versus not treating someone's pain [35] (physician, USA)

There were additional concerns about prescribing opioids to older adults because of the potential severity and impact of adverse effects. In theory a person's age should not affect decisions, but in practise, there was a sense that it does.

> But there are safety issues, and at the end of the day if they came to grief and fell over, fell down the stairs and broke something, died, then, you know, you'd feel guilty about giving them adequate pain relief in your view, but excessive side effects, drowsiness, what have you, that contributed to some major event on their part. So we walk at a fine line sometimes between giving adequate pain relief and giving safe treatment [39] (GP, UK)

Although HCPs felt that opioids should be used to manage older peoples' pain, they also discussed how the risks and benefits of prescribing opioids would require assessment on an individual basis.

> Older people metabolize medication differently than younger people, so you don't want to give them medication that's going to impair their ability to function ... A lot of them drive even though they may be even much older, so you don't want falls. You don't want automobile accidents. You don't want injuries. You don't want to interfere with their ability to make judgments and so on, so I don't like using opioids in elderly people at all ... *[however]* my feeling is that they should be used, but we need to, again, look at each person individually, and then determine which person benefits from opioid therapy [45] (HPC not stated, USA)

Social guardianship

The theme 'social guardianship' describes a culture hostile to opioid use and the professional taboo of prescribing opioids. HCPs compared their own prescribing practise to their colleagues and were concerned over being judged by their peers. Some felt that they had a personal responsibility to protect society from the consequences of opioid misuse and viewed patients with suspicion, particularly if they requested opioids. To protect society, some implemented strategies to control patients' behaviour (for example: bottle checks, opioid contracts, background checks). HCPs also described concerns over diversion of opioid prescriptions to others.

> I am a naysayer on opiates ... too much of my day is spent policing how many [opioids] have been prescribed and how many times a patient is a return patient and how often they visited requesting opiate prescriptions [41] (emergency physician, USA)

> If you prescribe to a population where you think diversion is going on, you definitely have a responsibility. I also worry about who is getting the drug, is it my son? I mean, we are members of society after all... . I think it is okay to go into a relationship with some mistrust. It is survival in the business we are in [38] (advanced practice nurse, USA)

Some HCPs discussed indicators of potential abuse (for example: lost prescriptions, early requests for medication, frequent attendance), although acknowledged that these might actually indicate poorly managed pain.

> If people are taking it genuinely for pain they tend to stick to the prescribed dosage ... addicts tend to be the ones who are always ordering early ... you don't lose your tablets if you are ... getting great benefit from them for pain [33] (physician, UK)

> The concern would be is this pain real, or is it just put on to obtain opioid? ... I mean, an assessment of the pain and whether I think it's genuine or not. I think it's very difficult; it's something I'm currently dealing with at the moment, and not very successfully [46] (GP, UK)

Moral boundary work

The theme moral boundary work is underpinned by the clinical work of deciding whose pain is 'real' and thus who should be prescribed opioids. HCPs described ideal patients (for example, those that made appropriate demands, took advice and did not cause trouble) and 'difficult' patients (the demanding, non-adherent and trouble-making). They made judgments based on non-clinical factors about whether or not a patient was 'legitimate'.

> For those patients that have a legitimate reason for wanting to take it and if I can trust them—that they are not selling, they're not abusing, and most of these are older patients of mine. They never request early refills, they don't go to the [emergency room] in between visits to get them—there's no need for me to do periodic drug screenings and so forth (primary care physician, USA) [43]

Pain with no biomedical diagnosis, vague symptoms or dissonance between a patient's report of pain and professional observation could trigger suspicion.

> A lot of patients you can tell ... that they really need it ... based on their underlying pathology, for example, a patient who has a cancer or a real anatomic foundation for it ... now this is not 100% reliable, but you have to count on more observation, combined with other clinical data. So after 2 or 3 visits, you pretty much know who is abusing and who is not [43] (primary care physician, USA)

> I think for patients who have chronic pain it's more challenging and I think that's the place where I'm constantly rethinking my practice... You're always on the fence: am I doing the right thing for my patient? [41] (Emergency physician, USA)

Non-clinical moral judgments or *gut-feelings* contributed to prescribing decisions. HCPs recalled episodes when they had made a mistake by trusting 'the wrong' patient. Over time they described how they had become better at making the *right* decision.

> The way I behave now prescribing for everything is a sort of rather woolly, nebulous product of everything I've done... You just pick it up over the years, so I'm sure I've been moulded by the successes and the failures which have come my way ... we all learn on the hoof, don't we?' ... I think everybody's fingers get burnt with people who you give the opioids to with a more trusting attitude than maybe you should have [46] (GP, UK)

> I've had trust in people, and it's been betrayed ... I find I'm not always that great a judge of who to trust and who not to trust... . I think people feel like they've been violated, you know, cheated, like they've been taken advantage of. I feel some of that, too. Ultimately you feel you've made a poor judgment, and you get mad at yourself ... My impression was that he had a true ankle problem. Then you find out it was all lies ... you're allowed to make mistakes [35] (physician, USA)

However, some sensed the dangers of judging a book by its cover and acknowledged that basing clinical decisions on their gut feeling was not fair or accurate.

> There's a disconnect ... even if it's the sweetest little 85-year-old woman who looks like your grandmother,

> versus, you know, some guy from the ghetto wearing his pants down at his knees ... it shouldn't really matter [49] (physicians, USA)

Regulations and guidelines

The theme regulations and guidelines depict HCPs' views about external regulation of opioid prescription (specifically guidelines, opioid agreements and drug screening). Some described a negative view of prescribing guidelines and felt that they interfered with professional autonomy; an example of the 'legislature practising medicine without a licence' [41].

> You're there to help them and they can tell you their deepest, darkest secrets, but yet you're policing them... . I'm not a big drug screen person, to be honest, because I like to see the person as a person. I'm not clouded by all this other stuff ... You can't do your job when you are thinking about these things [43] (primary care physician, USA)

> There could be negative implications to that if patients are actually leaving the emergency department because of the way they interpret that [regulations] poster ... there's potential that sick patients could actually leave your emergency department when they need help [41] (emergency physician, USA)

HCPs described fears legislative reprimand.

> My name is on that bottle. If they lose it and someone else takes it and they die, who do you think they are going to come to? What if it is a kid who takes it just for fun—my name is on that, not yours. ... I had a patient die. He took the entire bottle, and the police came to see me because they found him dead with the empty bottle with my name on it, and I say to patients now, 'I am only going to give you a small amount, because I don't want you found dead with my name on your bottle.' [38] (Advanced practice nurse, USA)

Others described a negative view of opioid prescribing agreements and drug screening as striking a blow at the heart of a patient-clinician relationship by creating mistrust and hostility.

> It can really strike a major blow to trust in the doctor patient relationship when you ask someone to sign a piece of paper ... A huge power play on the part of the doctor ... if there is already mistrust between the patient and the doctor, it could heighten that mistrust ... .It takes work on the provider's part, to make it an alliance-building instrument instead of a punitive contract [49] (physician, USA)

Some HPCs described a more positive attitude to regulation. For example, opioid agreements could be useful in establishing boundaries and opening up honest discussion.

> I think it improves the care, because you are able to then have more open and frank discussions around their pain ... . and [about] other things going on in their life ... In the best of circumstances it actually will make for a deeper more trusting relationship [49] (physician, USA)

Some used guidelines as leverage or to justify decisions and thus help them to deal with 'challenging' patients.

> I tell them this is standard protocol. I'm not singling you out. I'm not picking on you. I'm not treating you like an addict. This would happen to anybody. If you take our chronic pain meds long enough, anybody will become physically dependent on them [43] (primary care physician, USA)

> [An agreement] gives me leverage or comfort in discontinuing the medication if the patient violates the agreement, because we've kind of laid it out from the beginning that those behaviors were not okay... . it made my life a little easier, but I'm not sure it did the patients a giant service [49] (physician, USA)

Summary and conceptual framework

We developed six themes that help us to understand HCPs experience of prescribing opioids to patients with chronic non-malignant pain:

> *'Should I, shouldn't I?'* demonstrates feelings of ambiguity about describing opioids for chronic non-malignant pain; *'Pain is pain'* demonstrates that although the ideal aim is to alleviate pain, in practice there are reasons why a HCP might not prescribe opioids to people with chronic non-malignant pain; *'Walking a fine line'* describes the need to balance the benefits and adverse effects of opioids; *'Social guardianship'* describes a culture hostile to opioid use and a feeling of personal responsibility to police and protect society; *'Moral boundary work'* describes the work of deciding whose pain is 'real'; *'Regulations and guidelines' describes* ambivalence towards external regulation and guidelines.

Our conceptual model hinges on the HCPs need to decipher the ambiguity surrounding opioid prescription for chronic non-malignant pain and (*Should I, shouldn't I?*) (Fig. 2). Social suspicion and hostility toward opioids (*social guardianship*) will tip the balance for prescribing towards the negative, whereas the pre-eminence of pain (*pain is pain*) might tip the balance toward prescribing.

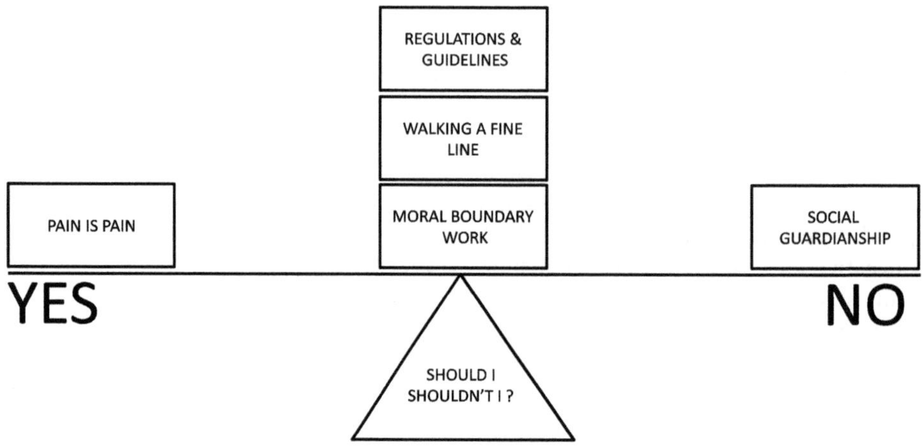

Fig. 2 Conceptual framework: this figure illustrates the conceptual framework that demonstrates the complex decision 'Should I shouldn't I?' prescribe opioids for chronic non-malignant pain. The decision is underpinned by the need to decipher ambiguity. 'Social guardianship' tips the balance against a decision to prescribe, whereas a sense that 'pain is pain' tips the balance towards prescribing. However the decision is not straightforward. The influence of the themes, 'moral boundary work', 'walking a fine line' and 'regulations and guidelines' are not clear-cut and add complexity to the decision

The decision is not clear-cut. Firstly, HCPs might make non-clinical judgments about the person (*moral boundary work*), thirdly, they must determine the balance of positive and adverse effects for each individual (*walking a fine line*) and finally there is a sense of professional ambivalence towards prescribing guidelines (*regulations and guidelines*). This conceptual model demonstrates the complexity of making a decision to prescribe opioids to someone with non-malignant pain. It also demonstrates that the decision is influenced by intra- and interpersonal factors and broader external concerns.

Discussion

This exploration of HCPs experience of prescribing opioids is embedded within a wider qualitative evidence synthesis that aims to further understand healthcare professionals' experience of treating patients with chronic non-malignant pain [20]. The findings of qualitative research are an interpretation of data. The centrality of interpretation to qualitative research is also its strength; it aims to challenge and develop ideas rather than test theories. In collaborative projects *individual* interpretations enter into a dialectic process where they are challenged and modified. Our model is based on a rigorous collaborative process that included the research team and an advisory group that included patients and clinicians. The innovation of our study is to identify concepts that explore HCPs' experience of prescribing opioids and to provide a conceptual framework to help us to understand its complexity. This topic is important because an increasing number of HCPs are prescribing opioids despite very limited evidence for long-term opioid therapy for chronic non-malignant pain outside of end-of-life care [18]. In light of recent USA Guidelines [11] and UK [12] resources, our conceptual model can help us to try and unpick why HCPs prescribe opioids for chronic non-malignant pain. Understanding that this process is complex and that guidelines are only one aspect of the process can help suggest how we can address changes to opioid prescribing. Ten out of the 17 studies explored experiences in the USA where the recently introduced bill to congress on opioid abuse prevention and treatment suggests a move towards tighter controls (https://www.congress.gov/bill/115th-congress/house-bill/993/text). Their guidelines [11] conclude "evidence on long-term opioid therapy for chronic pain outside of end-of-life care remains limited, with insufficient evidence to determine long-term benefits versus no opioid therapy ... and extensive evidence shows the possible harms of opioids". Similarly, a UK resource to support the prescribing of opioids [12] stated "there is little evidence that they [opioids] are helpful for long term pain." There is thus a drive to move away from prescribing opioids for chronic non-malignant pain.

Our conceptual model demonstrates that opioid prescription is underpinned by the therapeutic aim of alleviating pain. HCPs reported a professional duty to get rid of pain (*'pain is pain')*. However, recent guidelines are clear that patients who do not achieve useful pain relief from opioids within 2–4 weeks are unlikely to gain benefit in the long term [11, 12]. It might be anticipated that reported inefficacy of opioids for chronic non-malignant pain would be a significant reason for *not* prescribing. However, our findings do not indicate that the limited efficacy of opioids for chronic non-malignant pain is a barrier to prescribing. This has clear implications for education, policy and practice. That professionals expressed the importance of alleviating pain suggests the necessity of an intervention that discontinues opioids if they show no benefit. A study is underway in the UK that is testing an intervention to reduce opioid use and provide other support for people with chronic non-malignant pain. The primary studies in this review were published between 2007 and 2015, thus pre-dating the recent guidelines [11, 12]. It is therefore important to consider any potential delay, inherent in systematic reviews, between publication and impact on practice.

Findings demonstrate that although some HCPs were aware of the adverse effects of opioids ('walking a fine line'), they remained concerned that deciding not to prescribe would lead to unnecessary suffering. In addition, although HCPs discuss potential harm from opioids, the focus was on preventing abuse and addiction. It could be argued that the elephant in the room is the increasing death rate from opioid-related prescription [50, 51]. Between 2003 and 2013, the age-adjusted drug poisoning death rate involving opioid analgesics in the USA increased from 2.9 to 5.1 deaths per 100,000 population [51]. In a Canadian study (1997–201), 1.8% of those prescribed opioids escalated to high dose therapy and 2% died of opioid-related causes while on treatment [50]. Our findings also support a feeling of ambiguity about the efficacy of opioid medication for people with chronic non-malignant pain ('Should I, shouldn't I?'), which indicates a gap in knowledge to be filled.

We found that a strong antagonist for prescribing opioids was a feeling of *personal* responsibility to police and protect society from opioid misuse ('social guardianship'). This was aligned with the '*Moral boundary work*' of determining who had 'real' pain and who might potentially be playing the system. A qualitative evidence synthesis of patients' experience of living with chronic non-malignant pain [21] has shown they struggle to prove their legitimacy and experience their pain as adversarial and contested; patients with chronic non-malignant pain often experience the shame and stigma of not fitting the medical model and struggle to *prove* their credibility to others [21]. An environment of mistrust and suspicion is likely to add to this negative experience of healthcare. A more positive and collaborative frame for making the decision to prescribe, or not, might be useful. For example, emphasising the limited efficacy and serious adverse effects of opioids [11, 12].

Finally, our findings demonstrate ambivalence towards the external regulation of opioid prescription. There was a sense that regulation limited professional autonomy and that there should be freedom to prescribe. Some felt that regulation could lead to mistrust and hostility. Others felt that opioid agreements could help to open up honest discussion. Others used them to justify difficult or unpopular decisions. Our search strategy focused generically on chronic non-malignant pain. Further research might usefully focus on specific diagnoses, such as osteoarthritis or rheumatoid arthritis, in order to explore potential similarities and difference in HCP experience of treating these conditions.

Conclusion

The innovation of this study is to provide a synthesis of qualitative research that helps to explain the challenges involved with prescribing opioids to patients with chronic non-malignant pain. We demonstrate that syntheses of qualitative research can help us to understand complex processes of care and for the first time uncover a new overarching concept of "ambiguity" that explains the balancing required around many of the factors HCPs take into account when prescribing opioids for chronic non-malignant pain. Our findings can inform HCPs dealing with these difficult decisions. Findings demonstrate that the decision is influenced by intra- and interpersonal factors and broader external concerns. Although opioid prescription is underpinned by the therapeutic aim of alleviating pain, this aim may be misplaced. In view of the rise of opioid prescription and recent guidance, further research to explore HCPs' experience and view of guidelines would be useful. Research to explore patients' experience of deciding to take opioids for chronic non-malignant pain is also timely. This would help us to understand the motivations and experiences of those with chronic non-malignant pain, and the HCPs trying to manage that pain.

Acknowledgements

Thanks to the authors of the qualitative studies included in the meta-ethnography and all the healthcare professionals who shared their stories. Thanks also to our project advisory group of patients and healthcare professionals.

Funding

This study was funded by the National Institute for Health Research Health Services and Delivery Research Programme 14/198/07. The views and opinions expressed therein are those of the authors and do not necessarily reflect those of the HS&DR Programme, NIHR, NHS or the Department of Health.

Authors' contributions

I would like to confirm that all authors have read and approved the final manuscript. FT, KB and KS made a substantial contribution to the design, acquisition, analysis and interpretation of data. ST made a substantial contribution to the analysis and interpretation of data. FT drafted the first, subsequent and final versions. KS, KB and ST revised all versions for important intellectual content and approved the final version. All authors agree to be accountable for the accuracy and integrity of the work.

Consent for publication

Not applicable.

Competing interests

The authors declare that they have no competing interests.

Author details

[1]Nuffield Orthopaedic Centre, Oxford University Hospitals NHS Foundation Trust, Windmill Road, Oxford 0X3 7HE, UK. [2]Warwick Research in Nursing, Warwick Medical School, University of Warwick, Coventry CV4 7AL, UK. [3]Nuffield Department of Orthopaedics, Rheumatology and Musculoskeletal Sciences (NDORMS), University of Oxford, Windmill Road, Oxford 0X3 7LD, UK.

References

1. Breivika H, et al. Survey of chronic pain in Europe: prevalence, impact on daily life, and treatment. Eur J Pain. 2006;10(4):287–333.
2. Elliott AM, et al. The epidemiology of chronic pain in the community. Lancet. 1999;354:1248–52.
3. König HH, et al. Comparison of population health status in six European countries: results of a representative survey using the EQ-5D questionnaire. Med Care. 2009;47:255–61.
4. Covinsky KE, Lindquist K, Dunlop DD, Yelin E. Pain, functional limitations, and aging. J Am Geriatr Soc. 2009;57:1556–61.
5. Croft P, Peat G, Van-der-Windt D. Primary care research and musculoskeletal medicine. Primary Health Care Res Dev. 2010;11:4–16.
6. Smith B, et al. The impact of chronic pain in the community. Fam Pract. 2001;18:292–9.
7. Department-of-Health, Pain breaking through the barrier. Chief Medical Officer's report, 2009. 150th annual report of the Chief Medical Officer.
8. Toye F, Jenkins S. 'It makes you think' – exploring the impact of qualitative films on pain clinicians. Br J Pain. 2015;9(1):65–9.
9. Parsons S, et al. The influence of patients' and primary care practitioners' beliefs and expectations about chronic musculoskeletal pain on the process of care: a systematic review of qualitative studies. Clin J Pain. 2007;23(1):91–9.
10. Breen A, et al. "you feel so hopeless": a qualitative study of GP management of acute back pain. Eur J Pain. 2007;11(1):21–9.
11. Dowell D, TM. Haegerich, and R. Chou, CDC (Centers for Disease Control and Prevention) Guideline for Prescribing Opioids for Chronic Pain — United States, 2016. Morb. Mortal. Wkly. Rep, 2016. Report 65, March 15: p. 1–49.
12. Royal-College-of-Anaesthetists, Opioids Aware: A resource for patients and healthcare professionals to support prescribing of opioid medicines for pain. 2016(8th November 2016).
13. Ruscitto A, Smith BH, Guthrie B. Changes in opioid and other analgesic use 1995–2010: repeated cross-sectional analysis of dispensed prescribing for a large geographical population in Scotland. Eur J Pain. 2015;19:59–66.
14. Zin CS, Chen L-C, Knaggs RD. Changes in trends and pattern of strong opioid prescribing in primary care. Eur J Pain. 2014;18:1343–51.
15. Levy B, et al. Trends in opioid analgesic-prescribing rates by specialty, U.S., 2007–2012. Am J Prev Med. 2015;49:409–4013.
16. Paulozzi LJ, Mack KA, Hockenberry JM. Vital signs: variation among states in prescribing of opioid pain relievers and benzodiazepines—United States, 2012. MMWR Morb Mortal Wkly Rep. 2014;63(26):563–8.
17. Fredheim O, et al. Prescription pattern of codeine for non-malignant pain: a pharmacoepidemiological study from the Norwegian prescription database. Acta Anaesthesiol Scand. 2009;53(5):627–33.
18. Chou R, et al. The Effectiveness and Risks of Long-Term Opioid Treatment of Chronic Pain. The Evidence Report/Technology Assessment, Number 218, 2014. Prepared by the Pacific Northwest Evidence-based Practice Center under Contract No. 290–2012-00014-I (Agency for Healthcare Research and Quality (AHRQ) Publication No. 14-E005-EF). https://effectivehealthcare.ahrq.gov/topics/chronic-pain-opioid-treatment/research/.
19. Daubresse M, et al. Ambulatory diagnosis and treatment of nonmalignant pain in the United States, 2000-2010. Med Care. 2013;51:870–8.
20. Toye F, Seers K, Barker K. 2015–17. www.journalslibrary.nihr.ac.uk/programmes/hsdr/1419807/#/.
21. Toye F, et al. A meta-ethnography of patients' experiences of chronic non-malignant musculoskeletal pain. Health Services and Delivery Res. 2013; 1(12):1–189.
22. Noblit G, Hare R. Meta-ethnography: Synthesising Qualitative Studies. Qualitative research methods series 11. 1988. California: Sage Publications.
23. Wong SS, Wilczynski NL, Haynes RB. Developing optimal search strategies for detecting clinically relevant qualitative studies in MEDLINE. Medinfo. 2004;11(1):311–6.
24. Wilczynski NL, Marks S, Haynes RB. Search strategies for identifying qualitative studies in CINAHL. Qual Health Res. 2007;17(5):705–10.
25. McKibbon KA, Wilczynski NL, Haynes RB. Developing optimal search strategies for retrieving qualitative studies in PsycINFO. Eval Health Prof. 2006;29(4):440–54.
26. Walters LA, Wilczynski NL, Haynes RB. Hedges team., Developing optimal search strategies for retrieving clinically relevant qualitative studies in EMBASE. Qual Health Res. 2006;16(1):162–8.
27. Toye F, et al. Meta-ethnography 25 years on: challenges and insights for synthesising a large number of qualitative studies. BMC Med Res Methodol. 2014:**14**(80).
28. Campbell R, et al. Evaluating meta-ethnography: systematic analysis and synthesis of qualitative research. Health Technol Assess. 2011;15(43)
29. Dixon-Woods M, et al. Appraising qualitative research for inclusion in systematic reviews: a quantitative and qualitative comparison of three methods. J Health Serv Res Policy. 2007;12(1):42–7.
30. CASP. Critical Appraisal Skills Programme: making sense of evidence about clinical effectiveness: 10 questions to help you make sense of qualitative research. 2010. http://www.casp-uk.net/casp-tools-checklists.
31. Toye F, et al. Trying to pin down jelly' - exploring intuitive processes in quality assessment for meta-ethnography. BMC Med Res Methodol. 2013;13:46.
32. Lewin S, et al. Using qualitative evidence in decision making for health and social interventions: an approach to assess confidence in findings from qualitative evidence syntheses (GRADE-CERQual). PLoS Med. 2016;12(10): e1001895. doi:10.1371/journal. pmed.1001895.
33. Baldacchino A, et al. Guilty until proven innocent: a qualitative study of the management of chronic non-cancer pain among patients with a history of substance abuse. Addict Behav. 2010;35(3):270–2.
34. Barry T, et al. Opioids, chronic pain, and addiction in primary care. J Pain. 2010;11(12):1442.
35. Berg M, et al. Providers' experiences treating chronic pain among opioid-dependent drug users. J Gen Intern Med. 2009;24(4):482.
36. Briones-Vozmediano E, et al. Patients' and professionals' views on managing fibromyalgia. Pain Res Manag. 2013;18(1):19–24.
37. Esquibel AY, Borkan J. Doctors and patients in pain: conflict and collaboration in opioid prescription in primary care. Pain. 2014;155(12):2575–82.
38. Fontana JS. The social and political forces affecting prescribing practices for chronic pain. J Prof Nurs. 2008;24(1):30–6.
39. Gooberman-Hill R, et al. Professional experience guides opioid prescribing for chronic joint pain in primary care. Fam Pract. 2011;28(1):102.
40. Kaasalainen S, et al. Pain management decision making among long-term care physicians and nurses. West J Nurs Res. 2007;29(5):561.
41. Kilaru S, et al. How do physicians adopt and apply opioid prescription guidelines in the emergency department? A qualitative study. Ann Emerg Med. 2014;64(5):482.
42. Kaasalainen S, et al. An action-based approach to improving pain management in long-term care. Can J Aging. 2010;29(4):503–18.
43. Krebs E, et al. Barriers to guideline-concordant opioid management in primary care—a qualitative study. J Pain. 2014;15(11):1148.
44. McCrorie C, et al. Understanding long-term opioid prescribing for non-cancer pain in primary care: a qualitative study. BMC Fam Pract. 2015;16:121.
45. Ruiz JG, et al. Primary care management of chronic nonmalignant pain in veterans: a qualitative study. Educ Gerontol. 2010;36(5):372–94.
46. Seamark D, et al. GPs prescribing of strong opioid drugs for patients with chronic non-cancer pain: a qualitative study. Br J Gen Pract. 2013;63(617)
47. Siedlecki L, et al. Exploring how bedside nurses care for patients with chronic pain: a grounded theory study. Pain Manag Nurs. 2014;15(3):565.
48. Spitz A, et al. Primary care providers' perspective on prescribing opioids to older adults with chronic non-cancer pain: a qualitative study. BMC Geriatr. 2011;11:35.
49. Starrels L, et al. It made my life a little easier: primary care providers' beliefs and attitudes about using opioid treatment agreements. J Opioid Manag. 2014;10(2):95.
50. Kaplovitch E, et al. Sex differences in dose escalation and overdose death during chronic opioid therapy: a population-based cohort study. PLoS One. 2015;10(8):e0134550. doi:10.1371/journal.pone.0134550.
51. National-Center-for-Health-Statistics, Health, United States, 2014: With Special Feature on Adults Aged 55–64. Hyattsville: 2015.

Permissions

All chapters in this book were first published in FP, by BioMed Central; hereby published with permission under the Creative Commons Attribution License or equivalent. Every chapter published in this book has been scrutinized by our experts. Their significance has been extensively debated. The topics covered herein carry significant findings which will fuel the growth of the discipline. They may even be implemented as practical applications or may be referred to as a beginning point for another development.

The contributors of this book come from diverse backgrounds, making this book a truly international effort. This book will bring forth new frontiers with its revolutionizing research information and detailed analysis of the nascent developments around the world.

We would like to thank all the contributing authors for lending their expertise to make the book truly unique. They have played a crucial role in the development of this book. Without their invaluable contributions this book wouldn't have been possible. They have made vital efforts to compile up to date information on the varied aspects of this subject to make this book a valuable addition to the collection of many professionals and students.

This book was conceptualized with the vision of imparting up-to-date information and advanced data in this field. To ensure the same, a matchless editorial board was set up. Every individual on the board went through rigorous rounds of assessment to prove their worth. After which they invested a large part of their time researching and compiling the most relevant data for our readers.

The editorial board has been involved in producing this book since its inception. They have spent rigorous hours researching and exploring the diverse topics which have resulted in the successful publishing of this book. They have passed on their knowledge of decades through this book. To expedite this challenging task, the publisher supported the team at every step. A small team of assistant editors was also appointed to further simplify the editing procedure and attain best results for the readers.

Apart from the editorial board, the designing team has also invested a significant amount of their time in understanding the subject and creating the most relevant covers. They scrutinized every image to scout for the most suitable representation of the subject and create an appropriate cover for the book.

The publishing team has been an ardent support to the editorial, designing and production team. Their endless efforts to recruit the best for this project, has resulted in the accomplishment of this book. They are a veteran in the field of academics and their pool of knowledge is as vast as their experience in printing. Their expertise and guidance has proved useful at every step. Their uncompromising quality standards have made this book an exceptional effort. Their encouragement from time to time has been an inspiration for everyone.

The publisher and the editorial board hope that this book will prove to be a valuable piece of knowledge for researchers, students, practitioners and scholars across the globe.

List of Contributors

Melissa Dominicé Dao, Patricia Hudelson and Noëlle Junod Perron
Department of Community Medicine, Primary Care and Emergency Medicine, Geneva University Hospitals, rue Gabrielle Perret-Gentil, CH-1211 Geneva, Switzerland

Cédric Lanier
Department of Community Medicine, Primary Care and Emergency Medicine, Geneva University Hospitals, rue Gabrielle Perret-Gentil, CH-1211 Geneva, Switzerland
Primary care unit, University of Geneva, Centre Médical Universitaire de Genève, Geneva, Switzerland

Bernard Cerutti
Faculty of Medicine, University of Geneva, Geneva, Switzerland

Enrique de la Peña
Sondika Primary Health Care Center, Uribe Integrated Care Organization - Osakidetza, Lehendakari Agirre 41, 48160 Sondika, Spain

Justo Mugica
Beasain Primary Health Care Center, Goieri-Alto Urola Integrated Care Organization - Osakidetza, Bernedo s/n, 20200 Beasain, Spain

Esther Gorostiza
Matiena Primary Health Care Center, Barrualde-Galdakao Integrated Care Organization - Osakidetza, BioCruces Health Research Institute, Trañabarren 13-Bajo, 48220 Abadiño, Spain

Natalia Zarbailov
Family Medicine Department, State University of Medicine and Pharmacy "Nicolae Testemitanu", Bd. Stefan cel Mare 165, MD-2004 Chisinau, Republic of Moldova

Stefan Wilm
Institute of General Practice, Heinrich-Heine-University, Werdener Str. 4, D-40227 Düsseldorf, Germany

Francesco Carelli
University of Milan, Francesco Sforza 35, Milan, Italy

Mette Brekke
Department of General Practice, Institute of Health and Society, University of Oslo, Blindern, Norway

Kristy Payne, Tegan Dutton, Ross Wilson and Jannine Bailey
Bathurst Rural Clinical School, School of Medicine, Western Sydney University, Bathurst, NSW, Australia

Kate Weal and Maree Earle
Marathon Health, Bathurst, NSW, Australia

Anthony Dowell, Caroline Morris, Lindsay Macdonald and Maria Stubbe
Department Primary Health Care & General Practice, University of Otago, 23a Mein Street, Wellington, New Zealand

Alvaro Sanchez, Gonzalo Grandes, Haizea Pombo and Catalina Martinez
Primary Care Research Unit of Bizkaia, Basque Healthcare Service - Osakidetza, BioCruces Health Research Institute, Luis Power 18, 4ª planta, E48014 Bilbao, Spain

Josep M. Cortada
Deusto Primary Health Care Center, Bilbao-Basurto Integrated Care Organization– Osakidetza, BioCruces Health Research Institute, Luis Power 18, E48014 Bilbao, Spain

Mary Helen Corrales
La Merced Primary Health Care Center, Bilbao-Basurto Integrated Care Organization - Osakidetza, Luis Iraurrizaga 1, 48003 Bilbao, Spain

Anja Maria Brænd, Jørund Straand and Atle Klovning
Department of General Practice, Institute of Health and Society, Faculty of Medicine, University of Oslo, N-0318 Oslo, Norway

Tessa Magnée and Derek P. de Beurs
Netherlands Institute of Health Services Research (NIVEL), BN Utrecht, The Netherlands

Xiaolin Wei
Division of Clinical Public Health and Institute of Health Policy, Management and Evaluation, Dalla Lana School of Public Health, University of Toronto, 155 College St, Toronto, ON M5T 3M7, Canada

Martin C. S. Wong
The Jockey Club School of Public Health and Primary Care, Faculty of Medicine, The Chinese University of Hong Kong, Hong Kong, SAR, China

Bertolt Kuhn, Kim-Sarah Kleij, Sebastian Liersch and Volker Amelung
Medical School Hannover, Institute for Epidemiology, Social Medicine and Health Systems Research, OE 5410, Carl-Neuberg-Str. 1, D-30625 Hannover, Germany

Jost Steinhäuser
University Hospital of Schleswig-Holstein, Campus Lübeck, Institute of Family Medicine, Lübeck, Germany

Irene Svenningsson, Dominique Hange, Nashmil Ariai, Shabnam Nejati and Carl Wikberg
Department of Primary Health Care, Institute of Medicine, The Sahlgrenska
Academy, University of Gothenburg, Gothenburg, Sweden

Eva-Lisa Petersson
Department of Primary Health Care, Institute of Medicine, The Sahlgrenska Academy, University of Gothenburg, Gothenburg, Sweden
Region Västra Götaland, Närhälsan Research and Development Primary Health Care, Gothenburg, Sweden

Cecilia Björkelund
Department of Primary Health Care, Institute of Medicine, The Sahlgrenska Academy, University of Gothenburg, Gothenburg, Sweden
Department of Primary Health Care, Institute of Medicine, The Sahlgrenska Academy, University of Gothenburg, 40530 Göteborg, Sweden

Camilla Udo
School of Education, Health and Social Studies, Dalarna University, Falun, Sweden

Lars Wallin
School of Education, Health and Social Studies, Dalarna University, Falun, Sweden
Department of Health and Care Sciences, The Sahlgrenska Academy, University of Gothenburg, Gothenburg, Sweden
Division of Nursing, Department of Neurobiology, Care Sciences and Society, Karolinska Institute, Stockholm, Sweden

Catrin Wessman
Health Metrics Unit, Sahlgrenska Academy, University of Gothenburg, Gothenburg, Sweden

Malin André
Department of Public Health and Caring Sciences - Family Medicine and Preventive Medicine, Uppsala University, Uppsala, Sweden

Jeanette Westman
Division of Family Medicine, Department of Neurobiology, Care Sciences and Society, Karolinska Institute, Stockholm, Sweden

Mark Porcheret, Chris Main, Peter Croft and Krysia Dziedzic
Arthritis Research UK Primary Care Centre, Research Institute for Primary Care & Health Sciences, Keele University, Staffordshire ST5 5BG, UK

Andrew O'Regan, Louise Hickey, David Meagher and Ailish Hannigan
Graduate Entry Medical School, Faculty of Education and Health Sciences, University of Limerick, Limerick, Ireland

Walter Cullen
School of Medicine, University College Dublin, Health Sciences Centre, Belfield, Dublin, Ireland

Damien Contandriopoulos
School of Nursing, University of Victoria, STN CSC, Victoria, British-Columbia V8W 2Y2, Canada

Mélanie Perroux, Aurore Cockenpot and Arnaud Duhoux
Faculty of Nursing, Université de Montréal, C.P. 6128 succ. Centre-ville, Montréal, Québec H3C 3J7, Canada

Emmanuelle Jean
School of Nursing, Université du Québec à Rimouski, 300, allée des Ursulines, C. P. 3300, succ. A, Rimouski, Québec G5L 3A1, Canada

Denise Y. S. Tam and Wendy Tsui
Department of Family Medicine and Primary Healthcare, Hong Kong West Cluster, Hospital Authority, North Wing, Room 601, 6/F, Tsan Yuk Hospital, 30 Hospital Road, Hong Kong, Hong Kong

Yvonne Y. C. Lo
Wellness Family Medical Practice, Room 605, Hang Seng Tsim Sha Tsui Building, 18 Carnarvon Road, Hong Kong, Hong Kong

Emily J. Cameron
Faculty of Medicine, Dalhousie University, Halifax, NS, Canada

Susan K. Bowles
Department of Pharmacy, Nova Scotia Health Authority-Central Zone, Halifax, NS, Canada
Department of Medicine (Geriatrics), Dalhousie University, Halifax, NS, Canada

Emily Gard Marshall
Department of Family Medicine, Dalhousie University, Halifax, NS, Canada

Melissa K. Andrew
Department of Medicine (Geriatrics), Dalhousie University, Halifax, NS, Canada

Rebecca Elvey, Simon Bailey, Kath Checkland, Anne McBride and Damian Hodgson
The University of Manchester, Oxford Road, Manchester M13 9PL, UK

Stephen Parkin
Radcliffe Observatory Quarter, University of Oxford, Woodstock Road, Oxford OX2 6GG, UK

Katy Rothwell
NIHR Collaboration for Leadership in Applied Health Research and Care (CLAHRC), Salford Royal Foundation Trust, Stott Lane, Salford M6 8HD, UK

Katja Krug, René Alexander Ballhausen, Regine Bölter, Peter Engeser, Michel Wensing, Joachim Szecsenyi and Frank Peters-Klimm
Department of General Practice and Health Services Research, University Hospital Heidelberg, Im Neuenheimer Feld 130.3, 69120 Heidelberg, Germany

Todd R. Fredricks, Andrew Leubitz, Benjamin R. Oldach and Daniel Kana
Department of Family Medicine, Ohio University Heritage College of Osteopathic Medicine, Athens, OH 45701, USA

Elizabeth A. Beverly and Emily H. Guseman
Department of Family Medicine, Ohio University Heritage College of Osteopathic Medicine, Athens, OH 45701, USA
The Diabetes Institute, Ohio University, Athens, OH 45701, USA

Michael D. Grant
Department of Psychology, Ohio University, Athens, OH 45701, USA

Jonathon Whipps
The Graduate College, Ohio University, Athens, OH 45701, USA

Julia Hackett
Martin House Research Centre, Social Policy Research Unit, University of York, York YO10 5DD, UK

Lucy Ziegler and Michael I. Bennett
Academic Unit of Palliative Care, Leeds Institute of Health Sciences, University of Leeds, Level 10 Worsley Building, Clarendon Way, Leeds LS2 9NL, UK

Mary Godfrey
Academic Unit of Elderly Care and Rehabilitation, Bradford Institute for Health Research, Temple Bank House, Bradford Royal Infirmary, Duckworth Lane, Bradford BD9 6RJ, UK

Robbie Foy
Academic Unit of Primary Care, Leeds Institute of Health Sciences, University of Leeds, Level 10 Worsley Building, Clarendon Way, Leeds LS2 9NL, UK

Charlotte F. Davies and Charlotte Chick
Bristol Medical School, University of Bristol, Canynge Hall, 39 Whatley Road, Bristol BS8 2PS, UK

Margaret T. May
Bristol Medical School, University of Bristol, Canynge Hall, 39 Whatley Road, Bristol BS8 2PS, UK
National Institute of Health Research (NIHR) Health Protection Research Unit (HPRU) in Evaluation of Interventions, Bristol Medical School, University of Bristol, Oakfield House, Oakfield Grove, Bristol BS8 2BN, UK

Joanna M. Kesten
Bristol Medical School, University of Bristol, Oakfield House, Oakfield Grove, Bristol BS8 2BN, UK
National Institute for Health Research Collaborations for Leadership in Applied Health Research and Care West (NIHR CLAHRC West), University Hospitals Bristol, NHS Foundation Trust, 9th Floor, Whitefriars, Lewins Mead, Bristol BS1 2NT, England
National Institute of Health Research (NIHR) Health Protection Research Unit (HPRU) in Evaluation of Interventions, Bristol Medical School, University of Bristol, Oakfield House, Oakfield Grove, Bristol BS8 2BN, UK

Jeremy Horwood
National Institute for Health Research Collaborations for Leadership in Applied Health Research and Care West (NIHR CLAHRC West), University Hospitals Bristol, NHS Foundation Trust, 9th Floor, Whitefriars, Lewins Mead, Bristol BS1 2NT, England

Mark Gompels
Department of Immunology, Southmead Hospital, North Bristol NHS Trust, Westbury-on-Trym, Bristol BS10 5NB, UK

Megan Crofts
Genitourinary medicine, Unity Sexual Health, Bristol Sexual Health Services, Tower Hill, Bristol BS2 0JD, UK

Annette Billing
NHS Bristol, North Somerset and South Gloucestershire CCG, South Plaza, Marlborough Street, Bristol BS1 3NX, UK

Haitao Li
School of Medicine, Shenzhen University, Shenzhen, China

Howard Tandeter
Department of Family Medicine and Siaal research center for family medicine and primary care, Ben-Gurion University of the Negev, Beer-Sheva, Israel

Peter F. Verhaak
Netherlands Institute of Health Services Research (NIVEL), The Netherlands
Department of General Practice, Groningen University, Groningen, The Netherlands

Richard Boxem
The Dutch Healthcare Authority, Utrecht, The Netherlands

Elisabeth Mangrio and Karin Persson
Department of Care Science, Faculty Health and Society, Malmö University, Jan Waldenströms gata 25, 205 06 Malmö, Sweden

Natalia V. Lewis, Eszter Szilassy and Gene S. Feder
Centre for Academic Primary Care, School of Social and Community Medicine, University of Bristol, Canynge Hall, 39 Whatley Road, Bristol BS8 2PS, UK

Cath Larkins and Nicky Stanley
School of Social Work, Care and Community, University of Central Lancashire, Harrington Building, Preston PR1 2HE, UK

William Turner
School for Policy Studies, University of Bristol, Social Science Complex, 8 Priory Road, Bristol BS8 1TZ, UK

Jessica Drinkwater
Leeds Institute of Health Sciences, Charles Thackrah Building, 101 Clarendon Road, Leeds LS2 9LJ, UK

Dinny H. de Bakker
Netherlands Institute of Health Services Research (NIVEL), The Netherlands
Tilburg University, Scientific Centre for Transformation in Care Welfare (TRANZO), Tilburg, The Netherlands

Fran Toye
Nuffield Orthopaedic Centre, Oxford University Hospitals NHS Foundation Trust, Windmill Road, Oxford 0X3 7HE, UK

Kate Seers and Stephanie Tierney
Warwick Research in Nursing, Warwick Medical School, University of Warwick, Coventry CV4 7AL, UK

Karen Louise Barker
Nuffield Department of Orthopaedics, Rheumatology and Musculoskeletal Sciences (NDORMS), University of Oxford, Windmill Road, Oxford 0X3 7LD, UK

Index

CPSIA information can be obtained
at www.ICGtesting.com
Printed in the USA
LVHW061254231121
704237LV00003B/11

9 781639 274536